PSYCHOPHYSIOLOGY OF RESPIRATION IN HEALTH AND DISEASE

APPLETON-CENTURY-CROFTS
EDUCATIONAL DIVISION
MEREDITH CORPORATION
New York

PSYCHOPHYSIOLOGY OF RESPIRATION IN HEALTH AND DISEASE

DONALD L. DUDLEY, M.D.

In Collaboration With

C. J. MARTIN, M.D.

MINORU MASUDA, Ph.D.

HERBERT S. RIPLEY, M.D.

THOMAS H. HOLMES, M.D.

669-1

Library of Congress Catalog Card Number:
76-85884

PRINTED IN THE UNITED STATES OF AMERICA
390-27675-8

DONALD L. DUDLEY, M.D.

*Instructor, Department of Psychiatry,
University of Washington School of Medicine,
Seattle, Washington*

C. J. MARTIN, M.D.

*Director, Institute of Respiratory Physiology, Virginia
Mason Research Center, and Firland Sanatorium;
Clinical Associate Professor, Department of Physiology and
Biophysics, and Department of Medicine, University
of Washington School of Medicine, Seattle, Washington*

MINORU MASUDA, Ph.D.

*Associate Professor, Department of Psychiatry, University of
Washington School of Medicine, Seattle, Washington*

HERBERT S. RIPLEY, M.D.

*Professor, Chairman, Department of Psychiatry,
University of Washington School of Medicine,
Seattle, Washington*

THOMAS H. HOLMES, M.D.

*Professor, Department of Psychiatry,
University of Washington School of Medicine,
Seattle, Washington*

To the patients and subjects who donated time and effort to a demanding experimental program, and to the following for support on this endeavor:

Public Health Service Undergraduate Training in Psychiatry Grant No. 5-T2-MH-5939-18, Graduate Training in Psychiatry Grant No. 5-T1-MH-5557-19, and Undergraduate Training in Human Behavior Grant No. 5-T2-MH-7871-06 from the National Institute of Mental Health; O'Donnell Psychiatric Research Fund; Firland Exchange Incorporated; National Tuberculosis Association; and Boeing Employees Good Neighbor Fund.

PREFACE

Psychophysiology is generally defined as the study of psychologic and physiologic components and their interrelationships in biologic functions. As such, it represents a bridge between medicine and psychiatry. This monograph is an attempt to integrate psychologic, medical, and physiologic data into a unique view of the respiratory system. To call it the psychophysiology of respiration is an oversimplification, but, perhaps best communicates the contents. Both the clinical and basic scientific approaches are utilized and are integrated as closely as possible.

This monograph is a product of the combined efforts of five investigators who have an average of over 20 years of experience in applying their particular approach to research. The material was gathered over a ten-year period of continued work on the respiratory system which utilized all of the biases inherent in each investigator's particular field. More data are continuing to develop and hopefully, will continue to do so for another ten years.

Division of the monograph into five sections was done to facilitate its use. Each section is relatively independent of the others. A reader is thereby able to follow his own interests in selecting parts of the monograph which are of particular interest without having to read the preceding material.

We are appreciative of the many patients and supportive personnel who have contributed time and effort, but who are too numerous to mention individually. There are many who are omitted in the bibliographies who have contributed significantly to the general field of study. We wish to extend our appreciation to the Departments of Medical Illustration and Medical Photography for the illustrations.

Finally, we extend our sincere thanks to Marion Amundson and her colleagues for the difficult task of typing, proofreading, and correcting the copy.

CONTENTS

PSYCHOPHYSIOLOGY OF RESPIRATION IN HEALTH AND DISEASE

Section I

Background Information

This section provides an introduction to the monograph. Contained in it are the historical, medical, psychologic, anatomic, and physiologic data necessary for a basic understanding of the psychophysiology of respiration in health and disease. In addition to providing an introduction to the monograph, however, this section can also be used as a general introduction to pulmonary anatomy and physiology and to the diffuse obstructive pulmonary syndromes. The last chapter provides pertinent details regarding the various experimental studies which make up the monograph.

1

Introduction

The often repeated adage to "treat the whole man" is exceedingly difficult to apply and even more difficult to understand. What is the whole man —and, even if we knew, how would we treat him? Medical knowledge is complex in breadth and depth and yet it is evident that the surface has barely been scratched. This monograph is intended to be a *small* scratch on the surface of knowledge aimed at the evaluation and treatment of patients with psychophysiologic respiratory reactions, clinical emphysema, and, to a lesser degree, other chronic lung disease entities. As such it tells a story.

The story begins with the normal physiology and psychophysiology of respiration and extends to respiratory disease as seen through the eyes of psychiatrists, physiologists, and internists. The diseased individual is one who has developed—for largely unknown reasons—a condition of undetermined or questionable etiology which decreases the function of the pulmonary system and poses a threat to life and productivity. Once the disability and insufficiency appear, the person struggles to adjust his behavior to the failing system in order to retain some degree of comfort. It is soon evident to the patient that the experts have little of lasting value to offer: it dawns on him that, indeed, no one has any answers and that he is incapacitated for life. The patient then has increasingly severe emotional problems. He may become angry and self-destructive, accepting, or overwhelmed and depressed. He may decide the struggle to breathe is not worth it and wish to die, or he may live in constant fear of death. Regardless of his response, he pays a psychologic and physiologic price.

The development and progression of a disease obviously have some psychophysiologic effect on the patient. Personality changes may be caused by the physical or mental limitations imposed by the disease, by the realization that he is failing, or by direct effects on the central nervous system.

However, they represent only a portion of the toll exacted by chronic lung diseases. As lung function deteriorates, the patient's respiratory system becomes less and less able to respond to environmental inputs. Emotions which previously had little or no effect now produce disability. The patient has little understanding of this and his physician is ill-equipped to help him. At this point the patient may become a "problem patient" or a "hypochondriac." There may be a flood of telephone calls from the frightened, angry, anxious, or depressed and dyspneic patient. The physician may have little to offer, and the situation seems hopeless and overwhelming. Because of the chronic, seemingly hopeless, time-consuming and expensive nature of the problem, the patient may end up without a doctor. He may then go to emergency rooms and public hospitals, or he may learn to adapt to his disease without professional care. If he is lucky, he may be directed to one of the few hospital units which are designed to care for chronic lung disease.

The above represents the predicament for the majority of patients with emphysema. However, the treatment of these people does not seem quite so hopeless with a combined medical, physiologic, and psychologic approach.

The theoretical approach utilized in the studies to be outlined is based on work first published in the 1800s by Bell and by Darwin. Examples of their observations illustrate their point of view and the point of view finally adopted by current investigators.

According to Charles Darwin, during grief "The breathing becomes slow and feeble, and is often interrupted by deep sighs," and during anger "the chest heaves, and the dilated nostrils quiver." Sir Charles Bell, in work published in 1806, arrives at similar observations:

> In the expression of the passions, there is a compound influence in operation. Let us contemplate the appearance of terror. We can readily conceive why a man stands with eyes intently fixed on the object of his fears, the eyebrows elevated to the utmost, and the eye largely uncovered; or why, with hesitating and bewildered steps, his eyes are rapidly and wildly in search of something. In this, we only perceive the intent application of his mind to the object of his apprehensions—its direct influence on the outward organ. But observe him further; there is a spasm on his breast, he cannot breathe freely, the chest is elevated, the muscles of his neck and shoulders are in action, his breathing is short and rapid, there is a gasping and a convulsive motion of his lips, a tremor on his hollow cheek, a gulping and catching of his throat; and why does his heart knock at his ribs, while yet there is no force of circulation?—for his lips and cheeks are ashy pale.
>
> So in grief, if we attend to the class of phenomena, we shall be able to draw an exact picture. Let us imagine to ourselves the overwhelming influence of grief on woman. The object in her mind has absorbed all the powers of the frame, the body is no more regarded, the spirits have left it, it reclines, and the limbs gravitate; they are nerveless and relaxed and she scarcely breathes; but

> why comes at intervals the long-drawn sigh?—or why is the hand so pale and earthy cold;—and why, at intervals, as the agony returns, does the convulsion spread over the frame like a paroxysm of suffocation?

Henry found that the basal metabolic rate was elevated with elated, overactive, overtalkative, apprehensive, tense or agitated states, and was lowered by depressed, underactive, undertalkative, or apathetic states.

From the observations of the above-mentioned three investigators, it is suggested that if the individual is preparing or prepared for some type of physical activity, then ventilation and oxygen consumption increase. If no action is called for, or if, in fact, the individual is withdrawing from action, ventilation and oxygen consumption decrease. These situations point to two general types of emotional response to stimuli; this type of approach is suggested in Bell's writings. If the following quotation is integrated with the preceding one, these two types stand out clearly:

> In pain, the body is exerted to violent tension, and all the emotions and passions allied to pain, or having their origin and foundation in painful sensations, have this general distinction of character, that there is an energetic action or tremor, the effect of universal excitement. . . .
>
> On the other hand, as pleasure is characterized by languor, tranquility, and relaxation, all the emotions related to it, or deducible from pleasurable sensations, are felt in the prevailing state of the system—a degree of inaction, and as it were forgetfulness of bodily exertion, and an indulgence of mental contemplation. The contemplation of beauty, or the admiration of soft music, produces a sense of languor; the body reclines; the lips are half-opened; the eyes have a softened lustre from the falling of the eyelids; the breathing is slow; and from the absolute neglect of bodily sensation, and the temporary interruption of respiration, there is a frequent low-drawn sigh.

The above data indicate that there is biologic utility in psychologically induced ventilatory and metabolic changes. The effects upon the respiratory system of naturally occurring environmental stimuli, experimental head pain, and hypnotic and nonhypnotic suggestion of these stimuli were investigated and provided the framework for this monograph. Psychologic aspects of respiration have been reported from clinical, x-ray, bronchoscopic, spirographic, and pneumonographic observations. Until recently, no psychophysiologic study has directly measured the ventilation and gas-exchange variables concerned with respiration.

The study of the psychophysiology of respiration has progressed significantly since the studies of Sir Charles Bell and Sir Charles Darwin, who simply observed breathing patterns and recorded their impressions of the psychologic state. Despite their lack of equipment they made fundamental observations which were instrumental in the development of the particular psychologic approach used in this monograph. The current electronic sophistication in physiology provides us with elegant tools to document and extend concepts which are otherwise unacceptable because of our current insistence on statistical maneuvers and quantification of observations. Thus, although the following chapters are filled with scientific information largely unobtainable in the 19th century, most of the conclusions drawn are similar to those observed by workers such as Bell and Darwin. However, psychologic evaluation has not progressed to the degree of quantification manifested by the physiologic sciences and we still depend upon clinical evaluations derived from interviews. These types of data are also amenable to statistical treatment, which adds to the degree of comfort we experience in accepting it.

In addition to the normal psychophysiology of respiration, there will also be emphasis on psychophysiologic changes in the diseased pulmonary system. For example, emotions associated with physiologic change similar to that found in exercise might produce pulmonary disability by the same mechanisms as exercise. On the other hand, emotions which produce physiologic change similar to that found during sleep might produce disability by the same mechanism operating during sleeplike states.

The primary focus of attention will be on ventilation and metabolism. However, it should be kept in mind that there are simultaneous changes occurring in the nasal mucus membrane, tracheobronchial tree, chest, and diaphragamatic musculature.

The action-orientation/nonaction-orientation approach to the investigation of respiration is consistent with the integrative approach to emotions and behavior utilized by Gellhorn with neurophysiologic techniques. He found that direct or indirect stimulation of the parasympathetic or sympathetic divisions of the hypothalamus on hypothalamic reactivity led to a predictable responsiveness of these divisions. He used the term "tuning" for these reversible changes. A state of sympathetic tuning was said to exist when the sympathetic division of the hypothalamus was augmented and the parasympathetic division attenuated. The opposite was found to occur in states of parasympathetic tuning. The changes consequent to hypothalamic tuning were not confined to the autonomic nervous system.

To designate the autonomic plus somatic changes occurring, Hess's terminology was adopted. Thus states of ergotropic and trophotropic tuning were distinguished. Ergotropic tuning is characterized by increased sympathetic and somatic discharges and reciprocally attenuated trophotropic activity. Trophotropic tuning is characterized by increased parasympathetic discharges and reciprocally attenuated sympathetic and somatic activity.

Gellhorn's conceptualization of the integrative functioning of the nervous system is based on a considerable body of psychologic and physiologic data. His observations in the laboratory confirm and expand the clinical psychiatric observations concerning action-orientation and non-action-orientation reported in the studies of the respiratory system. Thus action-orientation is hypothetically synonymous with ergotropic activation while nonaction-orientation is hypothetically synonymous with trophotropic activation.

REFERENCES

Alexander, F., and Saul, L. J. Respiration and personality, Psychosom Med, 2:110, 1940.

Ames, F. The hyperventilation syndrome, J Ment Sci, 101: 466, 1955.

Baker, D. M. Sighing respiration as a symptom, Lancet, 1:174, 1934.

Bell, Sir C. The Anatomy and Philosophy of Expression, 4th ed. London, John Murray, 1847.

Bulow, K. Lung function in cardiac neurosis, Acta Med Scand, 169:1, 1961.

Christie, R. V. Some types of respiration in neuroses, Quart J Med, 28:427, 1935.

Clauson, J. Respiration movement in normal, neurotic and psychotic subjects, Acta Psychiat Neurologica (Supp.), 68, 1951.

Darwin, C. Expression of Emotions in Man and Animals. New York, Philosophical Library, 1955.

Dudley, D. L., Holmes, T. H., Martin, C. J., and Ripley, H. S. Changes in respiration associated with hypnotically induced emotion, pain, and exercise, Psychosom Med, 27:46, 1964.

——— Martin, C. J., and Holmes, T. H. Psychophysiologic studies of pulmonary ventilation, Psychosom Med, 26:645, 1964.

——— Masuda, M., Martin, C. J., and Holmes, T. H. Psychophysiologic studies of experimental action oriented behavior, J Psychosom Res, 9:209, 1965.

Faulkner, W. B., Jr. The effect of the emotion upon diaphragmatic function, Psychosom Med, 3:187, 1941.

——— Influence of suggestion on size of bronchial lumen: Bronchoscopic study and report of one case, Northwest Med, 40:367, 1941.

Finesinger, J. E. Effect of pleasant and unpleasant ideas on respiration in pseudoneurotic patients, Arch Neurol Psychiat, 4:425, 1939.

——— The spirogram in certain psychiatric disorders, Amer J Psychiat, 100: 159, 1943.

——— and Mazick, S. G. The effect of a painful stimulus and its recall upon respiration in psychoneurotic patients, Psychosom Med, 2:333, 1940.

Gellhorn, E. The tuning of the nervous system: Physiological foundations and implications for behavior, Perspectives Biol Med, 10,559, 1967.

Goldberg, C. J. Psychiatric aspects of the hyperventilation syndrome, South Afr Med J, 32:447, 1958.

Henry, G. W. Basal metabolism and emotional states, J Nerv Ment Dis, 70: 598, 1929.

Holmes, T. H., Goodell, H., Wolf, S., and Wolff, H. G. The Nose: An Experimental Study of Reactions Within the Nose in Human Subjects During Varying Life Experiences. Springfield, Ill., Charles C Thomas, Publisher, 1950.

Kerr, W. J., Dalton, J. W., and Gliebe, P. A. Some physical phenomena associated with the anxiety states and their relation to hyperventilation, Ann Int Med., 11:961, 1937.

Kissin, B. Psychogenic "dyspnea" and the hyperventilation syndrome, Amer Practitioner, 8:1537, 1957.

Landis, C. Studies of emotional reactions: IV. Metabolic rate, Amer J Physiol, 74:188, 1925.

Lewis, B. R. Chronic hyperventilation syndrome, JAMA, 155:1204, 1954.

McFarland, R. A., and Barach, A. L. Response of psychoneurotics to variations in oxygen tension, Amer J Psychiat, 93:1315, 1937.

Mezy, A. G., and Copper, A. J. Respiratory adaptation to exercise in anxious patients, Clin Sci, 20:171, 1961.

Segal, H. L., Binswanger, H. F., and Strouse, S. The effect of emotion on basal metabolism, Arch Int Med, 41:834, 1928.

Stevenson, I., and Ripley, H. S. Variations in respiration and respiratory symptoms during changes in emotion, Psychosom Med, 14:476, 1952.

Stevenson, I. P., and Wolff, H. G. Life situations, emotions and bronchial mucus, Psychosom Med, 11:223, 1949.

Wolf, G. A., and Wolff, H. G. Studies on the nature of certain symptoms associated with cardiovascular disorders, Psychosom Med, 8:293, 1946.

Wolf, S. Sustained contraction of the diaphragm, the mechanism of a common type of dyspnea and precordial pain, J Clin Invest, 26:1201, 1947.

Ziegler, L. H., and Levine, B. S. The influence of emotional reactions on basal metabolism, Amer J Med Sci, 169:68, 1925.

2

Historical Highlights

MEDICINE AND RESPIRATION THROUGH THE AGES

Prehistoric Man

In the dark, dim past of history, when man was slowly evolving from an instinctive animal to a thinking being, he adapted chipped flints to use as tools. These tools placed man on an extraordinarily competitive and then masterful position in terms of survival and flourishing. Man experiencing the vicissitudes of cold, heat, rain, snow, sleet, thunder, lightning, floods, drought, earthquakes, disease, pain, and hunger, as well as warmth of fire and the various aspects of life and death must surely have wondered at the cause and meaning of these natural phenomena. Being a realist he reacted to these situations with pragmatism—but also with fear, anger, and anxiety.

As he enlarged his tool-making capacities, learned to cultivate the soil, domesticated animals, and evolved into a tribal social being, he must have reasoned that there were higher powers which controlled and directed his destiny; that there were mysterious unknowables that manifested themselves in many natural phenomena, especially those of disastrous and awesome character. To defend himself against these unknown spirits and to ask protection from their anger or evil, he began to worship significant objects of nature: the sun, moon, stars, animals, mountains, volcanoes, rivers, fires—any object which was important he rationalized as having some power over him. From this nature worship he gradually evolved into the embrace of symbol or fetish worship in which the world was inhabited by many different gods that had invisible powers to benefit or to plague man.

From these beginnings of a rude polytheistic "religion" there appeared the shaman or witch doctor who became the expert in sorcery and communion with the gods. The witch doctor was the individual who knew best how to interpret natural signs and how to assuage the gods. Magic, witchcraft, sorcery, spells, sacrifices, and incantations were the means of dealing with the gods and warding off disasters and disease. Disease was seen as a manifestation of some god's displeasure, or of being possessed of evil spirits. At the same time, however, man was also accumulating experiences and observations which had practical value and these were the beginnings of herbal curative treatments for illness, some knowledge of bonesetting, and perhaps some rude surgery with flint instruments. Man had begun to recognize the difference between health and disease and that certain practices and behavior were conducive to well-being, a state to be eagerly sought.

The Beginnings of Civilization

The beginnings of civilization are recorded in clay tablets, papyrus, carved bone, stone, trephined skulls, clay artifacts, paintings—everything that tells the story of ancient people who lived together in a large community characterized by distinctiveness of culture. Whether one accepts the theory of "convergence" (the arising of separate civilizations in space and time) or "convection" (that none arises separately but rather from the influence of neighbors in space and time) is not important.

Our first definitive knowledge of the flourishing of ancient civilizations shows that along the basins and valleys of four rivers there arose distinct civilizations which were the first auspicious beginnings of social man. Along the Nile in Egypt, the Tigris and Euphrates in Mesopotamia, the Yellow River in China, and the Indus in India, there arose communities of people exhibiting a flowering of culture as if suddenly new breeds of men had sprung into being. To these ancient beginnings are added the Minoan civilization of Crete and, in the New World, the Mayan culture in Yucatan, and the Chavin and Mochica cultures in Peru—exciting discoveries made relatively recently. Savage man, primitive man, and prehistoric man in gradual evolution for many millennia are suddenly revealed in the trappings of "civilized" man as he told his story in written hieroglyphics, hieratic script, cuneiform tablets, dististinctive characters, or pictographs. In carvings, statues, drawings, cities, and temples, man left a visual record of how he lived, how he planned, how he worshiped, and how he regarded life and death.

These records show a mixture of animism, sorcery, and witchcraft blended into a concept of health and disease, but it is also evident that there is a parallel but growing development of empirical-rational medicine in the beginning concepts of the anatomy and physiology of man. While spirits were regarded as infesting men and causing all manner of disease, man himself was being observed and studied with emphasis on the illnesses that afflicted him. In ancient history we begin to see the separation of the priest from the physician, the exorcist from the healer, and the philosopher from the faith healer.

It is a curious and extraordinary fact about which Rhys David commented: "then suddenly and almost simultaneously and almost certainly independently, there is evidence about the 6th century B.C. in each of these widely separated centers of civilization of a leap forward in speculative thoughts, of a new birth in ethics, of a religion of conscience threatening to take place of the old religion of customs and magic." In China, along the Yellow River in the Chou Dynasty, in the flowering of Greek thought among the Ionians, along the banks of the Ganges, and in the rise of Buddha and Indian philosophy, there was a great intellectual ferment, spiritual revolt, and philosophical progress. It is almost incredible that from each of these widely separated cultures would arise almost simultaneously a leap forward that would affect the world and history for centuries to come.

Egypt

The ancient civilization of Egypt stands as the most impressive of antiqiuity. Millennia before the birth of Christ, the Egyptians flourished and built the grandeur that has come down through the centuries. Somewhere in Egypt originated hieroglyphics that would eventually culminate in the alphabetical script of the modern world. The use of rolls of Egyptian papyrus on which to write this script preserved for us the story of Egyptian medicine. Egyptian medicine existed long before Greek medicine and Saunders says "the philosophical and scientific revolution which occurred in Greece during the 6th Century B.C. was not born in a vacuum. Its antecedent was the inheritance not only of the prescientific beliefs, myths and cosmogonies of the Greeks themselves but also the accumulated treasures of two thousand years of Babylonian and Egyptian art."

The first figure in Egyptian medicine is Im-Ho-Tep, physician-vizier of King Zoser (2773 B.C.). His healing powers and medical knowledge led to his reverement and to the erection of sanctuaries of Im-Ho-Tep as temples of healing. It is probable that the Greek god Aesculapius was named after Im-Ho-Tep and the Aesculapian temples of healing were the Greek counterparts of the Egyptian temples of Im-Ho-Tep. It is the judgment of Ebbell, who translated the Ebers Papyrus, that "we ought not to set up the Greek Aesculapius as the patron genius of medicine, but rather the physician to whom the Egyptians gave this dignity, vis, Im-Ho-Tep."

The source books of Egyptian medical knowledge are manuscripts of papyrus. The three most important and their dating are: (1) the Kahun Papyrus (2100 B.C.), the first textbook on gynecology in medical history; (2) The Smith Papyrus (1550 B.C.), a textbook on surgical procedures; and (3) the Ebers Papyrus (1555 B.C.), the best-preserved, longest, and most important of medical documents concerning internal medicine, pharmacotherapy, and surgery.

The Egyptian scribes in the long-distant past had put down in hieratic script the medical knowledge and practices of previously existing and much older texts dating back to the Old Kingdom and the Archaic period of Egyptian history. These papyri give evidence of the parallelism of the empirical-rational outlook on disease, mixed with incantations and prescriptions of infinite variety. The physicians of the Nile had taken the first step from demonology toward rational medical treatment based on observations and empirical treatment.

The Smith Papyrus, the surgical treatise, consists of 48 instructions or articles each setting down the malady, diagnosis, and rules for treatment. The instructions fully reveal a great deal of medical knowledge of fractures, the stitching of gaping wounds, cauterization, the description and consequences of infection, etc. The most physiological of these instructions is found in the First Instruction, which revealed the rational thinking of the Egyptians. "The counting of anything with the fingers [is done] to recognize the way the heart goes. There are vessels in it leading to every part of the body. . . . When a Sachmet priest, any *swnw* doctor . . . puts his fingers to the head . . . through the two hands, to the place of the heart . . . to the two legs, then he is measuring the heart . . . it speaks . . . in every vessel, every part of the body . . . one measures the vessels of his heart to learn the information that is given by it." This is an astonishing cardiovascular observation made millennia before the Greeks.

The Ebers Papyrus is of the same age as the Smith Papyrus. It came into full recognition as a medical document of great importance with the translation by Ebbell in 1937. It contains 108 columns of beautiful script in a scroll which is more than 65 ft long and 12 in high. It is a great compilation of ideas and writings of previous periods, giving recipes against various diseases and symptoms. It is clear that the symptoms have been put together into syndromes as pathological disease entities—e.g., angina pectoris, hernias, appendicitis, varicose veins, etc. Its descriptions of the drugs used in treatment count into the hundreds and run the gamut from excrements of flies, urine, copper salts, and antimony to drugs currently available in modern pharmacies—e.g., juniper, pomegranate, turpentine, thyme, hellabore, opium, mandrake, henbane, etc. This remarkable compendium of medicines also includes drugs found only in India, China, and Malaya —indirect evidence of the antiquities of land and sea trade routes between the Far East and the Middle East. The use of medications was rational and depended on the symptoms exhibited.

In the Ebers Papyrus three different kinds of healers are described. These are the physicians, sachmet priests (surgeons?), and *s3w* (sorcerer or exorcists). As corresponding to these three kinds of healers, the Ebers Papyrus describes three kinds of treatment: medical, surgical, and spells. Concerning the last, however, it is evident to Ebbell that the use of spells and incantations was not meant in the sense of strong beliefs in magic and evil spirits but rather as a psychological method of helping the patient in pain or with intractable ailments. The Papyrus clearly indicates that the Egyptian healer looked on disease as a consequence of natural causes rather than demoniacal possession.

The anatomical and physiological section is a revelation of the extent and powers of observation of the Egyptian healers. From Section 99 of the Ebers Papyrus we take the following excerpts: "The beginning of the physician's secret: knowledge of the heart's movement and knowledge of the heart." This Papyrus goes on to explain, just as in the Smith Papyrus, that "the heart speaks out of the vessels of every lip."

The first definitive writing in history on respiratory physiology is seen in the Ebers Papyrus. We quote: "as to the breath which enters into the nose: it enters into the heart and lungs; these give to the whole belly." Further, "there are four vessels to his two ears together with the [ear] canal, [namely] two on the right side and two on his left side. The breath of life enters into the right ear, and the breath of death enters into the left ear; another lection: it [i.e., the breath of life] enters into the right side, and the breath of death enters into the left side." In considering further the vessels of the body, the Papyrus goes on to state, "there are four vessels to the liver; it is they which give to it humor and air which afterwards cause all diseases to arise in it by overfilling with blood." "As to the minds kneeling [breakdown ?]: this means that the mind is constricted, and its heart in its place in the blood of the lung becomes small through it. It is [due to the fact] that his heart is hot, and then his mind becomes weary through it; he eats little and is fastidious."

From these writings it is clear that certain ethical precepts, medical-physiological concepts, and knowledge of disease conditions and treatments clearly antedate the Greeks. The anatomy and physiology are faulty but placed in the context of time it is remarkable that Egyptians had definitive ideas about "breath of life" and how it was distributed by vessels to the heart, lungs, and body.

Mesopotamia

As the Egyptian dynasties were waxing and waning in the Valley of the Nile, in the delta of the Tigris and Euphrates Rivers and along the river banks in Mesopotamia, there came into parallel being the Assyro-Babylonian civilization. It began with the Sumerians and the development by these advanced peoples of pictographic writing (3500 B.C.) and the cuneiform tablet as a means of communication. The oldest medical textbook known (2200 B.C.) is such a tablet, which revealingly describes treatment methodology without any mention of magic spells.

The history of the Land of Two Rivers is a history of successive conquests and defeats in which great kings and cities flourished while Sumerians, Assyrians, and Babylonians fought for political domination. During this period there was a mingling of the various tribal cultures, assimilations, and progression of knowledge.

The early Babylonian literature shows a high degree of sophistication in philosophy and ethics. This is particularly evident in the Code of Hammurabi, a Babylonian King (1720–1686 B.C.) whose concepts and codes of justice are inscribed in a great black stone monument 8 ft high. The codes or laws ostensibly received by Hammurabi from the Sun God are revealing in the ethical, moral and legal principles of the times. Here are some examples:

Paragraph 3. If a man in a case [pending judgment] bear false [threatening] witness, or does not establish the testimony that he has given, if that case be a case involving life, that man shall be put to death.
Paragraph 141. If the wife of a man who is living in his house sets her face to go out and play the part of a fool, neglect her house, belittle her husband, they shall call her to account; if her husband says "I have put her away," he shall let her go. On her departure nothing shall be given to her for her divorce.
Paragraph 221. If a physician set a broken bone for a man or cure his diseased bowels, the patient shall give five shekels of silver to the physician [$5.50 at present price of silver].

The medical knowledge of Mesopotamia derives principally from the great library of King Assurbanipal (668–626 B.C.), which contained more than 20,000 clay tablets of which 660 tablets pertained to medical knowledge. This material reveals that there had been sophisticated physicians in Mesopotamia.

These tablets describe diseases such as tuberculosis, pleurisy, bronchitis, jaundice, gastritis, hemorrhoids, stroke, gonorrhea, etc. They tell of a huge pharmacopoeia similar to that described in Egyptian papyri. There are, however, many drugs which do not appear there and one of the most significant is Atropa belladonna, the deadly "night shade" and one of the most useful plants known to medical science. From the use of medications in various ailments, it is clear that rational drug therapy existed—e.g., belladonna was used for bladder spasms, persistent coughing, asthma, and excessive salivation.

It is also evident that to test the toxicity of such drugs, slaves were used as guinea pigs. The Assyrian herbal likewise lists many drugs which came to it from the Orient. The Assyrian medical texts are mixtures of rational medicine and magic rituals and exorcisms. The Assyro-Babylonian culture was rampant with gods and demons of both Sumerian and Semitic origin who could cause disease states. Often, at the invention of priests in order to explain disease states, rituals and appeals were made to various gods and incantations and spells were part of the medical treatment. Supplementary to these priests there developed singularly the Mesopotamian priesthood, a special group that studied the stars and the planets and developed astronomy and, as its offshoot, astrology. These priests strived to associate the movement of heavenly bodies to human fortunes and disasters: the beginning of "scientific" astronomy. The 12 signs of the Zodiac were astrological expressions of the attempt to connect human and natural events to certain heavenly movements and thus enhance human decisions into a favorable arrangement. Here, too, we find the first evidence of the snake as a symbol of healing from the legendary story of Gilgamesh (3000 B.C.), in which—while Gilgamesh is bathing in the river—the serpent finds and eats the precious herb of life which rejuvenates him and gives him henceforth the power and knowledge of perpetual life.

The description of empirico-rational medicine found in the Mesopotamian tablets is further elucidated by the knowledge that surgery was practiced in the second millennium B.C. This has been verified by the findings of ancient skulls with definitive signs of trephination and postoperative survival. To date, however, there has not been found a treatise which dealt specifically with anatomical and physiological observations.

India

To the east of Egypt and the Land of the Two Rivers, in the north of India along the valley of the Indus River, there arose a culture dating from 2500 (probably earlier) to 1500 B.C. The recent excavations at Mohenjo-daro and Harappa reveal a civilization that culminated into great cities which nowhere else in the world had such detailed planning and hygienic facilities. Unearthed in these great cities, easily the match of those found in Egypt and Mesopotamia, were evidences of a flourishing culture and an economic empire. These people knew cotton, wheat, barley, and sesame; they raised zebus, water buffalo, swine, horses, and donkeys; and they had tamed elephants.

The pictographic script unearthed from these cultures is similar to those of Egypt and Mesopotamia, but still remains undeciphered. Writing was apparently done on destructible material—not papyri or clay tablets. It is, however, probable that the subsequent records of Vedic and post-Vedic times reflect the persisting religious and medical beliefs of the Indus Valley civilization.

The sanitation in Harappa and Mohenjo-daro—baths, lavatories, fresh-water tanks, airy ventilation, street drains, etc.—reveals in its own way that good hygiene was linked with health. In Egypt and Mesopotamia, the paralleling of hygienic practices with empirico-rational medical practice indicates the high quality of Indus Valley medicine.

The invasion of the Indus Valley by Aryan hordes in 1500 B.C. left the civilization in ruins. The Aryans who came from the northwest were fair-skinned, tall, and mostly fair-haired. They later took the name Hindu, conquered the greater part of India, and fused their culture with that of the Indus Valley. They grew prosperous and developed great cities, Sanskrit writing, and a well-defined caste system. Also a great body of traditional verse was collected into the Vedas, the two most important for medical knowledge being the Rigveda and the Atharvaveda.

The first written records of post-Indus India were compiled around 800 B.C. from previous texts. Atharvavedic medicine is an amalgam of magical-religious and empirical-rational medicine containing much of gods, spells, and incantations. There were two kinds of healers: the priest-physician and the lay physician. The widespread use of drugs by medical practitioners in the treatment of illnesses is evidence of rational medicine.

In post-Vedic times there was a great growth of medical thought, and in 600 B.C. two great medical universities arose, one at Taxila in the northwest and one in the east at Benares. The schools were those of Atreya and Dharvantari, respectively, the fathers of Indian medicine. This was a time of great intellectual ferment as Buddhism rose to challenge Brahmanism and medical teachings developed to culminate in the two great classics of Indian medicine, Charaka Samhita (from the medical teachings of Atreya) and the Susruta Samhita (from the surgical teachings of Susruta). The Samhitas have multiple authorships and were compiled from previous teachings, treatises, and monographs. The exact dates are controversial, but the original teachings might well be placed around 600 B.C.

The Susruta Samhita is an ancient textbook that deals with surgical matters with medicinal and methodological overlay. The surgical ideas and practices mentioned in the Susruta are astounding. Surgery, says the Susruta, "is the first and highest division of the healing art. . . ." The earliest

Indian surgical instruments from the first millennium A.D. suggest the remarkable development of surgery in these ancient times.

In the Susruta, details are given for the couching of cataracts, plastic surgery with the aid of an attached flap, bladder surgery for the removal of stones, and the utilization of sutures of hemp, hair, and animal sinews placed with straight and bent needles of bone and bronze. There is a biological counterpart to the modern method of making a wound suture with metal staples. The Indians used large black Bengali ants for intestinal wound closures by allowing the ants to join the pressed edges with their powerful mandibles and then separating their bodies. The use of living clamps on the gut implied a knowledge of the chances of surgical infection. The Susruta, in its description of conception and obstetrics, describes clearly surgical intervention at delivery, later called Caesarean section, as a method of decreasing infant mortality in certain difficult cases.

To understand Indian medicine there must be an understanding of the philosophy of the meaning of the Ayurveda, the philosophic basis for the Samhitas. The Characa states succinctly that the Ayurveda is the science of life. Life is good, evil, happy, and unhappy. It is a union of body senses, mind, and soul which constitutes life. In life both health and disease coexist and the parity or the balance of these factors leads to health. The formalized doctrine of health was bound in certain basic elements and constituents which maintain the body. The five important elements were water, fire, air, earth, and ether. There were seven body constituents which were modifications of the five elements that had to be in proportion for proper body function. The Indians had three body humors, air, bile, and phlegm, the disarrangements of which caused disequilibrium and disease. Health and disease were therefore states of equilibrium or disequilibrium. Illnesses were characterized by excesses, deficiencies, wrong administration of sense objects, climate considerations, and the misuse of intelligence. Thus diet, daily regimen, right thoughts, and medicine were primary in the maintenance of health.

The Samhitas' lessons on physician's training, practice, and ethics reveal a remarkable advancement of the medical profession. There are discussions on the initial decision to become a physician, the proper kind of a person to be a physician, the selection of the proper textbook, the selection of a proper preceptor, the selectiveness in screening of candidates. The initial charge to students, the six years of instructions in the proper courses (including mastery in medicine and surgery), and the proper behavior of physicians were included. It will come as no surprise that the physicians also looked forward to considerable fees, rewards, and status.

The charge of the preceptor to his pupils contained admonishments and rules reminiscent of the ethics of Hippocrates. For instance, one must give up "lust, anger, avarice, folly, vanity, pride, envy, rudeness, deception, falsehood, idleness and all other reprehensible conduct." One should keep clean and neat (e.g., cut your hair and nails short) and avoid sexual intercourse. One should treat Brahmins, paupers, friends, ascetics, etc., gratuitously; but hunters, fowlers, outcasts, and sinners should not be treated. "By acting in this way one makes himself known and attains friends, fame, wealth and objects of desire." The Charaka adds, "thou shouldst with thy whole heart strive to bring about the cure of those that are ill." Also, one should not commit adultery, steal, be flamboyant, or consort with sinful people. The physician should speak with tender truth, display right conduct, devote a single-mindedness in doing good to the patient, and keep doctor-patient communications private. Nor should one be boastful, but rather physicians should know humility.

Although the information is often fanciful and wrong, the Samhitas have sections on anatomy, embryology, fetal development, osteology, myology, angiology, neurology, splanchology, pathology, physiology, obstetrics, gynecology, pediatrics, surgery, medical ethics, diagnosis, and prognosis. In fact, the Susruta contains the first known discourse on human dissection by a peculiar method of water immersion and the scrubbing away of tissues.

Cardiovascular circulation was a combination of truth and fancy. The lungs and their functions are little mentioned, although observations on respiratory diseases are made. However, Charaka says:

> . . . of the ducts that bear the life breaths the root is the heart, and the great duct [trachea]. Beholding a person inhaling and exhaling long breaths or breathing obstructively, or breathing furiously or drawing short or incessant breaths, or breathing with noise or pain, the physician should understand that those ducts [bronchi] of man that bear the life breaths have become disordered.

The Indian physicians thought that the air entered through the nose, mouth, throat, and the heart and lungs. Another interesting passage in another document says: ". . . after coursing through the interior of the lotus-like heart goes out through the throat to drink of the outside air and after taking up the nectar of the air it enters the body again to nourish the whole body, and to keep up the digestive fire." The Characa describes the functions of inhalation and exhalation; proper actions of speech, mind, and body; regulation of the mind; the origin of joy and cheerfulness; and the excitement of the body fire. The concept of respiration and body or digestive fire is interesting for it antedates the Greek idea of heat of the heart as requiring the cooling effect of respiration and the Galenical idea that respiration is required for innate heat. Body fire or heat was a source of longevity, good complexion, strength, health, exertion, growth, luster, energy, animal heat, and the life breaths. When it became extinct the person died. When it burned brightly one lived long in health; when vitiated one is afflicted with disease. It would seem that respiration, oxidative metabolism, and heat production are involved in a fanciful manner in these statements, although the Indians did not fully grasp this.

The Indian materia medica is a compendium of useful vegetable, animal, and mineral drugs which includes most of the medications seen in the Egyptian and Mesopotamian collections. We know also that most of the drugs of India found their way to the West. There is nothing distinctive in respect to Indian drugs except for the notable fact that while the West used opium, this valuable herb was not used in India until centuries later.

The relationship of emotion to illness is succinctly stated in the concept embracing the derangement of humors of the body—e.g., anger, fear, and indulgence in sexual intercourse cause derangement of the bile, while sleeping during the day and idleness derange phlegm. And when the bile is deranged the blood is deranged. These are derangements of the body, while "passion" and "darkness" are faults of the mind. Excessive anger, grief, fear, joy, malice, etc., lead to mental distempers. In the observation and examination of the patient the Indian physician is told not only to use all his senses but to note the patient's social status (caste) and his mental disposition.

From the foregoing it is clear that Indian medicine was a highly enlightened profession which taught established ethical rules relating to the conduct of physicians and to their training. The rationality of these ancient lessons shows how favorably the Indian physician compared with his Egyptian and Mesopotamian contemporaries.

China

In the northwest of China, through the fertile valley of the Yellow River, was arising a contemporary of the cultures along the Nile, Ganges, Tigris, and the Euphrates. There were three revered legendary Chinese Emperors—the symbols of Chinese medicine in antiquity. The first was Fu Hsi, the first emperor, founder, philosopher, and originator of the Eight Diagrams symbolic of the concept of Yin and Yang, the prime forces of nature. Next in line came Shen Ning, the Blazing Emperor, who related agriculture, herbals, and medicine. Then followed Huang Ti, the Yellow Emperor, to whom is attributed the Classic of Internal Medicine. These three emperors were said to have lived in the obscure prehistoric period of 3000 to 2200 B.C.

The first definitive evidence of Chinese history came with the finding of the tombs of the Shang rulers (1523–1028 B.C.), confirming ancient Chinese history. Here, too, there was a first discovery of Chinese character writing which was preserved for the ages by being incised in bone and writings on bamboo. The Shang rulers conquered the region with their war chariots and superior bronze weapons and built the capitol city of Anyang. As their power and civilization grew, they developed astronomy, a calendar, and arithmetic. The Shang dynasty people were god worshipers and the world was one populated with demons. In this period there were the beginnings of the formulation of the concept of the natural cosmology, the oneness of nature, and man's place in it. Here developed the concept of the world spirit—the way, Tao—which found expression in the concept of Yang and Yin.

However, it was during the Chou dynasty (1027–221 B.C.) that these philosophies found their greatest flowering. It was a period of feudalism and the time when scholars and sages as a class were coming into being as the wise men to guide Chinese destiny and shape its philosophies and history. It was a time when the courts of the Chou rulers produced the most important ancient books of China. It was the time of Lao-Tsu, the Venerable Philosopher, and the time of Confucius (sixth and fifth Century B.C.). From a contemplation of the thought of early sages, and being troubled by the warring struggles of feudal lords, Lao-Tsu formalized the concept of Tao, a philosophy which was to last for millennia.

Tao is the way of life combining the metaphysical and the material. Involved in it are two cosmic forces, Yin and Yang, the negative and positive principles of the universe. In the creative sense, from the Great Absolute Yin, the grosser and heavier part precipitated to form earth, while the finer light part the Yang became sublimated to form the heaven. The union and interaction of these two form both the soul and material basis of the universe. Yin is the passive or female element—also cold, darkness, disease, and death; Yang is the active or male element that represents warmth, light, health, and life. By these elements' order or disorder, all creation continues to be in balance or imbalance. In the rigid scheme of things that evolved from these basic concepts there was a parallelism of the macrocosm to the microcosm that is man.

Materially all things were seen as being composed of five elements: metal, wood, water, fire, and earth. There must be a balance in these five elements which are matched by five chief viscera—metal to the lungs, wood to the liver, water to the kidneys, fire to the heart, and earth to the spleen. Added to this were the complexities of five directions, five planets, five seasons, five times of the day, five colors and tones, five tastes, five human relations—all variables affecting man in his health. Such tremendously complicated relations set in a rigid schemata could only be an obstacle to a rational concept of physiology and disease. However, it is a fact that, whereas only priest physicians existed previously during the Chou dynasty the ritual provided for priests (sorcerers) to make drought offerings, while the doctor was designated to superintend matters of medicine, treatment, and herbal collections. This change was reflected in the ancient Chinese character for medicine, which contained the symbol for sorcerer; it was subsequently replaced by the word for wine, the latter symbolizing the utilization of elixirs in medical treatments.

One of the great source books of Chinese medicine is the Yellow Emperor's Classic of Internal Medicine. It has mysterious authorship but is legendarily attributed to Huang Ti, the Yellow Emperor. However, he lived around 2600 B.C. while the known archaeological evidence indicates 1500 B.C. as the earliest Chinese writing. Experts estimate that this book was actually compiled around the fourth or fifth century B.C. in the Chou era, after Lao-Tsu and Confucius. However, its contents reveal that it unquestionably reflects earlier thoughts and teachings—exactly how far back is speculative. It is in the form of a dialogue between Huang Ti and Ch'i Po, his sage minister, in which the latter responds in erudite discourse to the former's questions on man, his destinies, and his body functions. For example:

> The Emperor asks, "How can you explain the angry appearance of the viscera?" Ch'i Po answered, "the heart is the root of life and causes the versatility of the spiritual faculties. The heart influences the face and fills the pulse with blood. Within Yang, the principle of light and life, the heart acts as a Great Yang which permeates the climate of summer. The lungs are the origin of the breath and the dwelling of the animal spirits or inferior souls. The lungs influence the body hair and has an effect upon the skin. Within Yang, the lungs act as a great Yin which permeates the climate in Fall." . . . [Later] Ch'i Po answers, ". . . hence, when joy is felt it creates a large vacuum and thus the force of the kidneys can ascend. The emotion of anger rises from the fullness of the liver. The emotion of sympathy arises from the fullness of the lungs. The emotion of fear releases the impulses of the spleen. The feeling of worry releases the impulses of the heart. These are the ways of the emotion, and thus disease has five times five, twenty-five possible transformations. . . ."
>
> [Further,] "those who are about at midnight have difficulties in breathing emanating from the kidney. Those whose demeanor is dissolute and licentious get a disease of the lungs. Those who are lazy and full of apprehension and fear have difficulties in breathing emanating from the lungs. Those whose deportment is licentious and excessive will injure their spleen . . . and those whose demeanor is immoral and dissolute will injure their hearts. . . ."
>
> "Therefore it is said in order to examine the course of the disease one must investigate whether man is courageous or nervous and cowardly, and one must examine his bones, flesh and skin, then one can know the facts of the case which are necessary for the methods of treatment."

Confined and restricted to the philosophic concepts of Yang and Yin and an incredibly complex system of numbers of theorized variables, the

Chinese concept of anatomy and physiology was subordinated to the concepts of Tao. This led to a highly systemized and stylized but inaccurate view of anatomy and physiology.

The chief method of diagnosis was an extraordinarily complicated system of pulse taking based on Yang and Yin and its interaction with the harmony and disharmony of the five elements, five viscera, etc. In consideration of the great numbers of variations of the pulse was also the admonition to note the respiration—its quality and number—as related to the pulse beat. Acupuncture and its therapeutic counterpart, moxibustion, arose as a method of puncturing certain channels whose flux of Yang and Yin had been interrupted, thus allowing the "evil air," which was causing stagnation, to escape so recirculation could occur. It was also recognized that proper needle insertion must be adjusted to the time of inhalation and extracted with the next exhalation.

As can be seen, the Chinese placed a high value on proper breathing as being one of the cardinal rules for attaining Tao. The philosophical and metaphysical concept of proper respiration was bound in the cosmic idea that one breathed in the great spiritual soul of the universe to be transmuted into the human soul substance. Proper breathing then was considered essential to feed the soul, foster longevity, and to nourish life and human nature. These goals could be achieved by deeper breathing—drawing from the uttermost depths—and by holding the breath for up to 120 heartbeats and exhaling gently so as not to stir "the feather of a wild goose."

Because of the prohibition of human dissection by ancestor worship, the ancient Chinese had obscure knowledge of anatomy and physiology. Thus in their quest for medical knowledge they were driven largely to speculations. Some moderns have speculated that perhaps the ancient Chinese in their concentration on Yang and Yin as the determinants of health were antedating the modern knowledge of the sympathetic-parasympathetic system, the imbalance of which can cause a variety of illnesses. The relationship of Yang and Yin to the pulse, to various viscera, to respiration, and to emotions, points to the possibility of such astuteness, albeit cloaked in metaphysical complexity.

Mexico

The very recent discovery and recognition of the antiquity of the New World have brought exciting new outlooks on the state of Mayan and Peruvian medicine. In the Yucatan peninsula, the Mayan civilization—characterized by huge terraced temples and buildings—was flourishing far back in the first millennium B.C. and probably earlier. At this time these people possessed cities, imposing architecture, hieroglyphic writings, arithmetic, astronomy, a calendar, and paper.

Surpassing the Aztecs of Mexico and antedating them, the Mayan's and their accomplishments were lost even as their incomparable cities were buried in the lush jungles of Yucatan. Anthropologists believe that the Olmecs were the precursers and originators of the culture that the Mayans and Aztecs were to bring to further development. From clay statues and drawings there is unquestionable evidence that diseases similar to those of modern man also troubled the Central American ancients. Also unquestionable is the evidence of a plethora of gods and demons to whom these people made sacrifices and offered prayers. The Mayan people must have been haunted as were the Mesopotamians by the view that disease and disasters were interventions of supernatural beings who must be placated. We do not have definite evidence of the state of medicine in these cultures during this period. However, later knowledge gleaned from Spanish documents indicates that the people had a large compendium of herbal medicine—always a sign of empirical medicine—which agents were apparently utilized in a rational manner. Included were sarsaparilla, peyote (which we now know contains mescaline), the mushroom, hanocatl (which we now know contains psylocybin), camotl (a plant used as a sedative and analgesic), tobacco, and cocoa bean. According to the Spanish, the Aztecs also had—in addition to the priests and sorcerers—apothecaries who could be separated into surgeons and medical doctors. They utilized steam baths and massage as therapy for rheumatism, palsy, and neuralgia. They used special diets in internal medicine. We can deduce that in the early Mayan and Aztec cultures, medicine was compounded of religiomagic components. Also, along with these, was an empirical-rational concept which flourished along with the advancing of the civilization.

Peru

Farther south on the western Pacific rim, on the coast and in the highlands of Peru, there developed cultures about which later archaeologists were to be astounded, for the Spanish conquest of the Incas in the 16th century gave no clues of earlier civilizations. In recent times, however, the evidence shows that great cultures existed long before that of the Incas. No written records exist, but the grandeur of their cities, their paintings, and clay statues leave indisputable evidence of their existence and advanced knowledge. The ruins of the great temples in scattered places are dated now to 900–600 B.C. The artifacts found in them are the remnants of the first great Chavin culture. The architectural grandeur of the temples, and the layout of streets, houses, and squares reflect a civilization that cultivated cotton, maize, beans, and peanuts, and domesticated animals such as the llama. They were craftsmen in the arts of ceramics, weaving, jewelry, and carving. These artifacts indicate a predilection for terrifying-looking animal demons. Subsequent to the Chavin, to the south there developed a neighbor culture—the Mochican Nation (500 B.C.)—whose temples and cities rivaled the Chavin. Moreover, these people left behind a large collection of beautiful pottery which gives a marvelous view of the life and times of these advanced people. The Mochican Empire extended along the coast and valleys and included many villages.

The ceramics tell of demons, diseases, wars and strife, history, sacrificial priests, and peasant life in all its aspects. We see peasants and kings at work harvesting or at table. There are astronomers, artisans, weavers, and metalworkers. The works vividly portray Mochican life without the use of a single word. The clay statues tell strikingly of the diseases and afflictions of these people. Representations of exorcist-priests, gods, and demons tell of the magical-religious influence in medical treatment which continued down into Spanish observations of Inca medicine. However, perusal of these ceramic artifacts shows clearly that rational treatments were employed.

The use of drugs in these times indicated that along with the magician priests, were also healers and surgeons. Many drugs probably stretching into antiquity included purges, antidiarrhea agents, minerals for intestinal illnesses, intestinal worm repellents, antiseptics, ointments, and cocoa leaves found only in the Andes. The Incas knew well the properties of this latter drug, which was distributed once daily to highland workers as a stimulant. The practice of cocoa chewing is evident in the Mochican ceramics. Thus the use of cocoa leaves covers the long span of time from the first millennium before Christ to the present.

However, it is the amazing surgery of the Peruvians that best indicates the extent of medical knowledge in this ancient culture. There are many ceramics which show successful leg amputations, the use of suturing, and the use of wooden stumps. But the most exciting is the finding of a great number of skulls—more than 10,000—which show trephination. Skulls such as these, dating back to the Stone Age, have been found elsewhere throughout the world but nowhere in the numbers found in Peru. The skull openings clearly reveal that the Peruvian surgeons utilized a great variety of methods in opening windows into the brain. But even more astonishing is the fact that by far the majority of these people survived. How the surgeons accomplished this—controlling pain, hemorrhage, and infection—is an intriguing unanswered question. Sculptures depicting actual trephination operations have been found, as have the tools which the surgeon used, and even the cotton bandaging on skulls. These remarkable surgical interventions—for what purposes are only conjectural—are unmatched in any other ancient culture.

Greece

At the time that the Mochican surgeon was plying his trade in far off Peru, as the Chou Dynasty sages were evolving the philosophy of Yang and Yin, as the Indians were setting up their medical universities, as the glory of Egypt was facing to fall to the Persians, and while Nebuchadnezzar II tried to restore Babylon to its former greatness, there were coming into flowering from the roots of the Minoan civilization of Crete the foundations of Greek medicine.

In the land of the Ionians—the crossroads and travel lanes of the great civilizations to the East, Far East, and South—in the 6th century B.C. arose philosophers such as Thales, Anaximander, Anaximines, Heraclitus, Anaxagoras, Empedocles, and Pythagorus. In their writings are the beginnings of the Greek doctrine of "airs" as the primary principle and "pneuma" as the breath of life. Here, too, is the concept of four elements: fire, earth, air, and water, combined with four qualities reminiscent of Indian and Chinese concepts.

It was in the time of the golden age of Pericles that Athens reached her height of glory. It was also the time of Socrates, Hippocrates, Plato, and Aristotle. From the foundation of Minoan culture were added the fruits of interchange with Egypt, Mesopotamia, and India. In this time of intellectual ferment in widely separated cultures, the Greeks superimposed their crowning achievements in philosophical thought. Their philosophy reflected on concepts of truth, justice, ethics, and human freedom; it was a time for dialogues based on criticisms, logic, and scientific methodology. It is this sense of philosophical freedom which shaped the course of Greek medicine.

The fountainhead of Greek medicine was Hippocrates of Cos who gave to Greek medicine its scientific spirit and ethical ideals. The Hippocratean doctrines appeared from the magicoreligious influence of priest-physicians of the temples of Asklepios to the art of clinical inspection, observation, and treatment.

In his collection of writings Hippocrates crystalized these elements into a systematic science and harkened physicians to the moral and ethical dignities of the profession. In his "Epidemics" he gave a case history which illustrates the clarity and perspicacity of his observations:

> In Thasos the wife of Delearces, who lay sick on the plain, was seized after grief with an acute fever with shivering. From the beginning she would wrap herself up and without speaking a word pluck, scratch, pick hairs, weep and

then laugh. But she did not sleep; though stimulated the bowels passed nothing. She drank a little when the attendant suggested it. Urine, thin and scanty; fever slight to the touch; coldness of extremities.
Ninth day. Much wandering followed by return of reason; silent.
Fourteenth day. Respiration rare and large with long intervals becoming afterward short.
Seventeenth day. Bowels under a stimulus passed disordered matters, then her very drink passed unchanged; nothing coagulated. The patient noticed nothing; the skin tense and dry.
Twentieth day. Much rambling followed by recovery of reason; speechless; respiration short.
Twenty-first day. Death.
The respiration of this patient throughout was rare and large; she took no notice of anything; she constantly wrapped herself up; either much rambling or silence throughout.

Hippocrates in "On the Sacred Disease" had these words on the physiology and function of respiration:

For when a person draws in air by the mouth and nostrils, the breath (pneuma) goes first to the brain, then the greater part of it to the internal cavity, then part to the lungs, part to the veins and from them it is distributed to the other parts of the body along the veins; and whatever passes to the stomach cools and does nothing more; and so also with regard to the lungs. But the air which enters the veins is of use to the body (by entering the brain and its ventricles) and thus it imparts sensibility and motion to all the members, so when the veins are secluded from the air by the phlegm and do not receive it, the man loses his speech and intellect and the hands become powerless and are contracted, the blood stopping and not being diffused, as it was wont; and the eyes are distorted owing to the veins being excluded from the air; and they palpitate; and froth from the lung tissues by the mouth.

Further, he describes the various emotions as emanating from the brain and thus affecting behavior.

And men ought to know that from nothing but thence, from the brain, come joys, praise, delight, laughter, sports and sorrows, griefs, despondency, and lamentations. And by this, in an especial manner we acquire wisdom and knowledge, see and hear, know what are foul and are fair, what are bad and what are good, what are sweet and what unsavory; some we discriminate by habit and some we perceive by their utility. By this we distinguish objects of relish and disrelish, according to the seasons; and the same things do not always please us. And by the same organs we become mad and delirious, and fears and terrors assail us, some by night and some by day, and dreams and untimely wanderings, and cares that are not suitable and ignorance of present circumstances, dissuatude and unskillfulness. All these things we endure from the brain when it is not healthy, but is more hot or cold, more moist or more dry than natural, or when it suffers any other praeter-natural and unusual affection.

Finally, he describes the concept of the supreme function of the brain and the essentiality of air to the brain.

In these ways I am of the opinion that the brain exercises the greatest power in man. This is the interpreter to us of those things which emanate from the air, when it [the brain] happens to be in a sound state. But the air supplys its sense to it. And the eyes and the ears and the tongue and the feet administer such things as the brain cogitates. For inasmuch as it is supplied with air, does it impart sense to the body. It is the brain which is the messenger to the understanding. For when the man draws the breath (pneuma) into himself, it passes first to the brain and thus the air is distributed to the rest of the body, leaving in the brain its acme and whatever has sense and understanding.

It is clear from the record that the greatest contribution of Hippocrates to medicine was the clarity and simplicity of his observations, the systematizing of his medical ideas, the emphasis on the ethical aspects of medicine (divorced from the magicoreligious), and the formalization of ethical precepts.

The state of respiratory anatomy and physiology is clearly in a naive state in Hippocratic writings. Plato (427 to 347 B.C.), who came after Hippocrates, stated the prevailing doctrine of his times in his *Timaeus:*

But as the Gods foreknew, with respect for the palpitation of the heart under the dread of danger and the excitement of passion, that all such dwellings of the inflamed spirit would be produced by fire, they form the lungs to be a sort of protection thereto; first of all soft and bloodless, and next internally provided with cavities, perforated like a sponge in order to cool the breath which they receive, and give the heart easy respiration and repose in its excessive heat. On this account, the gods led the channels of the windpipe into the lungs which they placed like a soft cushion around the heart in order that anger rises in it to an extreme height it might fall on some yielding substance, and so getting cooled, yield cheerfully and with less trouble to the authority of reason.

According to the Greeks, the function of respiration was to cool the heart and this concept was to hold forth until its questioning by Galen five centuries later.

Aristotle (384–322 B.C.), student of Plato and tutor of Alexander the Great, was the great biologist and scientist of the times. In his De *Animus* he discoursed first on the body-mind dualism:

. . . most of them, anger, confidence, appetite, perception—involve a body; thought looks the most like being peculiar to soul, but if even thought involves imagination, even it involves a body—in fact all the experiences of soul (anger, etc.) seem to involve a body; for along with them the body suffers some change. This is shown by the fact that sometimes violence and manifest experiences do not lead to anger or fear, or sometimes we are stirred by trifling experiences when the body is in the state of tension that it is when we are angry. Indeed, we may have the experience of fear when nothing fearful is happening to us—to return to our starting point we were saying that the phenomenon of soul insofar as things like anger and fear are inseparable from matter in the way stated.

He went further on to state the function of respiration.

> Nature uses for two purposes the air that is in any case breathed in—while utterance is for the sake of well-being, so it uses breath both to preserve the inner heat as something necessary and to produce voice for the sake of well-being. The organ in breathing is the windpipe, and this exists for the sake of the lung which secures the land animals more heat than other creatures have. It is primarily the region of the heart that needs respiration and therefore the air has to come in by being breathed.

Erasistratus (310–250 B.C.), the Alexandrian anatomist and physiologist, brought his critical experimental methods and dissections to bear on the function of circulation and respiration. He clearly saw the heart as a pump, described its valves, and promoted the notion of a one-way circulation. In this radical concept the right ventricle brought blood to the lungs while the left ventricle supplied pneuma from the lungs. According to his theory, the veins held blood and the arteries air. The whole circulatory system of blood and air was interconnected through anastomoses of the fine branches of arteries and veins. The fact that air could never be found in the arteries was explained on the basis that the air escaped so rapidly that blood was instantaneously drawn into the arteries from the veins via the anastomoses.

The greatest name in Greek medicine apart from Hippocrates is Galen (131–201 A.D.). Born in Asia Minor, a student of Greek philosophy (especially Aristotle), he traveled widely—training at Smyrna, Alexandria, and other cities. It was in Rome that he achieved his greatest triumph, although he was once forced to flee the city because of medical opposition. Nevertheless, he returned to be appointed tutor to the son of Emperor Marcus Aurelius.

He left a great body of medical works the substance of which, in error or not, would stand for 15 centuries. He was an experimentalist and theorist whose voluminous writings had such an air of infallibility and authoritativeness as to effectively bar innovative thinking. He left behind a veritable encyclopedia of medical knowledge: 9 books on anatomy, 17 on physiology, 6 on pathology, 16 essays on the pulse, 14 books on therapeutics, 3 books on temperaments, and 30 books on pharmacy. It is a fantastic compendium which is somewhat marred by the teleologic characteristics of his experimental works.

It was Galen who specifically refuted the concept of Erasistratus that pneuma was contained in the arteries. He proved that blood, and not air, was invariably contained in the arteries. Because of this assertion, however, he was forced to the position of nonunidirectional flow of blood. It was Galen's view that air (together with blood) did, indeed, pass into the left side of the heart by the pulmonary vein, and that air did exert a cooling influence on the heart and then return back to the lungs together with waste substances. Air was drawn into the arteries from the surrounding air through pores in the skin when the arteries were dilated or contracted (pulse). He said:

As we have seen respiration in animals exists in the interest of the heart which both needs, the substance of the air and being consumed with heat desires in addition the refreshing coolness which it thereby obtains. Entering with its cooling power the air refreshes the heart. In passing out it carries with it effervescent burnt and smoky particles–the heart–in dilating draws toward itself and in contracting empties itself.

It was in the concept of the meaning of pneuma that Galen took a great stride forward from the previous Greeks. Of the vital psychic air (transmitted via nerves to the rest of the body for muscular contraction) he said: "it is not air per se but pneuma which was derived from blood under the influence of innate heat." This radical departure placed the primary function of respiration to be the maintenance of innate heat. As he reviewed the respiratory concept of previous physicians and teachers, he came to the conclusion that it was a quality of the air that was essential, and that this essentiality resided in the production of innate heat. He likened life and the innate heat of the heart to a flame burning in a perforated gourd, that the flame could not burn without a quality in the air and when the animal respired it was similar to the respiration of the flame. This was a remarkable analogy, for he went on further to consider the waste substances of the flame and theorized that "ashes, fumes and smoke—tend to extinguish the fire no less quickly than water." From this he derived the notion that waste material from the production of innate heat in the heart must be exhaled after return travel to the lungs. This prescientific analogy antedated the line of thought which was to come in the 17th century with Hooke, Mayow, Lower, and Boyle of the Royal Society. He further noted the difference in color of arterial and venous blood; the former, he said, was "thinner and more golden" and always "hotter." The term golden ("flavior" in Latin) is the same one that Michael Servetus—the mystic heretic of the 16th century—was to apply to the color of arterial blood when it was mixed with spiritual air.

More Recent Times

From the downfall of the Roman Empire and through the Byzantine, Mohammedan, and Jewish periods, the Galenic concepts of medical knowledge held sway—a period of fifteen centuries. One recently discovered, illuminating manuscript prepared by Ibn Nafis (13th Century), was the only challenge to Galen's circulatory concept. An Egyptian physician, Ibn Nafis disputed Galen's claim of invisible pores in the ventricular septum which allowed the mixing of blood between the ventricles. Instead, he said that blood from the right ventricle ". . . passes in the Vena arteriosa through the lungs to permeate its substance and mingle with the air, its thin parts purify and then passes in the arteria venosa to reach the left cavity of the two cavities of the heart; having mixed with the air and becomes fit with creation of the spirit." The function of the heart was the creation of the animal spirit and its distribution to the animal organ. Ibn Nafis took Galen's views, added his own observations of the pulmonary vessels, and came up with a more systemized, reoriented view of the pulmonary circulation.

The concept lay buried until the time of the Rennaisance and Reformation. Europe was in the midst of a great wave of intellectual, scientific, and religious ferment. It was a time of great discovery, explorations, and scientific thought. It was the time of Rabelais, Paracelsus, Da Vinci, Paré, Columbus, Da Gamma, Petrarch, Gutenberg, Boccaccio, Dante, Raphael, Titian, Michaelangelo, Copernicus, Brahe, Kepler, Luther, Bruno, De Medici, Erasmus, Shakespeare, Drake, and Milton.

In this great time of humanism and intellectual and scientific freedom flourished the anatomical genius of André Vesalius (1514–1564), who, despite his greatness, did not break away from the Galenic concept of circulation and respiration. Michael Servetus (1511–1563), a Galenist who incurred the wrath of the Catholic Church and was burned at the stake by Calvin, was no experimentalist or physician. Yet in his last work of religious fervor he equated the divine spirit of God to the breath and thus imputed to respiration the inhalation of the divine spirit: "Indeed, the fact indicates that the divine breath is in the air which the spirit of the Lord fills, and the spirit was formed from the mixing of blood with air in the lungs." Here, even as had Ibn Nafis in the 13th century, Servetus contradicted Galen and postulated the pulmonary circulation with blood flowing from the right ventricle to the left by the lungs and not through septal communications. He said, "Not merely air but air mixed with blood, is sent from the lungs to the heart through the pulmonary veins; therefore, the mixture occurs in the lungs. That reddish-yellow color is given to the spiritless blood by the lungs; it is not from the heart." This free-wheeling, brash theologian who dabbled in medicine hit upon a revolutionary idea. Achieving notoriety from his burning at the stake and the almost complete destruction of his manuscripts, he served to stimulate further thinking along this line of speculation.

It was William Harvey (1578–1657) who experimentally and quantitatively derived the concept of a continuous closed circulation of blood and clearly established the heart as the pump that produced the motive power (1628). It was a momentous discovery of the peripheral and pulmonary circulation, especially because of the quantitative implications for circulation physiology. However, Harvey, brilliant as he was, was frustrated by the meaning of the function of respiration. Not subscribing to the ideas of Galen, Ibn Nafis, or Servetus on respiration, innate heat, and life, he could not rid himself of the Platonic idea that the respiratory function was that of refrigeration of the heart.

Also at this time came the microscope—with Kircher in Italy, Hooke in England, Swammerdam in Holland, Leeuwenhoek of Delft, and Malphigi in Italy being the leaders. It was the latter who first described capillary circulation in the lungs of the frog (1661). This was the first demonstration of the arteriovenous anastomoses postulated four centuries earlier by Ibn Nafis.

In the 17th century, in the period after Harvey, an English group of scientists explored and expounded the biochemical nature of the respiratory process and laid the foundation for the eventual discovery of oxygen as the essential gas for life processes. The brilliant speculative analogy made by Galen in the second century was brought to comparative modern times by Robert Boyle (1621–1691), who demonstrated that air was as necessary for life as it was for fire. It was the ingenious Robert Hooke (1635–1703) who demonstrated that it was not the mechanism of respiration and the movement of the ribcage which was necessary for the maintenance of life, but "the want of a supply of fresh air."

Richard Lower (1631–1691), a practitioner and experimentalist, did the first animal blood transfusion. In addition, in his treatise on the heart, he said, "it [the heart] is perverted in emotional states such as anger, joy, and sudden fright, when the spirits fly to the heart in excessive and unwanted amounts, or with a greater rush than usual, accelerate its movements very greatly, and excite and convulse with bounding movements that are sometimes terrific." Further, he stated, "when the movement of the heart is weak and intermittent, it predisposes to such head affections as vertigo, scotoma, blindness, and fainting. The reason for these symptoms lies in the fact that the animal spirit and life itself depend on a continuous supply of blood to the brain." Then he proceeded to a discussion of experiments on the color of blood and the meaning of this. ". . . it is extremely probable that the blood takes in air in its course through the lungs and owes this bright color entirely to the added mixture of air. Moreover, after the air has in large measure left the blood again within the body and the parenchyma of the viscera, and has transpired through the pores of the body, it is equally consistent with reason that the venous blood, which has lost its air, should forthwith appear darker and blacker."

According to John Mayow (1643–1679), the change in color from dark to bright red on mixing with air in the lungs owed to "certain particles of a nitro-saline nature, and these very subtle, agile and in the highest degree fermentative, are separated from the air by the action of the lungs and conveyed into the mass of blood. For this aerial salt is so necessary to every form of life." This nitro-aerial spirit excited in the blood the necessary fermentation for the production of "animal spirits" which was necessary for life. Mayow, then, was coming close to the discovery of oxygen, postulating a gaseous exchange in the lung. He stated that the heart was really nothing but a muscular pump, and that muscular contraction was directly dependent on the "fermentation" produced by the nitro-aerial salt.

Lower's "nitro-spirit" and Mayow's "nitro-aerial spirit" of the air clearly indicated these investigators' concept of oxygen, but the actual elucidation and isolation of the essential gas had to pass through theories of Stahl's phlogiston, Black's fixed air (CO_2), and Priestly's dephlogisticated air until, in 1775, the brilliant Frenchman Antoine Lavoisier uncovered the real meaning of the vital gas and gave it the name of oxygen. This discovery marked the beginning of a new era in respiratory chemistry.

COMMENTS

The preceding history sets the stage for the development of current concepts of respiration and is seen as a necessary step in this development. Current concepts, however, will in all probability seem no more sophisticated in the year 3000 A.D. than the concepts of 500 A.D. seem today. The perspective by which we view bodily functions is only as sophisticated as the current level of intellectual development.

Psychophysiologic concepts of respiration were relatively primitive despite tremendous gains in physiology and anatomy until very recent times. The works of Darwin and Bell (quoted in the Introduction) probably represent the first systematic investigation into psychologic aspects of respiration which can be called scientific; they are seen as the precursors of modern respiratory psychophysiology.

REFERENCES

Adams, F. The Genuine Works of Hippocrates. Baltimore, The Williams & Wilkins Co., 1939.

Ebbell, B., tr. The Papyrus Ebers. Copenhagen, Levin and Munksgaard, 1937.

Garrison, F. H. History of Medicine, 4th ed. Philadelphia, W. B. Saunders Co., 1929.

Gottlieb, L. S. A History of Respiration. Springfield, Ill., Charles C Thomas, Publisher, 1964.

Granbard, M. A. Circulation and Respiration. New York, Harcourt, Brace & World, 1964.

Harper, R. F. The Code of Hammurabi, King of Babylon. Chicago, Univ. of Chicago Press, 1904.

Hume, E. The Chinese Way in Medicine. Baltimore, Johns Hopkins Press, 1952.

Kutumbiah, P. Ancient Indian Medicine. Bombay, Orient Longmans, 1962.

Ross, Sir D. Aristotle: De Animus, Clarendon Press, 1961.

Saunders, J. B., de C. M. The Transition from Ancient Egyptian to Greek Medicine. Lawrence, Kans., Univ. of Kansas Press, 1963.

Selwyn-Brown, A. The Physician Throughout the Ages, Vol. I. New York, Capehart-Brown, 1938.

Stubbs, S. G. B., and Bligh, E. W. Sixty Centuries of Health and Physich. London, Sampon, Low, Marston & Co., Ltd., 1931.

Thorwald, J. Science and Secrets of Early Medicine. New York, Harcourt, Brace & World, 1962.

Verth, I. Translation of Huang Ti Nei Ching Su Wen (The Yellow Emperor's Classic on Internal Medicine). Baltimore, The Williams & Wilkins Co., 1949.

Wilson, L. C. Erasistratus, Galen, and the pneuma, Bull Hist Med, 33:293, 1959.

3

Pulmonary Anatomy and Physiology

The respiratory system consists of a large airway that continues in a succession of branching tubes that end in millions of minute air sacs. Across the walls of these sacs, gases are exchanged with the blood. The primary function of this system is the transport of fresh air to the sacs, where oxygen is supplied to blood and carbon dioxide is removed. Housekeeping functions of the system include the regulation of the temperature and humidity of the air inhaled and the maintenance of tracheobronchial hygiene.

THE CONDUCTING AIRWAYS

The conducting airways lead to the gas-exchange areas of the lungs. They extend from the external nares to the terminal bronchioles. Some segments of these airways have special functions where differences in the structure appear. Such structural and functional differences are maintained within the commonality of overall purpose.

The Upper Airways. The upper airways include the nasal cavity and the pharynx. These airways may contain as much as 50 percent of the total airway volume (dead space) and approximately that much of the resistance to air flow as well.

The nasal cavity extends from the nares anteriorly to the opening into the nasal pharynx through the choana posteriorly (Fig. 1). The floor is formed by the hard palate and is approximately 50 mm in length. The floor is broad compared with the remainder of the cavity, there being 10 mm or more between the lateral walls. The roof of the nasal cavity is narrow

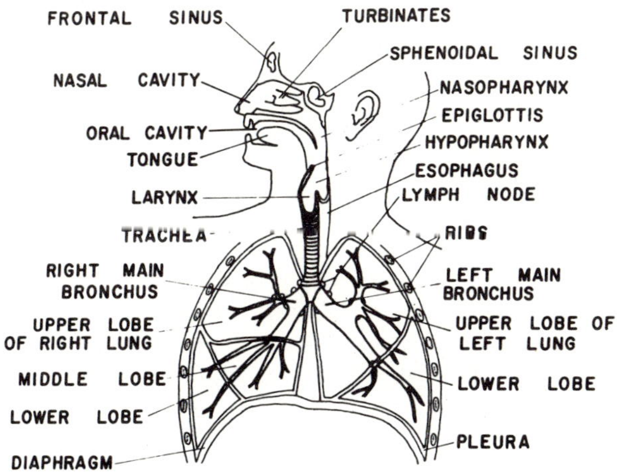

Fig. 1. Schematic representation of respiratory system.

(1 to 2 mm) and is formed from front to back by the nasal and frontal bones, the cribriform plate of the ethmoid, and the sphenoid bone. The roof is longer than the floor, being about 75 mm in length. The nasal cavity, although spoken of as being a single space, is actually two cavities. The dividing wall, formed by several bones, is collectively called the nasal septum. The lateral wall is covered for the most part by the superior, middle, and inferior turbinates (Fig. 1). These bones project into the nasal cavity and effectively double the surface area of this passage. They narrow the passageway to as little as 1 mm in some areas, with a widening to as much as 5 mm between the turbinates. A mucous membrane lines this cavity.

In the region of the turbinates the inspired air becomes turbulent, increasing the airway resistance but contributing to the surface contact necessary for regulation of the temperature and humidity. When one is at rest indoors, the inspired air is almost completely heated (37° C) and humidified within the nasal cavity. On cold, dry days the nose may add ½–1 pt of water to the inspired air, a part of which is recovered on expiration. If the recovery is excessive, pooling may occur, and a "runny nose" results. As much as 3,000 cal may be used in heating the cold air inspired in a 24-hr period.

The nares are directed inferiorly in the upright man. To enter the nasal passage, particulate matter must be of such a size and density that it is drawn in with the air stream. The nasal passage is guarded by coarse hairs just inside the nares and anterior to the mucocutaneous junction.

These hairs strain out as much as 50 percent of the inhaled particulate matter larger than 10 μ in diameter. The remaining particles of this size are removed within the nasal cavity by impingement and the effects of gravity. Many smaller particles (less than 10 μ) are removed in the nasal cavity as well.

The pharynx lies behind and communicates with the nasal cavity above, the oral cavity anteriorly, and the larynx below. It extends from the base of the skull to the esophagus (Fig. 1). Above the soft palate the nasal pharynx is a respiratory passage, while the middle portion or oral pharynx serves as a passageway for both air and ingested materials. The portion of the pharynx below the larynx is exclusively the domain of the gastrointestinal tract. The pharynx is a fibromuscular sac that forms a cavity that contains air in its superior and middle portions because of the bony attachments laterally. Below the glottis, however, the anterior and posterior walls approach one another and the structure is a potential tube, being closed except when occupied by ingested material.

The oral cavity can be isolated from the pharynx during mastication by the proximation of the soft palate and tongue. Breathing can continue without interruption. During swallowing, respiration must be interrupted while the food is forced to the back of the tongue and passed through the hypopharynx. A leaflike structure, the epiglottis, deflects the ingested stream away from the laryngeal opening and into the esophageal orifice.

The pharynx is important as a site for special sense organs (taste and the opening of the eustachian canals, which is essential to hearing), as a modulator of speech, and as a passageway for air and food. Its special function is the separation of the respiratory and ingested streams. A mixing of the contents occurs in certain conditions (such as paralytic diseases affecting the muscles of the throat), in coma, in certain emotional states, and in the aged. Air may be taken into the stomach in some emotional conditions through air swallowing. Gastric contents or food that may enter the respiratory tract may result in severe lung infections (aspiration pneumonia) or suffocation.

THE LOWER AIRWAYS. The larynx is a lumen, surrounded by cartilages for support, that communicates with the pharynx above and the trachea below. Muscles of the neck surrounding it are capable of raising, lowering, or tilting this opening. The opening is anterior to the esophagus or gullet and is at the base of the tongue beneath the epiglottis (Fig. 1). The triangular entrance is marked by the aryepiglottic folds that stretch from the lateral margins of the epiglottis anteriorly to the arytenoid cartilages behind. Closure of the laryngeal inlet approximates these margins. Piriform fossas, lateral to the aryepiglottic folds, form a gutter for food passing around the laryngeal opening to the esophagus. Within the laryngeal inlet is the vestibule, which is limited inferiorly by the vestibular folds (false cords). These folds of mucous membrane that project from the lateral wall of the larynx are close together anteriorly, but do not quite reach the posterior wall, so that they are considerably separated at this end. At laryngoscopic examination one can see the vocal folds, or the true vocal cords, between the vestibular folds. The vocal folds are fixed anteriorly on the thyroid cartilage and are inserted posteriorly on the mobile arytenoid cartilages. Changes in the position of the arytenoid cartilages cause the glottis opening to undergo changes—widening in inhalation and narrowing in exhalation. During phonation the true cords are approximated with a small linear chink remaining between them.

The larynx guards the opening of the lower respiratory tract. It functions as a valve to prevent contamination. In man it also serves as the organ of speech. It cooperates by obstructing the airway in any effort that requires fixation of the chest cage or increased intra-abdominal pressure (micturation, defecation, and parturition). Effective coughing and sneezing would be impossible without the larynx's capacity for being closed.

The trachea extends from the larynx to the bifurcation into the main stem bronchi below. It is approximately 2 cm in diameter and about 14 cm in length in the adult. Anteriorly the wall is supported by cartilagenous rings; but posteriorly, where it lies on the esophagus, the wall is membranous.

The bronchial tree begins with the dichotomous branching of the trachea into right and left main stem bronchi. Beyond this point a trichotomous branching is often seen. The major divisions of the right main stem bronchus include a right upper, right lower, and right middle lobe bronchus. On the left, two major branches are found, that to the upper and to the lower lobes. These lobar airways divide into approximately ten segmental divisions in the right lung, but on the left it is common for the apical and posterior segmental bronchi of the upper lobe to be fused so that only nine segmental bronchi are present. The branching continues through ever smaller divisions with as many as 16 generations between the lower end of the trachea and the respiratory bronchioles. In the course of these divisions cartilage is lost from the bronchial walls. The terminal bronchiole or the sixteenth division (internal diameter approximately 0.6 mm) has a muscular wall, stratified columnar epithelium, and is the smallest airway to have bronchial glands and goblet cells. It has no appreciable potential for gas exchange. The terminal bronchiole branches into the respiratory bronchioles, where alveolar sacs are found and gas exchange is possible.

Microscopic Anatomy of the Conducting Airways. The upper and lower airways, except for a few specific areas, are lined with a pseudostratified ciliated, epithelium that rests upon a well-defined basement membrane. This tissue covers a feltwork of collagen and reticular fibrils beneath which is the lamina propria—composed of loosely arranged collagen and elastic fibers, fibroblasts, macrophages, and cells of the lymphoid and myeloid series. An extensive capillary network as well as unmyelinated nerve fibers are seen in this layer. Extensive venous plexuses are present, particularly in the nose, overlying the turbinates. The erectile property of the nasal mucosa that may be seen following several means of stimulation has been attributed to the presence of this venous plexus. The submucosa contains bronchial glands of a mixed type, both serous and mucinous, and smooth muscle fibers as well in the lower airways.

Four cell types form the respiratory epithelium. Basal cells are polygonal and rest on the basement membrane. The walls of these cells are in contact with other cells and the basement membrane. They are poorly differentiated and may be replacements for the cell types described below.

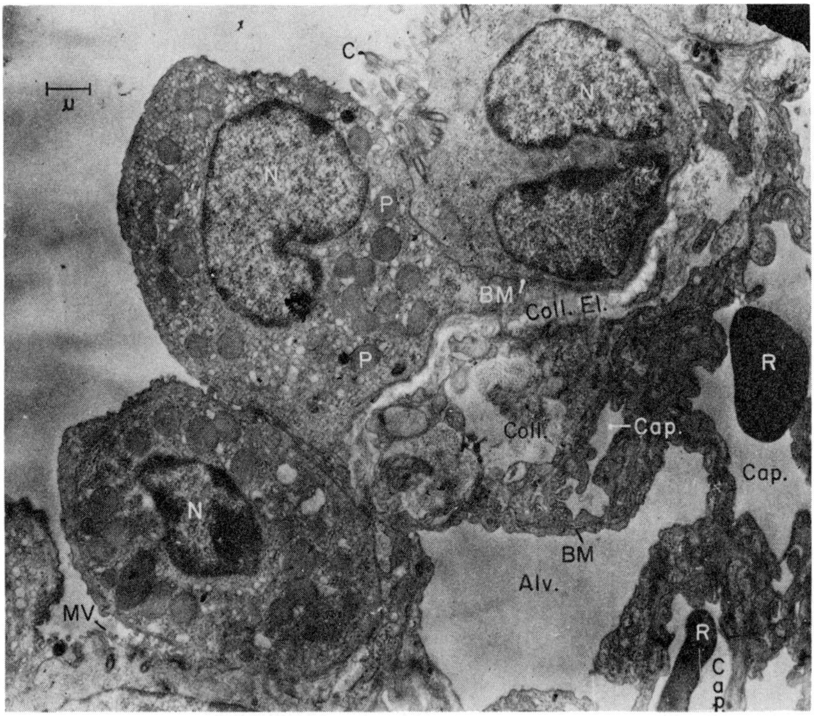

Fig. 2. Electron micrograph of normal human lung. Alv., alveolar space; B.M., basement membrane; C. cilia; Cap., capillary lumen; Coll., collagen; El., elastin; MV., microvilli, N., nucleus; P, premucous granule; R., red blood cell. Space at left is lumen of terminal bronchiole. Extending across left center of photograph are three large cells; uppermost cell is ciliated, lower two are goblet cells.

Intermediate cells are seen on some sections of the respiratory mucosa which are more elongated than the basal cells from which they are derived. These are apparently at an intermediate stage in the development between basal cells and those having specific function.

Goblet cells (Fig. 2) are mucous-producing cells that extend from the basement membrane to the surface of the epithelium. The darkly staining nucleus is located toward the base of the cell and a prominent golgi complex with secretory granules is seen. Premucous granules that are best seen by electron microscopy swell and collect in the upper part of the cell, later to form the typical goblet shape. These granules are formed within a membrane which they lose as the mucus coalesces before discharge from the cell.

For every goblet cell seen there are at least five ciliated cells present (Fig. 2). These also extend from the basement membrane to the epithelial surface. Concentrated toward the free cell surface is an abundance of mitochondria, while the large nucleus is usually located near the center of the cell. The free surface of the cell is adorned with cilia and microvilli (pellicular structures). Pellicular structures include three types of cytoplasmic extensions, one of which is the microvillus.

The cilia on these cells are small hairlike projections approximately 0.3 by 6 μ. Within each cilia there is a pair of central fibrils around which are nine paired peripheral fibrils. The fibrils end in the basal body at the cell surface within which the central pair cannot be distinguished.

The pharynx, epiglottis, sidewalls of the vestibule in the larynx, and the vocal cords are not covered with the pseudostratified columnar epithelium but with a stratified squamous epithelium. The layer of mucus overlying this area is provided by glands present in the submucosa. There are, of course, no cilia on this epithelium and the motion of the mucous stream is provided by gravity, friction (in swallowing), and by the pull of mucus from neighboring areas that is powered by cilia. The nares, of course, have no cilia anterior to the mucocutaneous junction.

FUNCTION OF THE CONDUCTING AIRWAYS. The volume of this system down to the terminal bronchiole approximates that of the subject's ideal body weight in pounds. A man weighing 150 lb has approximately 0.15 L of anatomical dead space. The amount of inspired air that may reach the alveolar sacs (V_A) is the volume of air inspired with each breath minus the volume of the conducting airways in this subject (0.15 L). With a tidal volume of 0.45 L, only 0.3 L reaches the area of gas exchange. A respiratory rate of 14 per min will result in a minute volume ($\dot{V}$) of 5.4 L and an alveolar ventilation ($\dot{V}_A$) of 3.3 L [5.4 L — 14 (0.15 L) = 3.3

L]. Shallow, rapid respiration that may occur with emotional stress, with pain in the chest wall, or with restriction of the chest may result in the frequency of respiration increasing (25 per min) without a change in the minute volume (5.4 L). The alveolar ventilation as a result is 1.65 L per min [5.4 L — 25 (0.15 L) = 1.65 L], or definite hypoventilation.

The volume of the conducting airway is affected by changes in lung volume. This relationship between lung volume and dead space volume is nonlinear, but as an approximation the anatomical dead space increases 2 to 3 ml for every 100 ml increase in lung volume. Emotional states that may result in the patient's breathing at high lung volumes will increase the volume of the conducting airway. There is bronchoscopic evidence that narrowing of the airways occurs with resentment and a loss of bronchial tone accompanies the recall of depressive incidents. The nasal mucosa has been shown to swell and become congested with increased secretion of mucus in certain emotional states. Similar changes have been described for bronchial mucous secretions. Measurement of the anatomical dead space is possible in these different emotional states, although it has not been specifically evaluated. Further study on the correlation between airway volumes and emotional states is warranted.

In dusty environments, a considerable number of particles less than 2 μ in diameter may enter the lower airways. Submicronic particles in fumes and smokes, as well as bacteria, may be carried into the area of gas exchange. Many of these substances are carried out in the following exhalation. The remainder of the inhaled foreign material, particularly that between 1 and 10 μ is deposited on the mucous membranes of the airways. This must be cleared from the respiratory tract by the mucous escalator covering the airways below the larynx. The ciliated cells lining the airways beat in a water medium beneath this mucous blanket. Some of this mucus is produced by the goblet cells in the respiratory epithelium but the majority of it comes from the submucosal bronchial glands. The cilia on the surface of the epithelium have a quick forward stroke in the direction of mucus flow—i.e., toward the larynx, and a slow return stroke. Mucus is moved by this means at a rate of 1 cm per min toward the larynx. Failure of the mucociliary escalator or a pile-up of mucus in one area may provoke coughing, which accelerates clearing.

Ciliary action depends, to a considerable extent, upon the viscosity of the fluid medium beneath the mucous blanket. It is therefore quite susceptible to drying. Dehydration of this medium by inhaling very dry gases or by means of an inadequate fluid intake will stop cilial action. In severe emotional or physical illness with mouth breathing and an inadequate fluid intake, the membrane in the upper airways and down into the lower airways may show considerable drying. Breathing cold, dry air aggravates this effect. If the patient is febrile, additional moisture will be required to humidify the inspired air.

The mechanism for the control of cilial action is unknown. Both humoral and nervous mechanisms have been suspected. Some control is evidenced as chilling the skin will stop cilial action. If a patch of respiratory epithelium is removed and grafted into place so that the cilia beat against the current of the adjacent epithelium, it takes but a short time for the beat to be altered to conform with the neighboring cilial action.

Many agents applied to isolated cilial preparations have been shown to slow or stop the motion. Tobacco smoke, other smokes, alcohol, dusts, and fumes, will all slow or stop cilial action when applied to the mucosa.

The cough mechanism, which aids in clearing the airway, is initiated by a mechanical stimulation of nerve endings in the epithelium of the large airways or may also be initiated by chemical action on endings in the smaller airways. The efferent limb of the reflex arc passes over the phrenic and intercostal nerves to innervate the bellows system. A cough center located in the medulla coordinates the sequence of action in the cough. A cough is preceded by an inspiration, the glottis is then closed, and intrapulmonary pressure is raised by the action of the expiratory muscles and fixation of the anterior abdominal muscles. The final act is a sudden opening of the glottis and a narrowing of the tracheobronchial tree, at which time the linear velocity of airflow may reach the speed of sound. Marked turbulence is generated and loose materials in the tracheobronchial tree are forcefully expelled. In man, the intrathoracic pressure may transiently rise to 300 mm Hg in the act of coughing, and it is doubtful if an effective cough can be generated with pressures less than 40 mm Hg.

THE AREA OF GAS EXCHANGE

The terminal bronchiole (0.6 mm in diameter) is the final division of the conducting airways. It commonly divides into three respiratory bronchioles which form two or more generations of respiratory bronchioles before ending in the alveolar ducts. These bronchioles and ducts have alveoli in their walls. The alveolar duct divides into three atria which have 20 or more alveoli in their walls.

The epithelium in the terminal bronchiole changes from a pseudostratified columnar epithelium to a low cuboidal epithelium within a few cells. In the respiratory bronchiole the epithelium becomes a flat plate. In the alveoli the distance between alveolar air and capillary blood may be less than 1 μ. This "membrane" consists of a mucoid or lipoprotein layer, a respiratory epithelial layer, a connective tissue layer, and a capillary endothelial layer. It forms the barrier to gas transport between the alveolar air and capillary blood.

Alveoli vary in diameter secondary to gravitational effects. The weight of the lung enlarges those alveoli that are high in the chest wall of upright man, while those at the bottom of the lung are smaller. Average alveolar diameters depend upon lung inflation but approximate 180 μ at the end of a tidal inspiration. The number of alveoli in normal man approximates 300 million, and the alveolar surface area for gas exchange may amount to 95 m^2.

Ventilation of the lungs is intermittent and alveolar gas composition varies with the frequency and depth of breathing. The lung volume is ventilated as a result of the bellows action of the chest wall and diaphragm. With inspiration, the chest cavity enlarges, which causes a drop in pressure within the pleural cavity surrounding the lung. A drop in the pressure within each alveoli causes air to enter. A positive transpulmonary pressure is generated which distends the viscoelastic parenchyma. Expiration is normally passive, the force being generated by the elastic recoil of the lung and chest wall.

The lungs are not ideally elastic, but a curvilinear relationship exists between the distending pressure and the volume change. The inflation pathway is not the same as the deflation pathway (hysteresis) so that a loss in energy occurs. Alveoli having different sizes, such as the differences owing to the effects of body position, may be at different points on their pressure-volume curves. As a result, there is a considerable variation in the amount of fresh air that each alveolar volume receives for the same distending pressure.

The transpulmonary or distending pressure is known to vary in different parts of the lungs. The pressure distending the lower lobes in normal man is greater than that distending upper lobes. It is probable that this results in greater movement of the lower chest and diaphragm with inspiration. Factors limiting chest wall action—such as pain, binding, splinting, or emotional states—may alter the mechanical properties of the chest wall. Changing the stresses applied to the lung will change the distribution of ventilation. The distribution of ventilation is more uneven with deep, and with more rapid breathing, and is also affected by irregular rhythms.

The distribution of ventilation to the gas-exchange area is affected by the preferential distribution of dead space gas. The upper lobe receives most of the dead space when inspiring at volumes below the midlung capacity. Inspiring from volumes above functional residual capacity causes the lower lobe to receive more of the dead space gas. The efficiency of regional lung ventilation is therefore affected by the volume at which inspiration starts.

Fresh air entering the alveolar volume dilutes the gas already present. Some mixing in this gas takes place by mass movement but most of it occurs by diffusion in the gas phase. This diffusion is complete within a fraction of a second and does not result in an uneven distribution of ventilation at physiological breathing rates. At rates above 200 per min, however, a diffusion gradient within the alveolar volume has been demonstrated.

Alveolar ventilation may vary within the lungs as a result of the uneven distribution of lung compliance (distensibility) or airway resistance. The compliance of lung changes with disease (see Chapter 4). Airway resistance varies with factors that affect bronchial diameter, which include the compliance of the wall, the action of bronchial musculature, swelling of the mucosa, and changes in bronchial secretions.

Some work is associated with the function of breathing. This results from resistance to airflow within the airways, the elastic recoil of the lung and chest wall, and inertia and tissue friction. The work of breathing is usually estimated indirectly through the increase in oxygen consumption at different ventilatory rates. In normal man, a liter increase in ventilation will require 0.5 to 1 ml of oxygen. The work of breathing is increased in those conditions that increase airway resistance, as well as those that increase the stiffness of the lung. In severe obstructive pulmonary syndromes, pulmonary fibrosis, pleural disease, and chest-wall fixation, the work of breathing may seriously limit the patient's tolerance to exercise. The work of breathing is most closely related to the symptom of dyspnea.

The resistance to airflow is reported as the pressure in centimeters of water required to get a flow of 1 L per sec. The pressure is that acting between alveolar and mouth to produce the flow of air. An average value at resting lung volumes is 1.3 cm of water per liter per sec. The resistance to airflow is more commonly estimated from a maximal flow rate, usually in expiration. The maximal driving pressure that can be generated within the thorax is adequate with a normal bellows system—so that a flow rate reduction is proportional to the rise in airway resistance. Peak flow rates, damped maximal expiratory flow rates, the maximal voluntary ventilation, and timed vital capacities are used in clinical laboratories for this purpose.

In a similar way a measure of lung distensibility or compliance requires an estimate of the transpulmonary pressure—i.e., the difference between pleural and mouth pressures at times when no air is flowing. Compliance is expressed as the volume change in milliliters for a change in pressure of 1 cm of water. Here again, if the maximal inspiratory pressures are normal, the vital capacity is some estimate of the compliance of the lung. Vital capacity is much more easily measured.

PULMONARY INSUFFICIENCY

Gas exchange is the primary function of the lung. Failure in this function is expressed as hypoxemia and hypercapnia. There are but four mechanisms for the failure of gas exchange in subjects breathing ambient air at sea level.

THE DISTRIBUTION OF VENTILATION IN RELATION TO PERFUSION. The uneven distribution of ventilation in the lungs must be matched by a similar distribution of blood flow for efficient gas exchange. The distribution of ventilation to perfusion ratios in lungs may vary from zero (shunts) to infinity (alveolar dead space); it is the commonest cause of pulmonary insufficiency in clinical medicine. This continuous distribution of ventilation

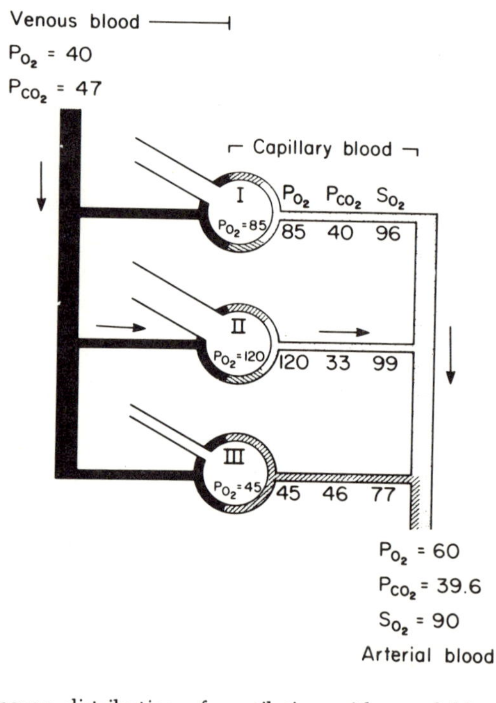

Fig. 3. Effect of uneven distribution of ventilation with equal blood flow on arterial blood oxygen and carbon dioxide. Units I, II, and III represent portions of lung which have similar blood flow but uneven distribution of ventilation as indicated by different values for P_{O_2}. Unit I, normally ventilated unit, and Unit II, overventilated unit cannot compensate for Unit III, the underventilated unit. End result is lowering of oxygen content of arterial blood.

to perfusion ratios may be depicted by three differently ventilated compartments having uniform blood flow (Fig. 3). Lung units with an optimum ventilation to blood flow ratio ($r = 0.83$) will have saturated end-capillary blood (S_{O_2}), and normal pressures for carbon dioxide (P_{CO_2}) (Fig. 3, Unit I). A second lung compartment, hyperventilated for the amount of blood flowing through it, has wasted ventilation (Fig. 3, Unit II). The amount of ventilation that is wasted has been called the alveolar dead space. These units will have high alveolar and end-capillary oxygen pressures (P_{O_2}) and low carbon dioxide pressures. On the other hand, those lung compartments with excessive blood flow in relationship to ventilation cannot maintain a normal P_{O_2} and have a high P_{CO_2} (Fig. 3, Unit III).

Because of the oxygen dissociation curve there is a nonlinear relationship between P_{O_2} and oxygen content (saturation) in the oxygen-carrying pigment, hemoglobin. As most of the oxygen is carried by hemoglobin, the dissociation curve influences the efficiency of oxygen transport. Relatively insignificant amounts of oxygen are dissolved in plasma. The hyperventilating unit (Fig. 3, Unit II) cannot supersaturate the blood. The poorly ventilated unit (Fig. 3, Unit III) with low oxygen cannot be compensated for by this hyperventilating unit. Hypoxemia is inevitable if as much as one-third of the lung has this distribution of ventilation-perfusion ratios. The arterial carbon dioxide content, however, is more linearly related to the arterial P_{CO_2} and the hyperventilating unit (Unit II) will blow off excess carbon dioxide to compensate for the compartment with a low ventilation-perfusion ratio (Unit III).

With progression of an obstructive pulmonary syndrome, or in any other disease state wherein this abnormality obtains, the hyperventilating compartments diminish in number—which increases the hypoxemia but, more importantly, the compensation for the carbon dioxide function fails. Deterioration in diseases marked by ventilation perfusion abnormalities is first manifested by hypoxemia, followed by the addition of hypercapnia, and finally, as the buffer-base system of the blood fails to compensate by respiratory acidosis.

HYPOVENTILATION. Hypoventilation produces pulmonary insufficiency and occurs when the respiratory center is poisoned (barbiturates, narcotics, tranquilizers, etc.) or damaged (excessive intracranial pressure, brain stem trauma, or vascular accidents), when there is a loss of respiratory muscle activity (myasthenia gravis, poliomeylitis, increased work of breathing), when there is a loss of chest-wall rigidity (severe trauma), in airway obstruction (foreign body, edema, tumor, etc.), or with certain emotional conditions.

Arterial hypoxemia and hypercapnia occur simultaneously in hypoventilation. Resting man uses approximately 6 L of fresh air each minute, providing approximately 240 cc of oxygen and removing approximately 192 cc of CO_2 per min. This minute ventilation includes the volume that is ineffective in gas exchange (dead space air). Anxiety may increase the frequency of respiration so that dead space volume is moved back and forth and forms a disproportionate part of the minute ventilation. The anxious patient may have a normal minute ventilation but a low alveolar ventilation, or hypoventilation.

MEMBRANE PERMEABILITY ABNORMALITIES. It has been calculated that 95 m^2 of alveolar membrane are available for gas exchange with a tissue barrier of 1 μ or less between gas and blood. In normal man this barrier results in no more than 1 mm Hg difference in oxygen pressure across the membrane, a function of the solubility of the gas and the distance traversed. Carbon dioxide is much more soluble than oxygen (25 times) and, therefore, reduction of CO_2 usually does not occur with membrane abnormalities. An arterial P_{O_2} at 75 mm Hg will saturate 94 percent of the hemoglobin in the blood. Alveolar P_{O_2} can reach 110 mm Hg with hyperventilation, allowing a membrane permeability gradient of 30 mm Hg before there is appreciable arterial unsaturation. The alveolar membrane in exercise can transmit as much as 60 cc of oxygen per min per milliliter of pressure difference across the membrane. A maximum oxygen uptake in this instance is 2,100 cc per min ($60 \times 35 = 2{,}100$ cc). Larger pressure differences across the membrane are possible and a larger membrane factor for permeability may be present in some individuals. Membrane permeability is lower than these values if measured at rest; it increases somewhat with hyperventilation and is maximal at severe exercise. In exercise, all the pulmonary vascular bed is perfused so that larger membrane factors are found than at rest or with hyperventilation.

SHUNT. Blood that passes from right to left—i.e., from pulmonary artery to pulmonary vein without contacting the gas-exchanging membrane—will be unoxygenated. No carbon dioxide retention occurs because the normal alveoli compensate by blowing off the carbon dioxide.

LUNG VOLUMES AND CAPACITIES

Conventionally the physiologist has viewed this functioning system in a static manner. The air contained in the lung is divided into volumes (or potential volumes called capacities) which have specific names and mean-

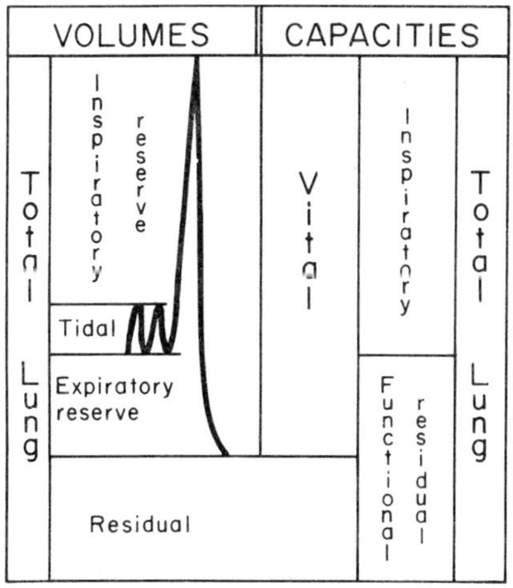

Fig. 4. Lung volumes and capacities (potential volumes). Tidal volume represents approximately 500 ml. Other volumes and capacities are roughly proportional to tidal volume.

ings (Fig. 4). The total lung capacity (TLC) is the total volume of the lung at maximal inspiration. The vital capacity (VC) is the maximal amount of air that can be expired following a maximal inspiration. The inspiratory capacity (IC) is the maximal amount of air which can be inspired after completion of normal expiration and the functional residual capacity (FRC) is the amount of air remaining in the lung at the completion of normal expiration.

The lung volumes are the inspiratory reserve volume, the tidal volume, the expiratory reserve volume, and the residual volume. The inspiratory reserve volume is the amount of air which can be inspired after the completion of a normal inspiration. The tidal volume is the amount of air inspired or expired during normal breathing. The expiratory reserve volume is the amount of air which can be expired after completion of a normal expiration and the residual volume is the amount of air which cannot be expired from the lung.

THE CONTROL OF RESPIRATION

Centers that control the frequency and depth of respiration are located within the reticular network of the pons and medulla (Fig. 5). The control network is composed of three areas that have different functions. In the medulla, below the origin of the tenth cranial nerve, there is an in-

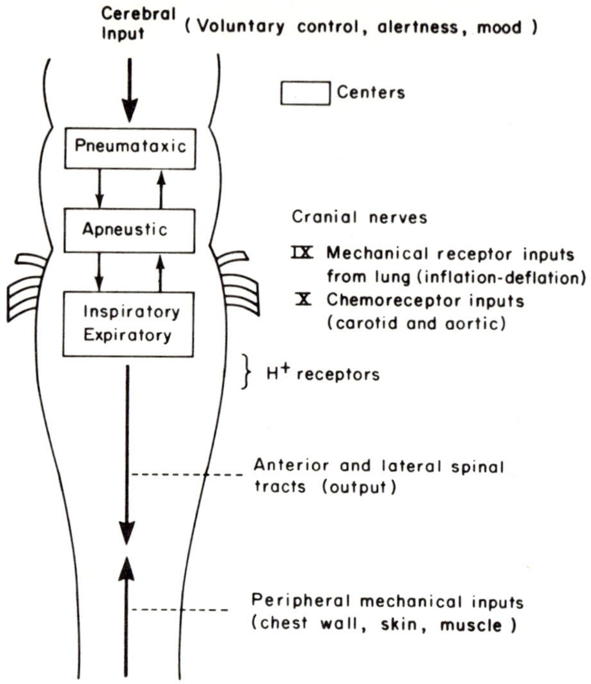

Fig. 5. Simplified diagram of central respiratory control network.

spiratory-expiratory center that is bilaterally innervated. This area, in the absence of all connections with the midbrain above, will initiate inspiration and continue a rhythmic respiratory effort. In the lower pons there is a loose collection of neurons that will, with unopposed action and in the absence of the vagus nerve, cause sustained inspiration even to death (apneustic center). Located in the upper part of the pons there is a center which controls the inspiratory activity of the two other areas described (pneumotaxic center). The output of the control network is carried through anterior and lateral tracts to the anterior horn cells of the cervical and thoracic spinal cord and through the motor neurons of certain cranial nerves (XI, XII). The respiratory muscles of the thorax, the diaphragm, and the accessory muscles of the neck and face are activated thereby.

Although respiration is initiated and rhythmicity is maintained by the network described, there is a feedback system which modifies the output considerably. Inputs of cerebral or somatic origin, the properties of blood perfusing the brain stem, and the carotid or aortic bodies are effective in altering respiration. The control network is not only responsible for initiating each breath and limiting the tidal volume and the respiratory rate but it also inhibits these functions for special purposes. Swallowing, coughing, sneezing, and breath-holding with great effort all require interruption of respiration and cooperation on the part of this network.

Inputs from Mechanical Receptors. Mechanical receptors, located in the bronchioles, sense the amount of tension in the pulmonary tissue. As inspiration increases lung volume, these receptors are progressively excited. They transmit this information via the vagus (Cranial Nerve X) to the control network where inspiration is inhibited (Hering-Breuer reflex). In the presence of intact vagi, the apneustic center cannot maintain an inspiratory effort, presumably because of this reflex.

Deflation Reflex. Mechanical receptors within the lung are also excited by low lung volumes. Volumes below normal end-tidal values produce a contraction of inspiratory muscles through the inspiratory-excitatory reflex of Hering-Breuer.

In addition to these intrapulmonary reflexes there are mechanical receptors located in the skin, the skeletal muscles, and the joints that will increase the respiratory rate and depth. The physician uses stimulation of the skin receptors to treat the depression of respiration following excessive use of drugs and to obtain the first breath in the newborn. Stretch receptors in the muscles of the chest wall have been described as acting in a servomechanism to regulate respiration. Stretch receptors in the carotid sinus (baroreceptors) activate circulatory mechanisms that affect respiratory control. Increased blood pressure leads to bradycardia and vasodilation as well as to a decrease in ventilation. A fall in carotid sinus pressure results in elevated blood pressure and hyperpnea.

Input from Humoral Receptors. The hydrogen ion concentration, the partial pressure of carbon dioxide, and oxygen are important in respiratory control. Chemoreceptors sensitive to the level of these agents in blood or tissue will cause an adjustment in respiratory minute volumes. As the hydrogen ion concentration decreases in alkalosis, hypoventilation ensues. An increase in the hydrogen ion concentration in acidosis results in hyperventilation. Increasing the inspired CO_2 concentration stimulates respiration as, to a lesser degree, does a low inspired oxygen concentration. The site of action of these humoral agents differs. Hydrogen ion and carbon dioxide concentration appear to act directly upon the respiratory control network, but oxygen is thought to have little effect there. Chemoreceptors located at the bifurcation of the carotid artery and in the arch of the aorta are more susceptible to oxygen deprivation.

Input from Cerebral Receptors. Poets have described these inputs more frequently than physiologists as in "the unconscious sigh" and "the bated breath." The voluntary control of respiration is so commonly practiced as to be overlooked. Speech is an integration of control network activity with several inputs of cerebral origin. Singing and playing a wind instrument are also good examples of the integration of several cerebral inputs. The maintenance of a proper carbon dioxide and oxygen pressure in arterial blood becomes of secondary importance during performance of these activities. Action-oriented behavioral states—such as anger, hostility, and anxiety—are associated with hyperventilation in some subjects, while those states having no action-orientation (such as apathy and depression) are accompanied by hypoventilation.

The threshold of the respiratory control network can be altered by altering the state of "alertness." Anesthesia and sleep are common means of changing the response of the centers. Some reflexes obvious during anesthesia (e.g., posthyperventilation apnea) are absent in conscious man. Ventilation decreases during sleep and a higher arterial P_{CO_2} is tolerated than when one is awake. The ventilatory response to a suggestion of exercise may be as marked as the response to exercise itself. The suggestion of sleep and sleep itself produce similar responses in ventilation. To susceptible individuals the suggestion of a depressive situation in which the individual cannot act results in hypoventilation. Hostile, angry individuals react with hyperventilation when conflict is suggested. In all of these instances the control network has been altered or cerebral input has been added to modify the humoral and mechanical inputs. This may be important to the patient with limited respiratory reserve, and to normal man in certain environments (e.g., in space and in deep diving).

REFERENCES

Comroe, J. H. Physiology of Respiration. Chicago, Yearbook Medical Publishers, Inc., 1965.

Dejours, P. Respiration. New York, Oxford University Press, 1966.

Dudley, D. L., Holmes, T. H., Martin, C. J., and Ripley, H. S. Changes in respiration associated with hypnotically induced emotion, pain and exercise, Psychosom Med, 24:46, 1964.

——— Martin, C. J., and Holmes, T. H. Dyspnea: Psychologic and physiologic observations, J Psychosom Res, 11:325, 1968.

——— Martin, C. J., and Holmes, T .H. Psychophysiologic studies of pulmonary ventilation, Psychosom Med, 26:645, 1964.

——— Verhey, J. W., Martin, C. J., and Holmes, T. H. Long-term adjustment in chronic lung disease: A prospective study of dying. Presented to the annual meeting of the American Psychosomatic Society March 29-31, 1968.

Faulkner, W. B. Influence of suggestion on size of bronchial lumen: bronchoscopic study and report of one case, Northwest Med, 40:367, 1941.

Fink, B. R. Influence of cerebral activity in wakefulness on regulation of breathing, J Appl Physiol, 16:15, 1961.

Holmes, T. H., Goodell, H., Wolf, S., and Wolff, H. G. The Nose: An Experimental Study of Reactions within the Nose in Human Subjects During Varying Life Experiences. Springfield, Ill., Charles C Thomas, Publisher, 1950.

Robin, E. D., Whaley, R. D., Crump, C. H., and Travis, D. M. Alveolar gas tension, pulmonary ventilation and blood pH during physiologic sleep in normal subjects, J Clin Invest, 37:981, 1958.

Webb, P. Air temperature in respiratory tracts of resting subjects in cold, J Appl Physiol, 4:378, 1951.

Wolff, H. G., Wolf, S., Grace, W. J., Holmes, T. H., Stevenson, I., Straub, L., Goodell, H., and Seton, P. Changes in form and function of mucous membranes occurring as part of protective patterns in man during periods of life stress and emotional conflicts, Trans Ass Amer Physicians, 61:313, 1948.

4

The Epidemiology of Diffuse Obstructive Pulmonary Syndromes

While the etiology may differ considerably, the mechanisms that produce increased airway resistance and reduction of expiratory flow are limited. The nature of the obstructing mechanism determines the effectiveness of therapy and the prognosis. In the reversible diffuse obstructive pulmonary syndromes that accompany bronchial asthma, for instance, the airway obstruction results from edema of the bronchial mucosa, increased tone of bronchial smooth muscle, copious viscid mucus, or a combination of these factors. In the irreversible diffuse obstructive pulmonary syndrome that is found in clinical emphysema or in chronic bronchitis, airway obstruction is secondary to pressure that acts upon bronchial walls and narrows the lumen during expiration.

REVERSIBLE DIFFUSE OBSTRUCTIVE PULMONARY SYNDROMES (DOPS$_R$)

Bronchial Asthma

Bronchial asthma may be defined as an episodic diffuse airway obstruction with complete remissions that occur spontaneously or with treatment. During the attacks there are retardation of expiratory flow and increased airway resistance. Commonly present are wheezing, coughing, and the production of thick, viscid sputum. A patient experiencing the changes described becomes short of breath and apprehensive. The attack may last from hours to days. Symptomatic relief follows the parenteral administration of aminophyllin or adrenaline, or the use of an aerosol containing isoproterenol or epinephrine, particularly if these medications are combined with reassurance. Two distinct types of bronchial asthma are recognized.

EXTRINSIC

The etiology of this disease is unknown. It is often referred to as "allergic asthma" and an eosinophilia of blood and sputum is often found. In these individuals there may be a characteristic intermediate whealing-type reaction to subdermally injected antigens, or atopy. Patients with atopy will demonstrate circulating reaginic antibodies. The atopic eczema occurring in infants is followed by a respiratory allergy in approximately 59 percent of the children. This hypersensitivity is peculiar to man and is not found in animals.

However, not all patients who demonstrate antibody formation have asthma, and antigen-antibody reactions are demonstrable in only 25 percent of those with the clinical disease. It is probable that bronchial asthma is the sum of genetic, constitutional, and environmental factors.

Precipitation of asthmatic attacks is known to occur more frequently following: (1) respiratory infection; (2) psychological stress; and (3) exposure to specific allergens, in patients shown to have an allergic diathesis. In most patients, more than one of these factors is at work.

The mechanism for producing bronchospasm, mucosal congestion, and sputum in asthma is unknown. Histamine has been implicated and studied extensively. However, antihistaminic drugs are not effective in bronchial asthma. Likewise, serotonin has not been proved to be responsible for the attacks. It is known that a parasympathetic discharge will induce bronchoconstriction and the secretion of mucus; this is relieved by the use of atropine. It has been postulated that, depending upon the balance between parasympathetic and sympathetic activity, small doses of histamine might be effective in provoking an attack. Therefore, the "vagotonic" patient might be affected by minimal doses of histamine or some other agent of this nature. However, anticholinergics do not help many asthmatic patients. The mucosal congestion and edema of the bronchial wall are the principal obstructive mechanisms in many of these patients. These conditions are not known to be affected by atropine administration.

The prognosis in patients with uncomplicated extrinsic bronchial asthma is excellent. Most patients have a decrease in the frequency of attacks with time and many are free of asthma by the time they reach middle age. Such a natural history may depend on the freedom of the tracheobronchial tree from chronic infection. Ogilvey has shown that the development of bronchitis in 43 percent of a population having intermittent asthma was a major factor in prognosis. While the intervention of chronic bronchial infection did not always result in the deterioration of the clinical condition, those deteriorating were more frequently in the infected group. By far the majority of asthmatics go through life without difficulty except at the time of attack. A small number develop irreversible airway obstruction and show a chronic and progressive retardation of expiratory flow.

INTRINSIC

A few patients have the onset of asthma after the age of 40—the intermittent DOPS of middle age. The attacks of cough, sputum, wheeze, and shortness of breath are relieved in a typical fashion by adrenergic drugs. Symptoms of cough and sputum have usually been present for years and persist between the attacks of bronchospasm. Nasal polyposis is found in some as additional evidence that such patients have a chronic respiratory disease. This illness has often been called "asthmatic bronchitis." While many of these patients have eosinophilia in the blood and sputum, an allergic state has not been established and antibodies can seldom be demonstrated.

The mechanism of bronchial narrowing is uncertain, however; bronchoconstriction and sputum production appear to be more important than edema of the mucosa. The importance of histamine, heparin, serotonin, and slow-reacting substances in producing this narrowing is unclear.

In very few patients is there a specific agent known to initiate the bronchospastic attacks. However, one form of community air pollution and some occupational pollutants appear to be associated with this illness. On the Kanto plain of Japan, an entity called "Tokyo-Yokohama asthma" has been seen in some American military personnel. This is evidently a reversible DOPS that may be aggravated by the air pollution in the area. Workers in certain occupations involving contact with vegetable dusts have a similar illness.

Histologically patients with intrinsic asthma show chronic bronchitis, but the disease is not consistently associated with emphysema. The administration of steroids to these patients will alleviate symptoms for several years. Flow rate determinations during this period, however, often show a gradual deterioration. With progression, complete reversibility of the airway obstruction cannot be obtained between attacks and the patient develops the irreversible diffuse obstructive syndrome.

Comment. In subsequent chapters some psychosocial factors thought to be important in the production and maintenance of asthma will be reviewed. A possible unifying concept of asthma has been presented by Graham in his "attitude hypothesis." The basic formulation states that specific symptoms are associated with specific attitudes which are peculiar to the symptoms. Without the attitude the symptom is thought not to appear, and vice versa. The attitude is specifically defined as the manner in which a person perceives his current situation and what he feels and wants to do about it. The asthmatic feels isolated and wants the person or situation producing this feeling to be shut out. He wishes to blot out the situation or person. The attitude is seen as being a necessary but not sufficient condition for the production of asthma. In other words, someone with no other predisposing factors could probably develop the attitude without developing asthma. However, someone with other predisposing factors may develop asthma whenever the attitude is developed. On the other end of the spectrum are patients who continually have the attitude but only develop asthma when specific antigens are present. In the absence of the attitude or the antigens they do not experience asthma. This concept is not seen as a final answer, but has heuristic value in any discussion of asthma. Also, it appears to be more applicable to extrinsic asthma than to intrinsic asthma.

IRREVERSIBLE DIFFUSE OBSTRUCTIVE PULMONARY SYNDROME ($DOPS_I$)

Irreversible obstructive pulmonary syndromes are the commonest cause of lung failure in clinical medicine. They are seldom seen before the age of 40. They may or may not be accompanied by cough, sputum, and wheeze. All patients with this difficulty show a persistent retardation of expiratory flow and increased airway resistance. As the airway obstruction progresses, the patient develops dyspnea, depending upon his level of activity. Patients with mild obstructive syndromes, or those with a maximal voluntary ventilation (MVV)* greater than 80 percent of predicted, are seldom symptomatic. In those with a moderate degree of airway obstruction (MVV 40 to 80 percent of predicted), approximately 50 percent complain of dyspnea. A significant percentage of these patients will have arterial hypoxemia and a few will have hypercapnia. When the airway obstruction is severe (MVV less than 40 percent of predicted), dyspnea is often present at rest and is always seen on exercise. Most of these patients have hypoxemia and many have hypercapnia. This syndrome is commonly called emphysema in the clinic. There is, however, a poor correlation with anatomical emphysema. Many patients who die with a progressive DOPS have no emphysema in their lungs. Also, some patients with a significant amount of anatomical emphysema have no airway obstruction. Chronic

* Also called maximal breathing capacity (MBC).

bronchitis has also been described as a cause of the narrowing of the airway lumen. However, chronic bronchitis is not found in all patients with DOPS and many patients have chronic bronchitis without DOPS. No consistent structural representation of the obstructive syndrome is known at this time.

The mechanism of the airway obstruction in irreversible DOPS is unlike that in reversible DOPS. Little or incomplete relief of the increased airways resistance occurs following the use of bronchodilators, anticholinergics, or antihistamines. Bronchoconstriction, mucosal edema, and sputum play a relatively small part in the narrowing of the airways in this condition. On the other hand, a remarkable narrowing of the large airways during deep expiration or cough can be demonstrated in these subjects at bronchoscopy. Not infrequently, a complete collapse of the cartilagenous main stem bronchi occurs with cough. The transmural pressure generated by the cough is so great that it overcomes the supporting structures in the bronchial walls.

A fall in expiratory flow rate unrelieved by adrenergic drugs accompanies the aging process. With age, man's lungs become more compliant—i.e., the elastic recoil of the lung is diminished, as in the ability of the lung to empty itself. The maximal lung volume is limited by the chest cage, so that with more easily distended lungs the maximal transpulmonary pressure that can be developed falls as well. Intrapleural pressures are higher for corresponding volumes than in normal young subjects.

In DOPS, these changes in lung compliance or elastic recoil are more marked. At maximal lung volume there is little distending pressure and the intrapleural pressures are not far below atmospheric levels. During expiration, the pressures within the alveoli must be above those within the airways for gas to flow. However, with the decreased elastic recoil, the tension within the alveolar walls is insufficient to drive the air out of the lungs. The only means the respiratory system has of emptying these inelastic lungs is to clamp the chest cage down upon the lung. During exercise and with more hurried expiration greater pressures are necessary. Such pressures applied to the lung are also applied to the small airways that have no rigid support. Thus higher pressures exist in the alveoli surrounding the airway than in the airway itself. The end result is a narrowing or collapse of the airway with resulting increased resistance and retardation of flow. Transmural pressures may become quite large, as demonstrated by the collapse of large, well-supported bronchi seen at bronchoscopic examination. Irreversible DOPS is lung failure that is associated with a reduction in the elastic recoil of the lung.

If the entire lung was equally involved in the change in lung compliance, the distribution of ventilation would be uniform. However, some areas of the lung become more compliant than others, and ventilation is preferentially distributed to these areas. Highly ventilated areas are inefficient and have more ventilation than necessary for gas exchange. Such highly compliant and highly ventilated areas have been found in the upper lobes in patients with severe DOPS. They have also been described in other locations. Wherever located, a relatively small, highly compliant area of the lung could contribute to the airway obstruction seen. Regardless of whether these are localized changes in compliance, the changes in airway resistance are distributed throughout the lung.

Nonuniform ventilation must exist in the smallest lung divisions. Unless matched by changes in blood flow, these units will have different ventilation-to-perfusion ratios. Hyperventilating units will have wasted ventilation (alveolar dead space), while those hypoventilating in relation to their blood flow will result in arterial hypoxemia or hypercapnia. As long as sufficient numbers of hyperventilating units are present to compensate for carbon dioxide exchange, arterial hypercapnia will not occur (see Chapter 3). However, as the number of respiratory units with low ventilation-to-blood flow ratios increases, the progression from hypoxemia to the stage in which hypoxemia is accompanied by hypercapnia cannot be prevented. With progression of the defect in the distribution of ventilation and blood flow, hypercapnia eventually results in acidosis as the compensation by the blood buffer base system fails. The course of these abnormalities is fixed in this group of diseases.

The cause of the change in elastic recoil is unknown. The alteration in lung mechanics probably results from changes in the properties of lung tissue, although an alteration in the surface film has been suggested. It is clear that it takes time, probably years, to develop these changes. While everyone has a decreasing expiratory flow rate—and it has been suggested that at 140 years of age everyone would have DOPS—the rate at which this condition appears varies considerably among individuals.

Several nonspecific factors play a part in the production of irreversible DOPS. It is seen more frequently in the aged, as stated above. Irreversible DOPS is more frequent in men than in women. Men are more likely to work in dusts, fumes, smokes, and use cigarettes that damage cilial action. They are more likely to get a respiratory infection and take less care of it than the female of the species. This sex incidence may reflect the mores of our culture more than a true sex-linked susceptibility.

Etiologic Factors

BRONCHIAL ASTHMA

As many as 5 percent of those with extrinsic bronchial asthma will lose the episodic character of their attacks and go on to irreversible DOPS.

Bronchial infection is frequently present in these patients and has been implicated as a cause of such deterioration.

INFECTION

Pulmonary tuberculosis is associated with an unusually high incidence of DOPS. Of the patients admitted to a tuberculosis sanatorium, 34 percent have obstructive airway syndromes. Of those with minimal and moderately advanced tuberculosis, 24 percent have airway obstruction—but as many as 57 percent of the patients with far-advanced tuberculosis have abnormal expiratory flow rates. The severity of the DOPS is more marked as well in those with far-advanced tuberculosis. The extent of the tuberculosis is also related to the prognosis of DOPS. Those with far-advanced disease and longer-activity disease are more likely to show deterioration of their flow rates in the follow-up period.

Chronic bronchities is a poorly defined entity. To the epidemiologist, it is diagnosed in patients presenting with cough and sputum for a three-month period in the preceding two years. The flora present in the tracheobronchial tree varies considerably. Hemophilus influenza is found in some patients with chronic bronchitis, but many have a sterile tracheobronchial tree. The structural counterpart of these symptoms is not well delineated. The bronchial-gland-to-wall ratio has been described as having a gross correlation with the amount of sputum produced. However, many patients with a high ratio have no cough or sputum, and the opposite is true as well.

Chronic bronchitis is often described as a cause of DOPS because chronic inflammation presumably narrows the airway lumen. However, the majority of patients who cough and spit do not have DOPS. A few have DOPS and deny having any cough or sputum. It seems doubtful, therefore, that chronic bronchitis is the only cause of DOPS, although there may be an association between the two.

AIR POLLUTANTS

Air pollutants may be categorized into three divisions. A personal form of air pollution occurs in smokers, a community form of air pollution occurs in urban areas, and air pollution occurs in certain occupations.

PERSONAL AIR POLLUTION. Personal forms of air pollution have been indicated as a cause of DOPS for many years. A correlation between airway obstruction and cigarette smoking has often been demonstrated. Any particulate matter inhaled may increase airway resistance in a reversible manner. If irreversible DOPS is caused by smoking, it must be a function of continued insults over a period of years. Irreversible DOPS is often, although not invariably, found in heavy smokers.

Many physicians believe that smoking is the major—and some believe it is the *only*—cause of DOPS. While important, it is not the only etiologic factor. Patients with tuberculosis show no relationship between the amount of smoking and the incidence of DOPS. Perhaps this is because tuberculosis is such a potent factor in the production of DOPS that smoking is of relatively little import. It has been shown that there is a marked difference in the personality and emotional traits between heavy smokers and nonsmokers. Therefore, the smokers and nonsmokers do not form a homogeneous population for direct comparison of incidence. All heavy smokers do not get DOPS and, therefore, an individual susceptibility or tolerance is thought to exist.

Patients with DOPS show an improvement in pulmonary function if they can be persuaded to cease smoking. As the patient has complete control over this form of air pollution, the condition would appear to be ideally suited for treatment. That this is untrue is a common experience. In many heavy smokers, smoking appears much like an addiction, even to having withdrawal symptoms. In others, the patient continuously rationalizes the use of cigarettes, in that it "helps to raise sputum" or "quiets my nerves," etc.

Community Air Pollution. A form of reversible bronchoconstriction also occurs in some of the American military personnel stationed in the Tokyo-Yokohama area. Usually it occurs in those over the age of 40, who have a heavy smoking history and symptoms of bronchitis. Episodic bronchoconstriction occurs which progresses to the irreversible form of DOPS if the patient stays on the Kanto plain. Usually upon leaving the area the patients are relieved of the difficulty, but if they are rotated back to the Tokyo area, they may develop irreversible DOPS. No other community in the world is known to have such a relationship with DOPS. New Orleans, Los Angeles, and London, as well as several other large centers, have reported periods of excessive pollution, at which times respiratory symptoms are aggravated, but these illnesses have not earned a sobriquet for themselves.

Occupational Pollutants. A disease of the carding room of cotton factories (byssinosis) begins as reversible DOPS. If the worker does not leave the industry, the disease continues to irreversible airway obstruction. In this, byssinosis is similar to "Tokyo-Yokohama asthma" in its capacity for moving from reversible DOPS to irreversible DOPS. Similar conditions afflict workers in flax, sisal, and hemp industries. The material in these vegetable fibers that are responsible for causing the airway obstruction is unknown.

The reversible airway obstruction that occurs in cotton factories has been shown to clear up when the worker is away from his occupation. Throughout the day on Monday, the worker's expiratory flow rates fall. Recovery is incomplete overnight and there continues a progressive fall in expiratory flow rates each day throughout the work week. By Friday night, the airway obstruction may be quite marked with wheezing, cough, and sputum. These symptoms and the airway obstruction clear over the weekend. For many years this may be a completely reversible DOPS, as demonstrated by the response to adrenergic drugs and avoidance of exposure. Reversibility is gradually lost unless the susceptible individual avoids the pollutant.

Workers with chronic poisoning from cadmium oxide fumes show a greater deterioration in respiratory function than do those who have no such exposure. The retardation in expiratory flow progresses even after the workers leave the industry.

Hard rock miners who develop silicosis have a higher incidence of DOPS than does the general population. In silicotuberculosis the incidence of DOPS reaches 66 percent of those examined.

DOPS has occurred in workers accidentally exposed to the fumes of rocket fuels (borane and diborane). The number of such incidents is quite small and only a suspicion concerning the activity of these agents is warranted. The dioxides of sulfur and nitrogen have also come under suspicion as being able to produce obstructive pulmonary syndromes.

Several of the specific dusts, fumes, or smokes described are present as particles of less than 10 μ. Inhaled inert particles of this size will increase airway resistance, and the question arises as to whether they may damage the lungs on chronic exposure. The effect of such agents is not universal and varies from subject to subject. Many workers in the carding rooms of cotton factories do not develop byssinosis. "Tokyo-Yokohama asthma" does not affect all our military personnel living on the Kanto plain but only certain susceptible individuals. It is quite likely that those afflicted are "respiratory reactors," the respiratory tract being a target organ for pollution, infection, and possibly emotional crises. The ability of particulate matter to enter the lungs varies considerably. Workers who get silicosis have an inefficient nasal straining apparatus and more dust is presented to the lung parenchyma; following inhalation of similar amounts of particulate matter, the degree of bronchoconstriction generated varies from subject to subject. Apparently some are more susceptible than others to the effect of particles on the bronchial mucosa. Some patients are particularly susceptible to respiratory infection, while others go through many successive winters without having colds. Holmes has demonstrated reddening and congestion of the nasal mucosa with mucus production following emotional stress in some individuals. Faulkner has observed similar effects in the bronchial mucosa. There would seem to be a considerable difference in the susceptibility of the respiratory tract to damage, and a considerable difference in the reaction of the tract between patients. Those susceptible subjects with great reactivity of the tract might be termed "respiratory reactors."

To accelerate the mechanism producing irreversible DOPS, one needs a respiratory reactor with exposure to allergins, infections, fumes, smokes, dusts, and environmental stress over a period of years. These respiratory reactors are susceptible to those pulmonary insults that result in a change in the mechanical properties of lung (tissue or surface film).

NATURAL HISTORY

The natural history of irreversible DOPS has been studied. The prognosis for life depends upon the severity of the airway obstruction (Fig. 1). The population described here had their DOPS found in the course of treating active pulmonary tuberculosis. Patients in Group I, who had normal flow rates during their hospitalization, had a life expectancy comparable to that obtained from Metropolitan Life Insurance figures—i.e., patients with inactive tuberculosis who have no obstructive pulmonary syndrome, have no different life expectancy than that of the general popu-

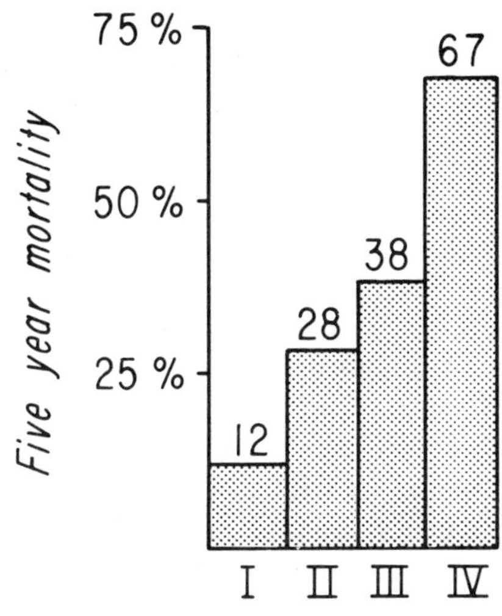

Fig. 1. Five-year mortality rate for patients with tuberculosis and no irreversible DOPS (Group I), with mild irreversible DOPS (Group II), with moderate irreversible DOPS (Group III), and with severe irreversible DOPS (Group IV). Patients in Group I have life expectancy comparable to that obtained from Metropolitan Life Insurance figures for the general population.

lation. The patients in Group II had mild DOPS, as defined by an MEF that was abnormal but above 180 L per min, or an abnormal MVV but one above 80 percent of that predicted. The patients in this group had no deaths that were described as caused by asthma, chronic bronchitis, emphysema, or cor pulmonale. Instead, the significantly greater death rate was due to the patients' inability to survive other illnesses. Surgical procedures, acute infection, and accidents proved to be more lethal in these people with mild DOPS than it did in the control group. In moderate DOPS or in those with an MEF between 105 and 179 L per min or an MVV 40–79 percent of predicted, there is an even higher death rate at five years than in either of the other two groups. In this group, a few death certificates showed diagnoses compatible with the diffuse obstructive pulmonary syndrome. The very high death rate in those who were severely obstructed (MEF less than 105 L per min or MVV less than 40 percent) is significantly different from that in the other groups. More people in this group died of asthma, cor pulmonale, chronic bronchitis, and emphysema. In this group, the risk of being dead within five years was almost seven out of ten.

COMMENT. As with bronchial asthma, a description of the physiologic abnormalities which occur with $DOPS_I$ can be made with scientific clarity. However, once again, when the question of etiology arises there is evidence to support almost any contention—depending on the population studied. It is evident that this syndrome is seldom the result of a specific isolated etiologic agent. The problem of predisposition to a particular disease has occupied the attention of numerous investigators. However, no unifying concepts have emerged. Physiology, anatomy, genetics, clinical medicine, and surgery all present their particular approaches to disease with little regard for the patient's environment and psychologic makeup. This divergency exists despite numerous studies indicating that psychologic and social variables are of the utmost importance in the treatment, prognosis, and etiology of disease.

Until recently there were little quantitative data which could be compiled from the psychologic and social areas. However, there are presently several tests of a psychosocial nature capable of providing data that will aid in predicting which patients will get well and which will get injured or diseased.* Future clinicians who can utilize advanced versions of the above type of test, plus data similar to that obtained from Graham's hypothesis of disease onset, as well as physiologic data, may be able to predict who will get sick and what they will get sick from.

* Information about the Schedule of Recent Experience (SRE) should be addressed to T. H. Holmes, M.D., Department of Psychiatry, University of Washington, Seattle, Wash. 98105.

REFERENCES

Bentivoglio, L. G., Bereel, F., Stewart, P. B., Byran, A. C., Ball, W. C. Jr., and Bates, D. V. Studies of regional ventilation and perfusion in pulmonary emphysema using xenon^{133}, Amer Rev Resp Dis, 38:315, 1963.

Berle, B. B., Pinsky, R. H., Wolf, S., and Wolff, H. G. A clinical guide to prognosis in stress diseases, JAMA, 149:1624, 1952.

Daymon, H. Mechanics of airflow in health and in emphysema, J Clin Invest, 30:1175, 1951.

Eriksson, S. Pulmonary emphysema and alpha^{1} antitripsin deficiency, Acta Medica Scand, 175:197, 1964.

Faulkner, W. B. Bronchoscopic observations of changes due to psychic factors, Pacific Coast Med, 8:22, 1941; also Northwest Med, 40,367, 1941.

Field, W. E. H., Davy, E. N., Reid, L., and Roe, F. J. C. Bronchomucous gland hypertrophy: Its relation to symptoms and environment, Brit J Dis Chest, 60:66, 1966.

Flick, A. L., and Patton, R. R. Obstructive emphysema in cigarette smokers, Arch Intern Med, 104:518, 1959.

Frank, N. R., Meade, J., and Ferris, B. G. Jr. Mechanical behavior of the lungs in healthy elderly persons, J Clin Invest, 36:1680, 1957.

Grace, W. J., and Graham, D. T. Relationship of specific attitudes and emotions to certain bodily diseases, Psychosom Med, 14:343, 1952.

Graham, D. T., Lundy, R. M., Benjamin, L. S., Kabler, J. D., Lewis, W. C., Kunish, N. O., and Graham, F. K. Specific attitudes in initial interviews with patients having different "psychosomatic" diseases, Psychosom Med, 24:257, 1962.

——— Stern, J. A., and Winokur, G. The concept of a differing set of physiological changes in each emotion, in Explorations in the Physiology of Emotions, Psychiatric Research Reports #12. American Psychiatric Ass, Washington, D.C., 1960, pp. 8–15.

Holmes, T. H., and Rahe, R. H. The social readjustment rating scale, J Psychosom Res, 11:213, 1967.

——— Goodell, H., Wolf, S., and Wolff, H. G. The Nose: An Experimental Study of Reactions Within the Nose of Human Subjects During Varying Life Experiences. Springfield, Ill., Charles C Thomas, Publisher, 1950.

Lenfant, C., and Pace, W. R. Jr. Alterations of ventilation to perfusion ratios distribution associated with successive clinical stages of pulmonary emphysema, J Clin Invest, 44:1566, 1965.

Martin, C. J., and Hallett, W. Y. The diffuse obstructive pulmonary syndrome in a tuberculosis sanatorium: II. Incidence and symptoms, Ann Intern Med, 54:1156, 1961.

——— Pardee, N., and Dominik, J. The diffuse obstructive pulmonary syndrome: I. Natural history, Amer Rev Resp Dis, 93:383, 1966.

——— and Young, A. C. Lobar ventilation in obstructive syndromes, Amer Rev Resp Dis, 96:929, 1967.

Ogilvey, A. G. Asthma: A study in prognosis of 1,000 patients, Thorax, 17:183, 1962.

Phelps, R. V. W., and Koike, S. Tokyo-Yokohama asthma, Amer Rev Resp Dis, 86:55, 1962.

Rahe, R. H., and Holmes, T. H. Life crisis and disease onset. I. Qualitative and quantitative definition of the life crisis and its association with health change. Unpublished data.

Schilling, R. S. F. The epidemiology of byssinosis–adventure and misadventure, J Occup Med, 1:33, 1959.

5

Material and Methods

The techniques for producing psychologic changes in physiologic studies are multiple. They vary from completely artificial induction of psychologic change to naturally occurring life stress. Regardless of the techniques employed the purpose is to elicit recognizable psychologic changes while measuring physiologic variables. The degree of physiologic and psychologic change supposedly depends on the significance, severity, duration, and type of initiating stimulus. This simple stimulus-response model is sometimes complicated by a further psychologic response to the physiologic change which may accentuate or minimize any physiologic and psychologic change. An example of this kind of "feedback" is provided by psychophysiologic back pain. The back pain attitude is followed by skeletal muscle spasm. The muscle spasm produces ischemia which in turn produces pain. The pain then provides a stimulus which accentuates the attitude, produces additional anxiety, and the patient experiences more muscle spasm, more ischemia, more pain, and so on. The original stimulus need not have been the back pain attitude but may have been a physical injury. This is illustrated in Figure 1. Thus a given stimulus may have far greater consequences than the initial physiologic and psychologic change. This is particularly true in respiratory disease and will be elaborated upon in subsequent chapters.

From our observations to date, the production of psychologic change would appear to be obtained best by the use of naturally occurring life events. This is probably the hardest method, but is more productive in terms of significant data. It is a frustrating experience to study a subject for a period of weeks, waiting for the occurrence of significant life events, but the resulting data are well worthwhile. If it is impossible to observe the naturally occurring event in the laboratory, the next best thing is the

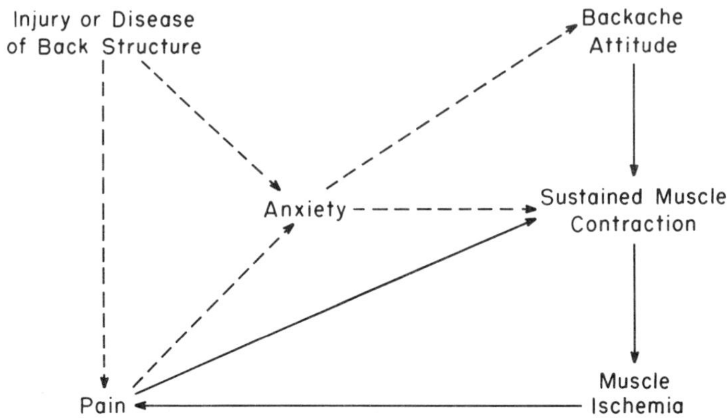

Fig. 1. Interaction of a number of so-called organic and functional variables which may work to initiate and/or aggravate a symptom or symptom complex. Backache is used as an example because it is a well studied phenomenon. (Previously published in *Northwest Med.*, 57:602, 1958, by Dorpat, T. L., and Holmes, T. H., and in *Postgrad. Med.*, 25:713, 1959.)

production of an event by direct suggestion with or without hypnosis, or with the use of an interview in which the event is reconstructed. The subject's response to such stimuli will be the result of a long-established life style, and detailed data about the subject's emotional response can be obtained. In addition to the above methods of producing psychologic and physiologic change, an artificial traumatic experience (noxious stimulation of the head) has been utilized.

SUBJECTS AND GENERAL PROCEDURES

The observations in the chapters to follow were based on 200 subjects who were studied in eight, sometimes overlapping, experimental groups. The observations are presented in 16 chapters. In addition to the organized group studies, many patients were studied individually to obtain specific types of data.

Group 1. Group 1 consisted of 22 hospital outpatients who complained of respiratory symptoms. Fifteen had bronchial asthma and the remainder anxiety states. There were 11 females and 11 males in the study.

For the purposes of the study a recording technique was needed which was as unobtrusive as possible and permitted the subject to talk. The rubber tube (Manning) type of pneumograph fulfilled this requirement. The subject lay on a comfortable bed, and the pneumograph was attached to his chest around the lower ribs. A rubber tube connected the pneumograph with a tambour which activated an ink-writing pen on a continuous feed kymograph. The recording utilized the movement of the thorax as an indicator of respiratory function. The method cannot be standardized and allows no comparison between the depths of respiration in different subjects. As no measurements were made of gaseous exchange, only inferential statements can be made about the volume of air respired and the metabolic state. However, the method does permit a comparison of the thoracic movement in the same individual at different times, and its disadvantages were compensated for by the fact that the subjects never complained, and were apparently rarely aware of the recording apparatus.

While recordings were being made the subject was interviewed by a physician who discussed various topics and attitudes known to be of relevance to his life and illness. Usually the subject was asked first to think about these topics which were suggested to him in groups of two or three and were followed by a suggestion of relaxation. After each group of thoughts, the subject was questioned about the exact content of his thinking at each time and the associated feeling state. The subject's statements concerning his feelings were related to the physician's observations of the subject's voice, facial expression, movements of his hands or body, and other indices of emotional change. A constructive discussion of the problem was encouraged before the next topic was taken up. From time to time, the subject was questioned about symptoms and sensations connected with his respiration. For the most part, the conversation was confined to matters of relevance to the subject's life and illness. In a few instances the effects of reading silently or aloud were studied, but this activity was invariably accompanied by emotional changes connected either with the tension of reading or with the material read. Each interview lasted approximately an hour.

The respirations of each subject during periods of relaxation or pleasant thoughts were compared to those during periods of emotional disturbance. Changes in rate, depth, expiration:inspiration ratio, and other variations were evaluated and related to the prevailing emotional state and occurrence of symptoms.

This pneumographic study provides the background for the study of Group 2. Fundamental observations were made which were further expanded with the use of quantifiable respiratory variables.

Group 2. Group 2 was composed of 11 male and 11 female subjects between the ages of 15 to 69 (mean age 36) who were selected because of mood fluctuations or troubled interpersonal adjustment. Three subjects had normal lungs and the remainder had pulmonary tuberculosis or obstructive airway disease. In 2 to 100 weeks these subjects had as few as 5 or as many as 45 studies. A total of 325 studies were made on this group. Naturally occurring adverse life situations were utilized to elicit psychologic change. The psychologic changes were then correlated with simultaneously measured respiratory and cardiovascular variables.

When psychologic changes occurred over periods of minutes they were called short-term. In most cases physiologic stabilization did not take place, and the calculation of carbon dioxide production could not be made because of the washout or retention of carbon dioxide that occurred with changes in ventilation. Measurements of carbon dioxide production taken during such "unsteady" states would give falsely elevated or lowered values. Psychologic changes which occurred over periods of days, weeks, or months were called long-term, and physiologic stabilization was attained. Carbon dioxide production measurements made during these periods reflect changes in metabolism.

The subjects were studied on alternate days or daily. When naturally occurring psychologic changes were present, the days on which the subject was relaxed and calm were used as controls. In addition, the psychologic change was usually terminated by verbal suggestion of relaxation, and the measurements repeated. In the absence of naturally occurring psychologic change, adverse life situations which were known to be present were often suggested after a control period. On each day of observation, the subjects were allowed to rest in the laboratory for 15 to 20 min (seated in a chair) before any measurements were made. A 5- to 15-min adjustment period on the equipment followed, after which control data were obtained over a period of 5 to 15 min.

Before, during, and after the experimental procedures the subjects were asked how they felt about the situation they found themselves in, and what they felt like doing about it. They were allowed to express themselves freely, and notes were taken of the interview content. The interview material was then evaluated in the light of behavioral observations made in the laboratory by the experimenter and on the ward by ward personnel. The psychologic data were compiled by one observer and submitted to a judge who was uninformed about the physiologic data. A conclusion about the subject's orientation toward action was arrived at by discussion between the observer and the uninformed judge.

The following experimental groups were used to validate and expand the observations made on Group 1 and Group 2.

GROUP 3. Group 3 consisted of 19 patients with a history of asthma who were currently in treatment. Two female subjects aged 43 and 64 were studied on a longitudinal basis, and 17 subjects (8 male, 9 female) ranging in age from 16 to 72 were studied on a cross-sectional basis during a standardized interview in order to confirm the relationships which were observed during the longitudinal study. Selection of subjects depended upon a history of intermittent asthmatic attacks, availability, and consent to participate in the study.

During the longitudinal study the two subjects were observed daily in their homes over a period of a month and catecholamine excretion (normetadrenaline and metadrenaline) in fractionated 24-hr urine samples was correlated with the subject's behavior before, during, and after asthmatic attacks. With the onset of an asthmatic attack the subjects were instructed to void and note the time. The next sample coincided with the duration of the symptoms and was collected at termination of the symptoms. A subsequent urine sample was collected for a period of time equal to that covered by the asthma attack. A diary kept by each subject focused attention on the events, attitudes, and feeling states of the day. These data were supplemented by a daily interview conducted at the subject's home.

For the 17 subjects in a response-to-interview situation, two urine samples were collected. The first was a pre-interview or control sample of 2- to 4-hr duration. The second or experimental sample was collected 20 min after termination of the interview. The tape-recorded interviews began with a discussion of the events occurring during the interval since selection for the study. Next, the subject was asked to give the history of his disease. From this the interview turned to a concentrated description of a typical asthmatic attack. This part of the interview was designed to elicit a discussion of the life setting in which symptoms occurred and the emotions, attitudes, and plan of action during an attack. Following this, the session gradually closed with a discussion of neutral topics.

At the beginning of the interview, and periodically thereafter, auscultation of the lung fields was performed. If wheezing developed or increased in intensity during the interview, that subject was designated an asthmatic reactor. An individual who manifested no asthmatic signs during interview was classified as an asthmatic nonreactor. In the longitudinal study the criteria used for determining an asthmatic attack were limited to the subject's subjective evaluation.

Group 4. Group 4 consisted of 26 subjects who volunteered for a total of 50 headband experiments. The number of experiments carried out on each subject varied from one to six. There were 3 females and 23 males in the experimental group. Their ages varied from 21 to 50 with a mean of 26. Among these subjects, 21 had normal lungs and 5 had tuberculosis. Of the 21 subjects with normal lungs, 19 were medical students, and 2 were laboratory technicians. The 5 tuberculosis subjects were participating in a parallel study (Group 2). The only criteria for selection of subjects were that they be available and willing to take part in the experiments.

Subjects were studied before, during, and after stimulation with a metal headband with 14 adjustable rubber-tipped screws around the edges. This device produced an aching pressure headache and mental discomfort when the adjustable screws were fixed tightly against the circumference of the head. As it was the object of the experiments to utilize the noxious stimulus to produce a significant change in behavior from the control state, time and magnitude of pressure were held as variables rather than constants. The end point of the observation was determined by the subject and was defined as that point at which he felt he could no longer tolerate the experience. All subjects were instructed to endure the stimulus as long as they possibly could, and when the stimulus was no longer tolerable it would be removed. Following application of the pressure device to the head, the screws were tightened at intervals of 5 to 8 min until the end point was achieved. Time required to reach the level of tolerance and termination of the noxious stimulus ranged between 11 and 39 min with a mean of 24 min.

GROUP 5. In Group 5 a total of 21 experiments were carried out on 11 male subjects ages 21 to 28. Ten were male medical students in normal health and one was a patient with tuberculosis. They were studied before, during, and after hypnotic suggestion of relaxation, depression, anxiety and/or anger, exercise, and head pain. Only one of the subjects had been hypnotized previously. The suggestion of anxiety or anger, exercise, and head pain was terminated with the suggestion of relaxation. Prior to the hypnosis experiments, 10 of these subjects were stimulated with a metal headband (see under Group 4). The results of the actual stimulation were compared with hypnotic suggestion of the experience. The eleventh subject was asked to recall a previously experienced migraine headache.

All subjects were interviewed prior to the experiments. Information was obtained about situations which had been accompanied by strong emotions of anxiety, anger, and depression, and about experiences which had included active participation in physical exercise. The hypnotic suggestion was based upon data gained in these interviews and was confined to these previous experiences. Emotion was defined as a state having both psychic and physiologic components. The ideation in anxiety was apprehension and tension; in anger, indignation and wrath; and in depression, dejection and hopelessness.

Hypnosis was induced by eye fixation on a light and the repeated suggestion of relaxation and drowsiness. After induction, the life situations and accompanying feeling states or head pain were suggested to the subjects. During hypnosis the subjects were questioned about their feelings, and observations were made of their overt behavioral responses. At the end of each experiment the subjects were questioned further about their sensations and emotional reactions during the experimental procedures. The psychological and physiological data were recorded by two investigators working independently.

In general, attention could be restricted under hypnosis so that life situations in which there had been active exercise and those accompanied by relatively pure emotion could be revived. However, in a number of instances, the intended uncomplicated single emotion was not produced. Instead, mixed or overlapping emotions—such as anxiety and depression or anger and depression—occurred.

GROUP 6. In Group 6, 339 studies were carried out on 25 subjects between the ages of 22 and 78 (mean age 45). These subjects were studied in an attempt to identify specific respiratory and emotional variables which are associated with dyspnea. The reporting of dyspnea by these subjects was strictly their own perception of breathing difficulty. All subjects were volunteers and were selected because of their availability and the fact that they experienced dyspnea. They were studied in two overlapping groups.

The first subgroup (Group 6a) was composed of 16 subjects (13 male, 3 female) who comprised a preliminary study group. Their ages varied from 29 to 78 with a mean of 54. Thirteen had DOPS (diffuse obstructive pulmonary syndrome or clinical emphysema) with tuberculosis, one had DOPS without tuberculosis, and two had tuberculosis without DOPS. Emotional and physiologic measurements made during days on which they complained of dyspnea were compared with days on which no dyspnea was reported. During these experiments the subject's mood was rated as good, average, or poor, and no data on specific emotions were collected. Thus a poor mood could mean anger, anxiety, depression, etc.

The second subgroup (Group 6b) consisted of 12 subjects: 5 were medical students with normal lungs, 2 were patients with DOPS and tuberculosis, and 5 were patients with tuberculosis without DOPS. Their ages ranged from 22 to 49 with a mean of 30. There were 5 females in this group. These subjects were studied during noxious stimulation of the head, during naturally occurring life situations, and during suggestion of stimuli which were known to be associated with dyspnea.

The hospitalized subjects were observed daily and naturally occurring variations in life situations were noted and correlated with dyspnea and measurements of respiratory function. The suggested stimuli consisted of life situations which the subjects had previously reported as being associated with the occurrence of dyspnea. They were first instructed to close their eyes and relax. After relaxation and the recording of control measurements these life situations were suggested. The suggestion was limited to asking the subject to free his mind of extraneous thoughts and to concentrate on the particular life situation which had been previously associated with dyspnea. The stimulus was then reinforced at 1- to 5-min intervals.

Of the 26 subjects in Group 4 who underwent the head pain experiment, 7 experienced dyspnea. These were matched as to age, sex, and disease with seven subjects who did not experience dyspnea in response to the head pain.

GROUP 7. Group 7 consisted of 40 hospitalized patients with severe clinical emphysema. They were followed over a 48-month period with repeated physiologic and psychiatric observations. With this study it was hoped that insight could be gained into the long-term adjustment of these subjects and the psychologic and/or social changes which preceded death. When possible, those subjects who died were studied up to the time of death with continuous psychiatric and physiologic measurements.

GROUP 8. Group 8 was composed of 51 asthmatics who were studied intensively in order to document their life styles and adjustment problems. There were 28 females and 23 males in the group. Skin tests were performed on them with extracts of six substances which are common causes of allergic reactions in the area: ragweed, kapok, dust, cottonseed, timothy, and feathers. In this group, 28 subjects had positive reactions to one or more of these substances, while 23 had negative reactions. Detailed histories were obtained from all subjects with emphasis on personal and family history and the past and present psychophysiologic aspects of the subject, so that a more complex understanding of psychodynamic factors might be gained. Attention was directed toward situations which might be threatening to the subject, his emotional response to them, and the relationship between his personality and the precipitation of his symptoms.

RESPIRATORY VARIABLES

Continuous measurements of respiratory rate (RR), minute ventilation ($\dot{V}$), and end tidal concentration of alveolar carbon dioxide were made by using a pneumotachograph and an infrared carbon dioxide analyzer. Intermittently, the anatomic dead space (V_D) was measured by graphic analysis of the expired carbon dioxide (or nitrogen) and volume curves. The measuring instruments were connected to a four-channel, direct-writing pen recorder. A description of these instruments has been previously published. The respiratory rate, minute ventilation, alveolar ventilation ($\dot{V}_A$), fractional concentration of alveolar carbon dioxide $F_{A_{CO_2}}$), oxygen uptake ($\dot{V}_{O_2}$), carbon dioxide production ($\dot{V}_{CO_2}$), and anatomic dead space are presented in the figures and tables which follow in the text. The experimental error varied with different equipments. It was usually less than 5 percent, but was considerably better than that in experiments in which each subject served as his own control. Standardization of the volume integrators of the pneumotachograph was carried out before and after each experiment by delivering a known amount of air from a spirometer at constant flow. The flow was standardized and the linearity of the system for flows between 8 to 70 L per min was checked daily. The infrared carbon dioxide meter was calibrated with four or five known concentrations of carbon dioxide before and after each experiment.

The anatomic dead space is an estimation of the amount of air in the conducting airways of the lungs. In analyzing for the dead space volume, five or more measurements were made in succession. The accuracy of this method was determined by measuring the volume in various lengths of ¾-in tubing and by using results calculated from the electronic instruments as compared with volume displacement. When necessary the dead space volumes measured on a given subject were corrected by means of these figures.

The alveolar ventilation represents an estimate of the amount of air reaching the alveoli. It is calculated from the following formula:

$$\dot{V}_A = \dot{V} - (RR \times V_D)$$

The end tidal carbon dioxide concentration is an estimation of the fractional concentration of alveolar carbon dioxide. This value is higher than the mean $F_{A_{CO_2}}$. However, for comparison purposes in the same individual, it is an adequate estimation. This also results in a high value for the $\dot{V}_{CO_2}$ which is calculated from the following formula:

$$\dot{V}_{CO_2} = (\dot{V}_A)\ (F_{A_{CO_2}})$$

The oxygen uptake represents the amount of oxygen removed from the inspired air per minute. In calculating oxygen uptake, the fractional concentration of expired oxygen and carbon dioxide is measured by using a Scholander gas analyzer. These values are then used in the following formula where $F_{E_{N_2}}$, $F_{E_{O_2}}$, and $F_{E_{CO_2}}$ are the concentration of expired nitrogen, oxygen, and carbon dioxide, respectively, and $F_{I_{N_2}}$ and $F_{I_{O_2}}$ are the concentration of inspired nitrogen and oxygen, respectively.

$$F_{E_{N_2}} = 1 - (F_{E_{O_2}} + F_{E_{CO_2}})$$

$$\left[\frac{F_{E_{N_2}}}{F_{I_{N_2}}} (F_{I_{O_2}}) \right] - F_{E_{O_2}} = \%O_2 \text{ extracted}$$

$$(\%O_2 \text{ extracted})\ (\dot{V}) = \dot{V}_{O_2}$$

The terms hyperventilation and hypoventilation, as used in the text, refer to changes in ventilation above or below the control values for a given subject. Hyperventilation was characterized by an increase in the alveolar ventilation and a decrease in the fractional concentration of alveolar carbon dioxide. Hyperventilation occurs when more oxygen is supplied and more carbon dioxide is removed than the metabolism requires; hypoventilation occurs when less oxygen is supplied and less carbon dioxide is removed than the metabolism demands. These conditions appear to occur when the organism is adjusting to new metabolic levels. Other terms which will be used to describe ventilation are increased and decreased ventilation. Increased ventilation refers to ventilation which has increased at a rate comparable to or behind metabolic rate, or to ventilation which has adjusted to metabolic rate at a higher level with no change in the $F_{A_{CO_2}}$. Decreased ventilation refers to ventilation which has decreased at a rate comparable to or behind metabolic rate, or to ventilation which has adjusted to metabolic rate at a lower level with no change in the $F_{A_{CO_2}}$.

CARDIOVASCULAR AND URINARY VARIABLES

Measurements of blood pressure, pulse rate, and fingertip skin temperature were made at 3- to 5-min intervals during many of the experiments. These variables were measured with the use of an aneroid sphygmomanometer, and electrocardiograph and/or manual palpation, and a McKesson Dermalor and/or thermistor, respectively.

Urinary 3-methoxy-4-hydroxymandelic acid (VMA) was measured by a method which combined and modified the methods of Armstrong et al. and Von Studnitz and Hanson. It involves ethyl acetate extraction of acidified urine, bidimensional chromatography of the extract, spraying and elution of the colored VMA complex, and photometric estimation. The procedure is specific, reproducible, and quantitative. VMA is a metabolite common to both noradrenaline and adrenaline. Its urinary titer has been used as an index of total catecholamine secretion and it is of value in the diagnosis of pheochromocytoma, as a measure of stress, and as an indicator of the effects of psychotropic drugs.

The recovery of VMA from urine was checked by the addition of known amounts to urine samples and analysis by the above method. The mean recovery of VMA added to 20 urine samples was 82.2 percent (S.D. ± 11.9). The reproducibility of the method was checked by duplicate determinations on 21 urine samples. The titers in these samples ranged from 1.46 to 6.70 μg per cc. The coefficient of variation of duplicate determinations was ± 2.2 percent. Replicate determinations on samples of untreated frozen urine indicate that VMA was stable over a period of at least six months.

Urinary metadrenaline (MA) and normetadrenaline (NMA), the 3-methoxy derivatives of adrenaline and noradrenaline, respectively, are the primary intermediates in catecholamine metabolism and are considered to be directly related to the secreted, physiologically active neurohormone. The method by which they were measured has been described in detail by Masuda. Briefly, the urine was acidified, hydrolyzed, and filtered through Dowex 50W-X2, 100-200 mesh resin. The solution was brought to a pH of 10.0 and evaporated with three drops of octanol. The residue was dissolved with 3 cc of ethanol and with an ethanol:acetone mixture. The total extract was then run bidimensionally in a paper chromatographic system. Spraying, elution, and photometry methods were identical to those used for the determination of VMA. Recoveries of standards added to urine and carried through the resin column processing were 70.9 percent (S.D. ± 9.4) for NMA and 83.8 per cent (S.D. ± 9.3) for MA. The standard deviation (coefficient of variation) of duplicate measurements (25 samples) was 8.7 percent of NMA and 14.6 percent for MA. All results reported are based on the mean of duplicate determinations and are not corrected for recovery.

CLINICAL EVALUATION

Clinical measurements used in assessing the respiratory function of the subjects were the standard gross ventilatory and blood gas measurements.

The gross ventilatory measurements consisted of the vital capacity (VC), the maximal breathing capacity (MBC),* and the maximal expiratory flow rate (MEF).

The vital capacity is the maximal volume that can be expired from

* Often called the Maximal Voluntary Ventilation (MVV).

the lungs after a maximal inspiration; it is expressed in liters. The maximal breathing capacity is the maximal volume of air that can be breathed in 1 min, and it is expressed in liters per min. Both of these variables were measured with a Collins 9-L respirometer. The maximal expiratory flow rate is a single breath test, which represents the maximal air flow during forced expiration. This variable correlates well with the maximal breathing capacity. The maximal breathing capacity and vital capacity are given as percent of predicted normal as well as in absolute measurements.

The blood gas measurements consisted of the partial pressure of oxygen expressed in mm Hg (Pa_{O_2}); the partial pressure of carbon dioxide, also expressed in mm Hg (Pa_{CO_2}); and pH. All were measured in arterial blood with a Beckman physiologic gas analyzer.*

Variations in method which apply to a particular experimental group will be mentioned in the text to follow. For more detailed physiologic data, see Chapters 3 and 4.

* Spinco Division of Beckman Instruments.

REFERENCES

Armstrong, M. D., McMillan, A., and Shaw, K. N. F. 3-methoxy-4-hydroxy-D-mandelic acid, a urinary metabolite of norephinephrine, Biochem Biophys ACTA (Amsterdam), 25:422, 1957.

Baldwin, E. DeF., Cournand, A., and Richards, D. W., Jr. Pulmonary insufficiency: I. Physiologic classification, clinical methods of analysis, standard values in normal subjects, Medicine, 27:243, 1948.

Berman, M. L., and Pettitt, J. A. Urinary excretion of 3-methoxy-4-hydroxy-mandelic acid after several stress situations, J Lab Clin Med, 57:126, 1961.

Comroe, J. H. Physiology of Respiration. Chicago, Year Book Medical Publishers, Inc., 1965.

——— Forster, R. E., Dubois, A. B., Briscoe, W. A., and Carlson, E. The Lung. Chicago, Year Book Medical Publishers, Inc., 1962.

Crout, J. R., Pisano, J. J., and Sjoerdsma, A. Urinary excretion of catecholamines and their metabolites in pheochromocytoma, Amer Heart J, 61:375, 1961.

Dorpat, T. L., and Holmes, T. H. Psychophysiologic aspects of backache. Postgrad Med, 25:713, 1959.

Fowler, W. S. Lung function studies: II. The respiratory dead space. Amer J Physiol, 154:405, 1948.

Goldsmith, J. R. A simple test of maximal expiratory flow for detecting ventilatory obstruction, Amer Rev Tuberc, 27:180, 1958.

Grace, W. J., and Graham, D. T. Relationship of specific attitudes and emotions to certain bodily diseases, Psychosom Med, 14:243, 1952.

LaBrosse, E. H., Axelrod, J., and Kety, S. S. O-methylation, the principal route of metabolism of epinephrine in man, Science, 128:593, 1958.

Martin, C. J., and Hallett, W. Y. The diffuse obstructive pulmonary syndrome in a tuberculosis sanatorium: II. Incidence and symptoms, Ann Intern Med, 54:1156, 1961.

Martin, C. J., and Young, A. C. Lobar ventilation in man, Amer Rev Tuberc Pulmon Dis, 73:330, 1956.

Masuda, M. Differing adaptive metabolic behaviors, J Psychosom Res, 10:239, 1966.

McDonald, R. K., and Weise, V. K. The effects of certain psychotropic drugs on the urinary excretion of 3-methoxy-4-hydroxymandelic acid in man, J Pharmacol Exp Ther, 136:26, 1962.

Pace, W. R. Pulmonary Physiology in Clinical Practice. Philadelphia, F. A. Davis Co., 1965.

——— Pulmonary physiology in clinical practice: V. Arterial blood gas analysis, Northwest Med, 62:350, 1963.

Von Studnitz, W., and Hanson, A. Determination of 3-methoxy-4-hydroxymandelic acid in urine by high-voltage paper electrophoresis, Scand J Clin Lab Invest, 11:101, 1959.

Wolff, H. G. Headache and Other Head Pain, 2nd ed. New York, Oxford University Press, 1963.

Section II

Naturally Occurring and Suggestion of Naturally Occurring Change

The four chapters in this section provide the basic information which led to the production of the monograph. Both normal subjects and subjects with diseased lungs were utilized in the belief that differences in the psychophysiology of respiration secondary to disease would be limited to the specific deficits, and the protective maneuvers made necessary by the deficits. By integrating the data on normal subjects with that of those experiencing asthma, emphysema, and tuberculosis, it was possible to arrive at a more inclusive view of the respiratory system. The specific protective defenses utilized by the patients with diseased lungs compose a good part of Section IV and will barely be mentioned in this section. It is recommended that this section be read with Section III—although, as with the other sections, it stands independently.

6

Pneumographic Observations

The relationships between emotional states and respiration have been explored by using several different approaches. A number of studies have been directed toward the discovery of relationships between breathing patterns and personality or constitutional types. A second group of studies has been concerned with alterations in pulmonary function with emotional changes. Marked variations in the respiration have been observed during sudden fright and after a painful injection. Finesinger made an exhaustive study of the influence of "pleasant and unpleasant ideas" upon the respiration measured with a spirometer. Faulkner and Wolf similarly studied variations in diaphragmatic action with changes in emotional state. A third series of studies has been directed toward the role of emotional states in respiratory diseases, especially bronchial asthma.

The present investigation of respiratory variations was undertaken to extend these observations and to explore further the relationship between emotional states and respiratory disorders. Attention was directed to breathing patterns associated with emotional states connected with the life situation of the subject and to symptoms associated with these situations and emotional states.

Twenty-two outpatients with chief complaints referable to the respiratory system were studied. Fifteen had bronchial asthma and the remainder anxiety states. There were 11 males and 11 females.

The rubber tube (Manning) type of pneumograph was utilized to measure chest excursions. The subject lay on a comfortable bed, and the pneumograph was attached to his chest around the lower ribs. A rubber tube connected the pneumograph with a tambour which activated an ink-writing pen on a continuous feed kymograph.

This chapter is adapted from an article originally published in *Psychosom Med,* 14:476, 1952, by Stevenson, I., and Ripley, H. S.

OBSERVATIONS

Alterations in the respiratory pattern accompanying changes in emotion were observed in all of the 22 subjects, although the nature of this variation differed among the subjects.

Changes in Rate. An increase in respiratory rate was observed in all of the subjects at one time or another. In 14 of them increase in rate was always noted during the periods of unpleasant emotion, while in the remaining 7 it sometimes decreased or remained unchanged in these periods. The extreme variation in respiratory rate occurred in a subject (Subject 3) who had at one time 4 and at another time 20 respirations per min during the interview. The former figure was the lowest rate observed while the highest was 26 respirations per min observed in another subject in whom the lowest rate was 12.

Changes in Depth. An increase in depth of respiration was observed in 16 of the subjects during some of the periods of emotional disturbance. In nine of these depth always increased during such periods, and in the remaining seven it sometimes decreased or remained unchanged. In three subjects, the depth always decreased, and in three subjects it sometimes decreased and sometimes remained unchanged. In general, the alterations in depth were more marked than those in rate. It was not uncommon for the depth of respiration to increase three- or fourfold with even greater increases during sighing or sobbing. In seven subjects the increase in rate and/or depth amounted to what was probably a marked hyperventilation.

Expiration:Inspiration Ratio. The proportions of each of the two components in the total respiration were found to vary. In the present group of 15 subjects with asthma, it was possible to ascertain changes in expiration:inspiration ratios in 11 subjects. In the remaining four, talking produced irregularities which prevented assessment of the ratio. Of these 11 subjects, all but one showed some prolongation of expiration during periods of emotional disturbance, although this feature was pronounced in only six subjects. In the seven subjects with anxiety, this finding occurred slightly in two subjects and to a marked degree in one other. In some of the asthmatic subjects the character of the pneumographic recording changed markedly with almost perpendicular inspiration lines and long sloping expiration lines. In other tracings there was a plateau with delay before effective expiration.

Other Qualitative Changes. Irregularity of the respiratory pattern during periods of unpleasant emotion occurred at some time or other in nearly every subject. It was a prominent feature in ten of them. Sighing respirations were likewise common and were a prominent feature of the pattern of nine. A deep inspiration similar to a sigh was observed in many subjects at any time the physician spoke to them.

Symptoms. During the interviews the subjects were almost entirely unaware of the recording and most of them were chiefly preoccupied with the discussion. It was found that the acknowledgment of symptoms depended much more on the attention of the subject to his body than on the objective changes in the respirations. Two subjects with extreme degrees of respiratory hyperfunction denied awareness of any variation whatsoever in their respirations, but they were intensely disturbed by the topics discussed. Other more sensitive subjects had complaints when only comparatively slight changes in the respiratory pattern were observed. Symptoms which arose during the interviews were always related to variations both in emotional state and in respiration.

The chief complaint was of difficulty in breathing—variously described by the subjects as a "need to take deeper breaths," "heavy breathing," or "shortness of breath." Several subjects were aware of increased breathing. One subject had fears that his breathing would stop. In all, nine subjects complained of dyspnea in one form or another. Three of the asthmatic subjects had wheezing during the interviews, which was related both to emotional changes and to changes in the pneumograph pattern. Three other asthmatic subjects had wheezing at the beginning of the interview. In two of them, it subsided shortly after the discussion began, and in the third it continued unchanged throughout an interview in which the subject showed little emotional change. In six subjects there were sensations of tightness or lumps in the chest. In all, 13 of the 22 subjects had some symptoms during the interviews.

Changes with Pleasurable Emotional States. In addition to the noted differences between periods of relaxation and emotional disturbance, in some subjects the respiratory pattern during periods of positively pleasurable emotion differed from that during periods of neutral thought content. Similar observations were made by Finesinger and Faulkner.

Associated Electrocardiographic Changes. In nine subjects on whom electrocardiographs were taken simultaneously with the pneumographs, there was an increase in heart rate during the periods of unpleasant emotions. Frequently there were changes in the configuration of the electrocardiographic complexes. These findings are reported more fully elsewhere.

Increases in Rate and Depth of Respiration. *Anxiety.* There was usually an increase in respiration function accompanying feelings of *anxiety*. Typical examples were found in the following subject.

subject 1. A 20-year-old man came to the hospital for the treatment of bronchial asthma. He had had asthma since the age of 5 and felt that it was related to his emotional state. His father and mother had both been hostile to him and to each other. Their marriage finally ended in separation. The subject felt tied to his mother and dependent upon her and lived with her after the separation. At the same time he despised her, thinking her dull and repulsive. He rejected her moral values with regard to sex and broke away from the tenets of her traditional church. He was the third of four boys. His oldest brother was patronizing to him and he resented this, but his relations with the others were

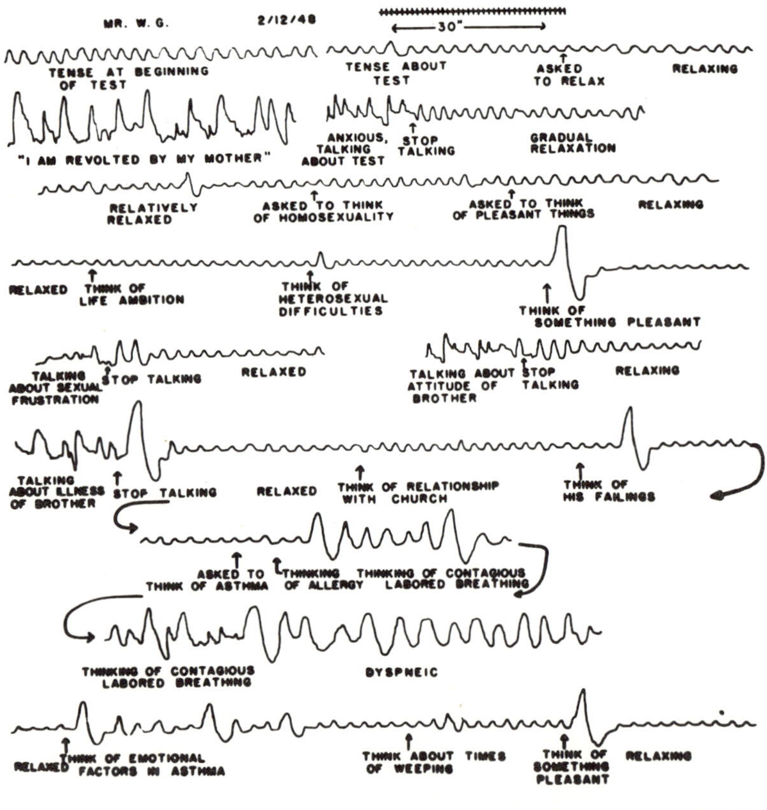

Fig. 1. Extracts of pneumographic tracings recorded during interview with Subject 1 shows increased rate and depth with anxiety and irregularities and increased depth with resentment. Hyperventilation and dyspnea occurred when subject thought of dyspnea. (Time in upper right hand corner. In this and succeeding figures, tracings are discontinuous where line is broken unless arrow indicates continuation on next line.)

good. He recalled that his asthma had occurred often in childhood when the oldest brother was receiving attention.

When he went to high school at 14, he had feelings of inferiority partly related to his brother's attitude and partly to his small stature and the feeling that his penis was "small and immature." At 15 he began to masturbate with considerable guilt and often had asthmatic attacks after masturbation. At 18 he attempted sexual intercourse but found himself impotent then and later. He also had some overt homosexual experiences. When he graduated from high school he took a job in a law office, and although the work was monotonous and promotion unlikely, he lacked initiative to go to college or to implement his ambition to be a writer. He had continued feelings of inferiority and at times felt dejected and wept.

Portions of the pneumograph tracing on this subject are shown in Figure 1. At the beginning of the interview, he was tense about the test and showed increased respiratory depth and rate. The heart rate was 100. When he was asked to think of his relationship with his mother, he had little reaction, but when he talked about this he expressed his dislike of her, saying "her presence repulses me." As he ventilated these feelings his heart rate increased to 124, and there was considerable acceleration of his rate of breathing. Increase in rate and, to a lesser extent, in depth occurred when he thought of his sexual problems and religious conflicts. After he stopped talking about the attitude of his oldest brother, toward whom he felt rivalry, relaxation was delayed. After talking about his younger brother, who was ill and for whom he felt sympathy, there was no delay in relaxation.

When the subject was asked to think about factors influencing his asthma, he first thought of possible allergic factors. Then he thought of the "contagious" nature of dyspnea and the fact that he had developed shortness of breath when he was aware of it in other people. As these thoughts entered his mind he expressed the need for more air, began to take deeper breaths and complained of a "hard, tight feeling," in his chest.

A little later depth of respiration increased again when he thought of emotional factors which made his asthma worse, such as his relations with his mother. Throughout the interview there were frequent sighs, especially when the subject was spoken to. The prevailing emotional state was one of anxiety. This was heightened during the discussion of the various topics mentioned and occasionally was mixed with irritation felt toward his mother and brother. At the end of the interview the subject was able to relax and the heart rate dropped to 85.

Anger. Increases in rate and depth were also observed during anger, as exemplified in the following subject.

SUBJECT 2. A 32-year-old Polish housewife had had dyspnea and palpitations for 18 months. Her early life was spent in Poland with her grandparents, who mistreated her. Her mother and younger sister were in the United States. Her long-standing desire to be with her mother was satisfied at 17 when she came to this country. Upon arrival she found herself at a disadvantage because of inability to speak English and her mother's favoritism toward her sister. She worked for a time as a servant and during this period felt lonely and became fearful that the isolated house where she worked would be broken into. After having very little association with men she married at 22. Her mother prepared her in no way for the sexual adjustments and intimacies of marriage, but her employer provided her with a little information a few days prior to her marriage. Her husband proved inconsiderate of her and she was rarely able to achieve sexual satisfaction. In addition, the husband gradually became less compatible with her in other respects.

Following the birth of her son a year after marriage, she devoted herself to the child and felt increasing hostility toward her husband. He, in turn, interested himself more in other women. In addition he was subject to violent outbursts and was frequently drunk and irresponsible financially. The subject assumed control of their mutual affairs. During one of his alcoholic sprees her husband almost killed a man and was sentenced to a year in prison but was permitted to join the army instead. While he was away she felt lonely, depressed, and anxious, and had palpitations, fatigue, chest pains, and dyspnea. Following the return of her husband she felt better for about a year. Later when he was working irregular hours at night she saw little of him and had a return of symptoms with generalized aches and more noticeable dyspnea. After being seen by a physician who told her she had rheumatic fever she became worried about her heart. Physical and laboratory investigations showed no evidence of structural disease, and it became clear that her symptoms were related to her emotional state. After expressing her feelings to the physician and receiving explanations and reassurance, she felt well for eight months. Then she found evidence of her husband's infidelity and with deep resentment and some anxiety made plans to divorce him. Under these circumstances her symptoms returned.

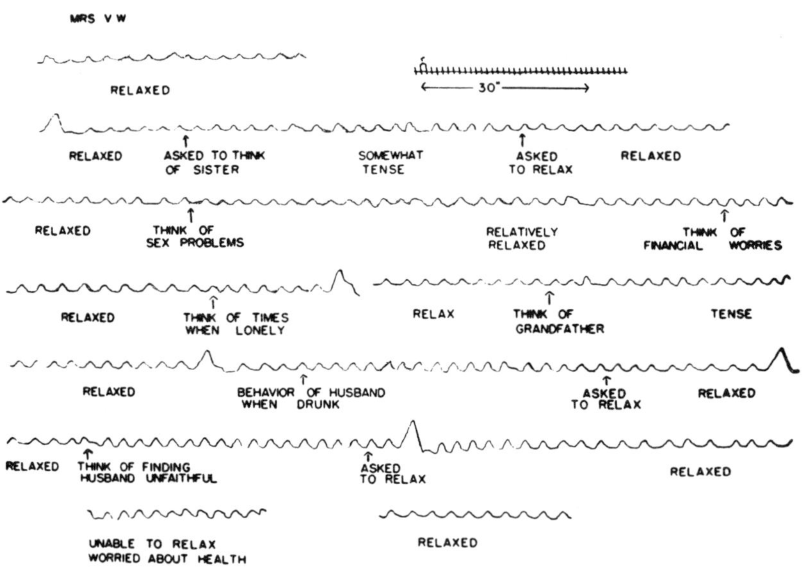

Fig. 2. Extracts of pneumographic tracings during interview with Subject 2 shows increases of rate and depth of respiration accompanying anxiety and resentment. There were frequent sighs.

At this time the subject was interviewed while pneumographic tracings were taken (Fig. 2). Respiratory changes were characterized by increased rate and depth of respiration. She showed both anxiety and anger at different times throughout the interview. The greatest reaction occurred when she thought of her husband's infidelity, and she described herself as feeling "mad" at this time. During this period there was an acceleration of the heart rate from 77 to 96. There were frequent sighs throughout the interview. During the interview the subject spoke of "getting shaky" and having "heavy breathing." These symptoms were related to increases in rate and depth of respirations.

Following this and other interviews, the subject was again able to see the relationship between her emotional state and her symptoms. She decided to try to make more of a success of her marriage. Her symptoms improved once more. The improvement was epitomized by the fact that dyspnea occurred only after she walked up five flights of stairs, whereas at the height of her symptoms she had noticed palpitations and shortness of breath after climbing only one flight of stairs.

COMMENT. Darwin related respiratory hyperfunction during anxiety and anger to primitive associations with appropriate action. "Men during numberless generations, have endeavored to escape from their enemies or danger by headlong flight, or by violently struggling with them; and such great exertions will have caused the heart to beat rapidly, the breathing to be hurried, the chest to heave, and the nostrils to be dilated. And now whenever the emotion of fear is strongly felt, though it may not lead to any exertion, the same results tend to reappear through the force of inheritance and association." Cannon and later authors have accepted this psychophysiologic view.

Sighing has been found to occur in subjects with anxiety or during periods of anxiety. Sighing is particularly common when a subject is asked a question or encouraged to relax after a period of tension. It was prominent in 5 of 15 subjects with asthma, and in 5 of 7 subjects with anxiety. Finesinger noted a higher incidence of sighing in subjects with anxiety than in those with hysteria, schizophrenia, or no illness.

DECREASES IN RATE AND DEPTH OF RESPIRATION. *Anxiety.* Decreases in respiratory function were associated with anxiety when the subject was "on guard" or overwhelmed by the situation or topic discussed. Two subjects showed shallower breathing when they thought of combat experiences. Such feelings of alarm were sometimes related to the interview situation itself, which some subjects regarded as a threat. One subject with asthma had been extremely guarded in her answers to all questions in the clinic. During the interview with the pneumograph tracings she displayed her usual reserve and, when questioned, obviously withheld her thoughts and showed diminished amplitude of respiration. Subjects 5 and 6 (Figs. 5 and 6) were similarly on guard and at the beginning of the interview showed shallow, rapid respirations which later, as they relaxed, yielded to slower respirations of considerably greater depth than the earlier ones.

The most striking instances of such respiratory depression were seen in the subjects who were asked to read. They interpreted this as an intellectual test of some kind and became extremely tense. One subject showed considerable diminution of respiratory amplitude while reading silently and another somewhat less decrease in amplitude but much irregularity. The following subject showed a variable amount of irregularity in having a pattern of either increased rate and increased depth or a decrease in depth with the rate remaining constant.

SUBJECT 3. A 32-year-old man was referred to the hospital because of episodes of "blacking out," weakness, and palpitations. His father had died when the patient was an infant. His mother was described as "nervous and emotional." Two brothers had peptic ulcers. One of them and two other brothers were alcoholics. Two sisters had had hyperthyroidism and another had had a "nervous breakdown." The subject was the youngest of eight children and there was considerable rivalry among the brothers.

In childhood the subject was shy and withdrawn and had enuresis until he was seven. Later, when he began to work, he changed jobs frequently and erratically. He had never married, ostensibly for economic reasons, but he was exceedingly dependent upon his mother. He had low heterosexual drive, and there was considerable evidence of latent homosexuality. During his army service he was found to have asymptomatic tachycardia and a systolic blood pressure of 160. While these findings were being investigated the subject developed symptoms of palpitation, sweating and "nervousness." He was finally discharged from the army with the diagnosis of psychoneurosis. Following discharge he again made no progress in his work, but felt obliged to persevere in a distasteful job. Attacks of palpitations and "blacking out" occurred particularly during emotional disturbances. He became intensely preoccupied with his heart, depressed, and at one point considered suicide.

At the beginning of the interview with this subject (Fig. 3) he was somewhat tense and anxious. Respiration was shallow with a rate of 13. When he was asked to relax the respirations became deeper and the rate slowed to 10. When the subject was asked to think of various topics which had been disturbing to him—such as his health, depression and suicidal thoughts, homosexual attractions, and relations with his brothers and mother—he showed increased anxiety and an increased respiratory function manifested chiefly by a rise in rate of respirations up to 20. When asked to relax the subject almost invariably showed deep respirations of a low rate. While thinking with anxiety and tension about his eldest brother his respiration rate was 16, and on his being asked to relax the rate fell abruptly to 4. These large slow respirations did not represent his breathing pattern when completely relaxed. The latter showed a depth of respiration somewhat less than that during the usual anxious periods. The irregularity in depth and rate of respiration in this subject during anxiety suggests that the periods of diminished respiration during initial relaxation were governed by chemical effects on the respiratory center as well as by nervous mechanisms.

One of the more marked changes in respiration occurred when he was

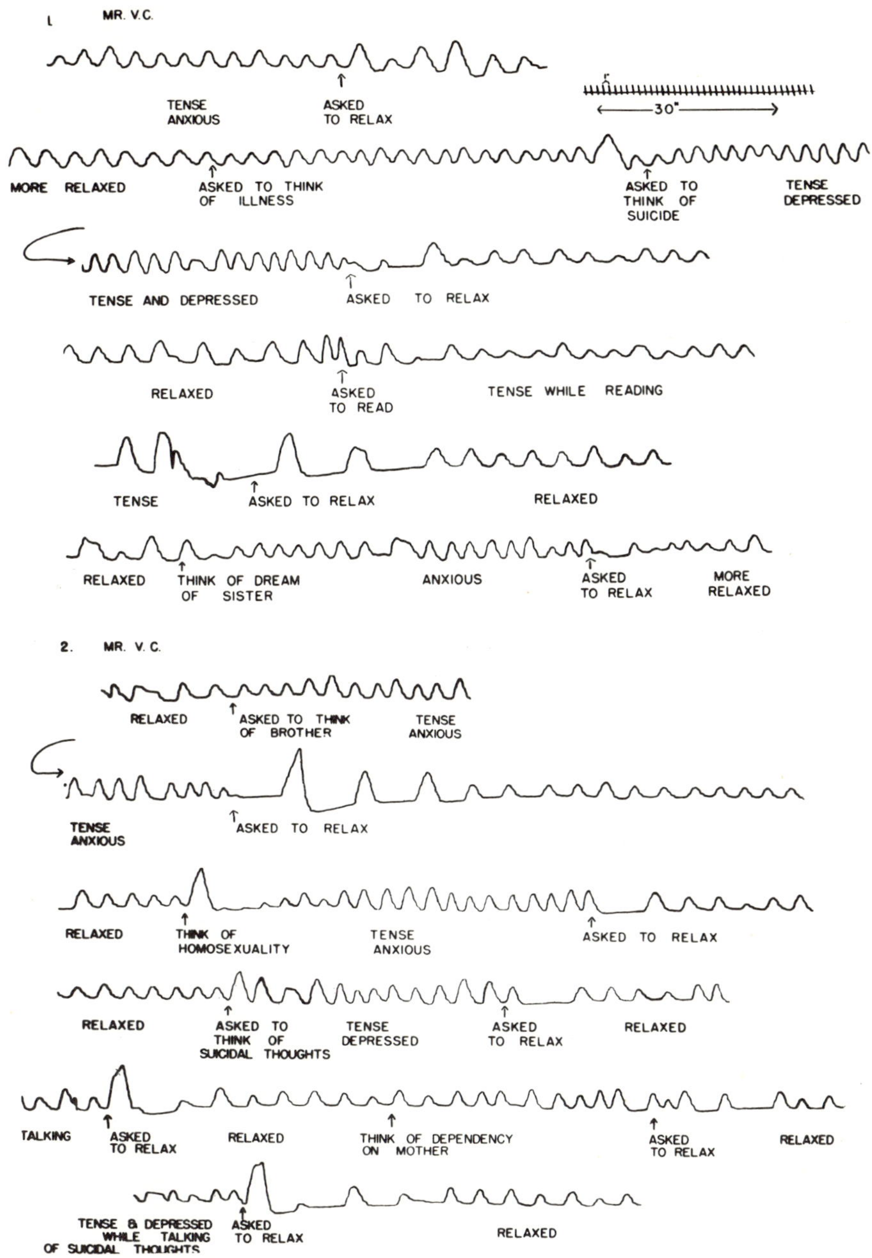

Fig. 3. Extracts of pneumographic tracings during interview with Subject 3. During anxiety the rate was rapid and was followed by slow, deep breaths on relaxation. Marked diminution in respiration occurred when patient felt he was being tested in reading. There were no symptoms despite marked changes.

asked to read silently and then aloud. Upon being handed the book he became tense and his respirations decreased abruptly in depth. (The tracing shown was recorded while he was reading silently.) The material read, a textbook on American government, was actually neutral to this subject, but the reading of it was not. He afterwards described himself as having felt great anxiety and tension and having been unable to recognize and integrate the words he was reading. In this situation, he evidently for a moment felt overwhelmed. It was at this point that his heart beat reached its greatest rate of 113. During periods of relative relaxation the heart rate was between 93 and 99 and during other periods of tension associated with the interview it rose to between 104 and 108. Despite the pronounced changes the subject had no symptoms of respiratory or cardiac dysfunction.

Anger. In a number of subjects, anger was associated not with increased but rather with decreased respiratory movements. This seemed to be more apt to occur when the resentment was unmixed with anxiety and the subject was not impeded in his resentful feelings by restraining fears. The following subject illustrates this type of reaction.

SUBJECT 4. A 42-year-old Negro woman came to the hospital for the treatment of asthma which she had had since the age of nine. Her father had been a kindly alcoholic. Her parents separated when she was six and she lived with her strict mother and a stepfather who was overly intimate with her.

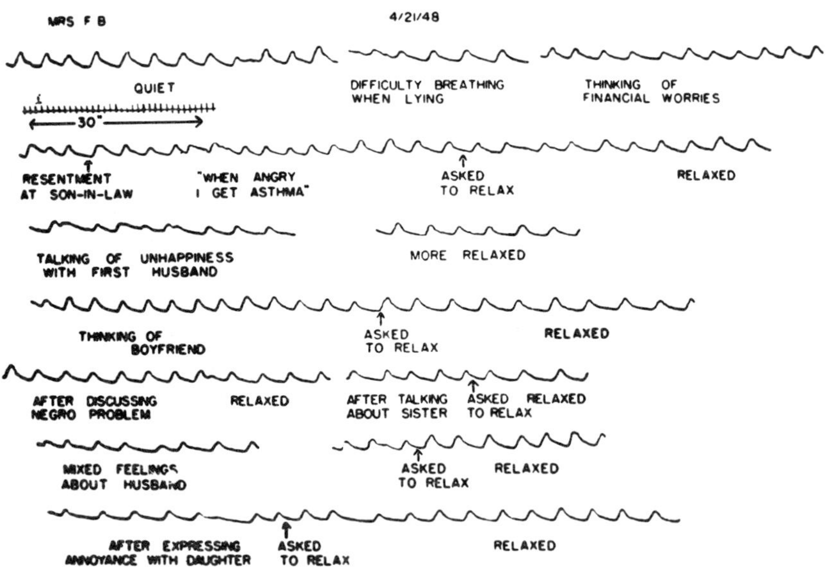

Fig. 4. Extracts of pneumographic tracings during interview with Subject 4. Diminution in amplitude occurred during most periods of emotional disturbance. Slowing of respiration rate occurred during sadness.

One of the subject's sisters died young in childbirth, and the other became an alcoholic and a burden on the subject who tried to help and reform her. The subject's first marriage was to a man who had little interest in her or in marriage, and they separated after a short time. A second marriage seemed successful to her until her husband went off with another girl. Later the subject began to have sexual relations with another man. She hoped he would marry her but he did not seem inclined to do so. The subject had endeavored to support herself, but her illness had forced her into unemployment and dependency on her daughter. She felt herself to be a burden and also resented the behavior of her son-in-law who had been obliged to marry her daughter when the girl became pregnant. The subject had befriended him at first, but later, when she was in need, he neglected her and would give her no financial assistance.

During the interview (Fig. 4) the subject's respirations showed noticeable diminution in amplitude during periods of resentment felt toward her son-in-law, daughter, and second husband. There was some diminution in amplitude associated with thoughts of financial worries which were, however, connected closely with her resentment toward her son-in-law. The rate did not change appreciably at these times. The patient had some wheezing throughout the interview and it remained unchanged during these discussions, which were not attended by as marked emotional changes as occurred in many of the other patients.

COMMENT. Diminished respiration (as indicated by the pneumograph) during anxiety and anger was associated with tension as if part of a preparation for action, analogous to the stillness of wild animals when about to spring or be sprung at. Henry V exhorted his soldiers at Harfleur:

> *Now set the teeth and stretch the nostril wide,*
> *Hold hard the breath, and bend up every spirit*
> *To his full height!*

Depression. Decreased respiratory function was also seen during periods of dejection or sadness evoked by the thoughts suggested or topics discussed. It was unusual to observe both a slowing of rate and diminution of amplitude. This occurred in Subject 4, whose respirations became slower and more shallow as she recalled the unhappiness of her first marriage (Fig. 4). Another subject showed shallow and rapid breathing when asked to think of his wife, with whom his relations were unsatisfactory; but when he was asked to think of his father, toward whom he felt affection and pity, breathing became shallow and was also appreciably slower as the subject fell into a mood of sadness. One subject with asthma showed a diminution in depth but an increase in rate as she thought with sadness of her father who, in her opinion, was her only friend of early life. Another subject showed an abrupt diminution in respiratory amplitude when he thought of the feeling of being different, which he had had in childhood. Dejection was accompanied by increased depth of respiration in Subject 6, but this was related to asthmatic breathing.

Respiratory Dysrhythmia. Irregularity of respiration was one of the most frequent findings. Irregularities in rate or depth occurred in 18 of the subjects, although it was a prominent feature in only about half that number. Three situations in particular—anger, guilt, and sorrow—were associated with gross irregularity of respiration.

Anger. Irregularity of respiration was uncommonly associated with anxiety, but it was frequently found with anger. Some of the more marked irregularities occurred when the subject felt obliged to suppress the expression of anger. In a number of instances the subject felt resentful at the interviewing physician because of the questions asked. Two subjects frankly admitted this feeling, but others did not express it verbally, although it was evident in their voices, bodily movements, and the general tenor of their remarks.

Irregularity of respiration was a pronounced feature in the following subject, who attempted to conceal his hostility throughout the interview.

SUBJECT 5. A 55-year-old man, who had long-standing bronchial asthma, came to the clinic at the insistence of his wife and his minister, who felt that he might be benefited by psychiatric help. He denied this but "went along with

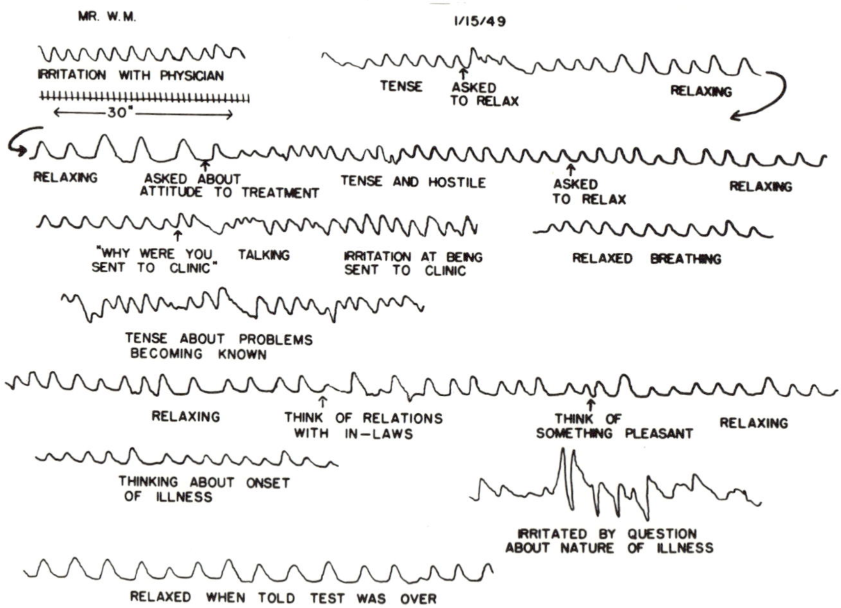

Fig. 5. Extracts of pneumographic tracings during interview with Subject 5. There was initially rapid breathing of low amplitude, marked increase in rate during irritation, and eventually gross irregularity. Note change in expiration:inspiration ratio.

them." Superficially he adopted an air of good-humored tolerance toward his physician and answered questions about his personal life with a complete denial that anything was troubling him or that any little thing which did come up could possibly be related to his asthma. The deep resentment which underlay this affectation was poorly concealed by a veneer of hearty good-fellowship. Because of the conscious resistance of the subject little could be learned about his personality or illness.

When he came for the pneumograph studies he assumed his usual attitude of indulging the physicians in their whims, but his voice and manner betrayed great irritation. At the beginning of the interview respirations were shallow but rapid. When the subject was asked to relax (Fig. 5), the respirations increased in rate but immediately reverted to the former pattern. They became more irregular when the subject was asked to think about the treatment he was receiving at the clinic. It happened that a slight acquaintance of his worked in the clinic and the subject might have been uneasy lest his problems be gossiped about. When asked if this possibility disturbed him, he insisted that this thought had never occurred to him and he expressed irritation at the question. His breathing became grossly irregular again.

When asked about relations with his in-laws, which were known to be unsatisfactory, breathing became slightly irregular, although the subject also denied that this matter disturbed him. When the physician asked him about the circumstances connected with the onset of his illness his breathing became slightly more shallow and shortly thereafter was grossly irregular. On this occasion the subject permitted himself to say that the question was foolish but did not further verbalize his resentment. During the periods of accentuated irritation there was a definite increase in the expiration:inspiration ratio. The subject denied any wheezing or other respiratory symptoms during the interview. Despite the background of continual irritation with the test, the subject still reacted to questions about his personal life. Thus his breathing showed a decrease in rate (not shown in Fig. 5) when he was asked to think about his son, with whom he had always had excellent relations, but no change when he was thinking about his daughter, with whom he had not been so close.

Guilt. Strong feelings of guilt occurred in four of the subjects, accompanied by gross irregularity in the respirations. When one subject thought with guilt of his sexual activities, his pattern became irregular. Marked irregularity of respiration was present in another subject when she thought with sadness and guilt of having parted in ill-humor from her daughter earlier that day.

In another subject, irregular respiration and symptoms of respiratory distress had begun in early childhood, were associated with strong feelings of guilt, and had persisted for 20 years. The subject had been quite jealous of his younger sister and had on several occasions told his mother that he wished his sister would die. When he was four years old, the girl did die of pneumonia, and at this time the subject began to sigh, feel choked-up, and fear that he might die because of inability to get his breath. He continued to feel guilty about the death of his sister. When discussing the matter during the early part of intensive psychoanalytic treatment, he had markedly irregular breathing and a feeling that he might not be able to continue breathing. A pneumographic tracing showed constantly irregular respirations with frequent sighs. During periods of emotional disturbance and tension, such as when thinking of his unsatisfactory relations with his wife and mother, his breathing became shallow. He was aware of this change and said afterward that he was afraid he might not be able to continue breathing. With improvement during his psychoanalysis respiratory symptoms disappeared.

COMMENT. The occurrence of irregular respirations in the situation mentioned may be related to mixed feelings and conflict of attitudes at such times. Anger or resentment was usually felt toward persons on whom the subjects were dependent and toward whom their feelings were markedly ambivalent rather than clearly hostile. This was brought out in the discussions when the subjects attempted to qualify their resentment or slightly praise the resented person. Similarly, guilt and sorrow were often accompanied by continued irritation. By contrast, anxiety and fear were felt often with respect to situations rather than to particular persons. In either case the feelings of anxiety were clearer and more acceptable. Respiratory irregularity was much less common with anxiety than with resentment.

PROLONGATION OF EXPIRATION. A relative prolongation of expiration is a characteristic feature of asthmatic dyspnea. Ziegler and Elliott observed a relative prolongation of expiration in asthmatic subjects occupied with thoughts of unpleasant emotional content. Similar results were obtained in this study. The observed changes occurred during periods of anxiety, resentment, guilt, or dejection. In several subjects these changes in expiration:inspiration ratio could be related to symptoms of dyspnea and wheezing. However, in some subjects dyspnea which resembled that of asthmatic attacks was present without wheezing. In several instances—as in the following subject—the occurrence of wheezing depended as much on the presence of bronchial mucus as on the changes in expiration:inspiration ratio.

SUBJECT 6. A 35-year-old housewife came to the hospital for the treatment of asthma which she had had since the age of 20. She was the eldest of six children. Her father was a kindly supporting figure. Her mother was a businesswoman who apparently used her career as an opportunity to escape from household duties and was frequently away from home. The subject longed for her mother and as she grew up became dependent upon her but at the same time resented her. She described herself as "withdrawn, shy and a daydreamer" in childhood. When she was 20 she had pulmonary tuberculosis and while in a sanatorium began to have asthma. When she was 25 she married a man whom she chose "with the head rather than the heart." He seemed to have qualities she admired in her mother. However, he turned out to be irritable and harsh. He drank excessively and was severe to their children. Sexual relations were usually unpleasant and never satisfying to her. The subject felt her efforts to get close to her husband were rebuffed by him, while he found her excessive dependency intolerable. The subject had three highly intelligent children who afforded her considerable satisfaction, but she felt that their lives were threatened with ruin in the present family setting. She was close to a younger brother whose company she found pleasant and relaxing. On the other hand, she identified herself more closely with an older brother who was, like herself, unsettled and unhappy.

The subject recognized three alternating emotional states in herself. She

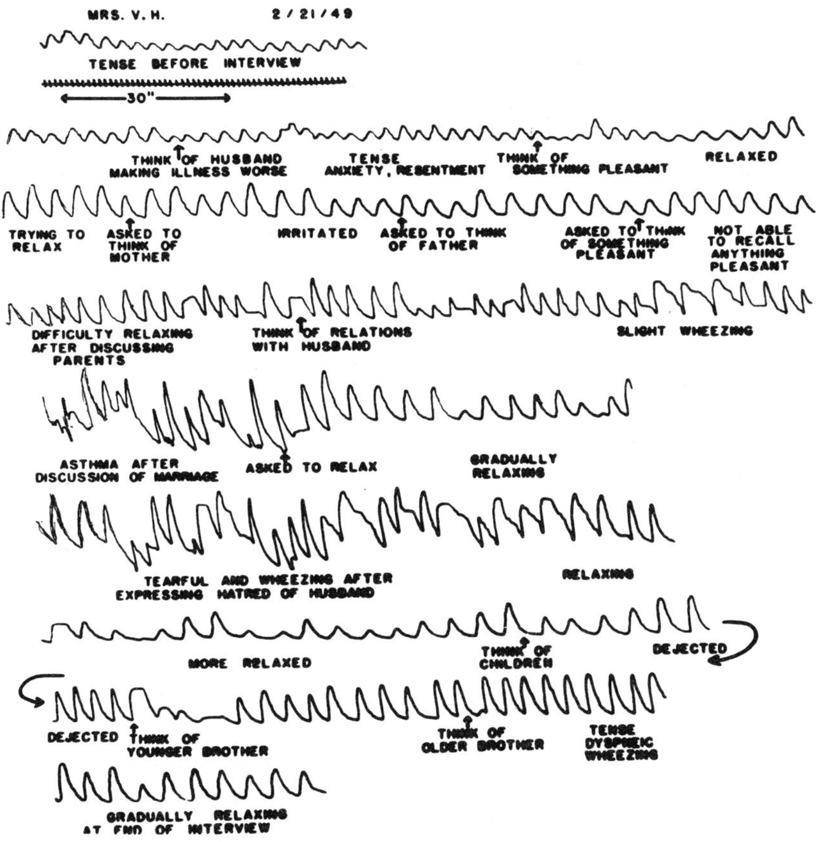

Fig. 6. Extracts of pneumographic tracings during interview with Subject 6. Note initial shallow rapid breathing compared with deeper, slower respirations at end when patient was relaxed. Periods of resentment and dejection were associated with changes in rate, depth, regularity, expiration:inspiration ratio, and at times were accompanied by dyspnea and wheezing.

rarely felt completely at ease and peaceful. At other times she felt great anxiety and depression. The third pattern, associated with asthma, she considered less unpleasant than the second one. Her asthmatic episodes were closely related to her life situations and certain feeling states associated with them. She said "the least thought" would bring asthma. She was particularly likely to have asthma when feeling anger and resentment toward her husband. At other times asthma occurred in conflictful situations or those which were overwhelming to her and from which she withdrew. She felt that asthma in such situations was a way of telling others that she could not cope with her problems and needed attention, help, and sympathy.

At the beginning of the recorded interview (Fig. 6) the subject was somewhat tense with rapid shallow breathing and a heart rate of 100. Breathing became deeper when she was asked to relax. When asked to think about things which made her asthma worse she thought of her husband's severity toward their children and became more tense with feelings of anxiety and resentment. Breathing became irregular and somewhat shallow. Upon being asked to relax she was able to do so, but after further discussion found this more difficult, and breathing was of greater depth. When asked to think of her mother she remembered a typical incident when her mother had irritated her while trying to please her. When she was diverted to thoughts of her father she relaxed somewhat but a little later was unable to recall anything specifically pleasant and relax further. After the discussion of her parents she was more tense.

By this time the pattern of breathing had definitely changed and inspirations were short with a relative prolongation of expiration. The heart rate was 115 during this discussion but fell to 97 afterwards. When the subject thought of relations with her husband, slight wheezing appeared. The subject then said she was "afraid to be happy" and that she and her husband were "worlds apart." She said, "I wanted to be close to him. I don't have a capacity to love except rarely." At the end of this discussion, in which the subject's mood was one of depression, she had frank asthma with plainly audible wheezes and she expectorated mucus. The heart rate during the discussion reached 121. When asked to relax she was slowly able to do so, and the wheezing subsided.

A little later the topic of sexual relations was touched upon and the subject expressed great resentment at her husband for his ineptitude in this sphere. She became tearful and developed relatively prolonged expirations. Breathing became irregular once more, with increased amplitude and with the reappearance of wheezes and expectoration of mucus. The heart rate was 125. After this the subject was again able to relax upon suggestion and the breathing became shallower with shorter expiratory phases. When she thought of her children she felt dejection and anxiety as she contemplated the ruin of their lives. When asked to think of her younger and more cheerful brother she felt a little more relaxed, and breathing became slower until she was asked to think of the other brother with whose miseries she identified herself. Abruptly she became tense again with dyspnea and a return of wheezing. Finally, the subject was able to relax at the end of the interview—saying that it had helped her to unburden herself. Her breathing became more shallow and slower, wheezing disappeared, and expiration became shorter. The heart rate slowed to 80.

COMMENT. In this subject the changes of breathing pattern were similar to those of Subject 5 and another subject whose pneumograph is not included in this report. Wheezing did not occur in either of these subjects. The occurrence of wheezing in Subject 6 may be largely attributed to the presence of mucus. She did not expectorate mucus nor appear to be aware of it except during periods of emotional disturbance. It appears likely, therefore, that it was secreted more abundantly at these times.

Extreme degrees of tachycardia occurred during asthma in this subject and during asthmalike breathing in the other two subjects with similar pneumographic tracings. This tachycardia cannot be attributed to anoxemia secondary to the respiratory changes because of its simultaneity with the latter, and because it was quite disproportionate to the respiratory embarrassment. Thus if the usual explanations of nervous mechanisms in asthma are accepted, it appears that an increase in vagal activity in one system may be associated with a decrease in another and closely related system.

DISCUSSION

Relation of Symptoms to Respiratory Changes Associated with Emotional Disturbances. When the respiratory changes accompanying emotional disturbances became sufficiently great, they obtruded on the attention of the subject and he became aware of symptoms. The complaint of dysfunction depended partly on the attention of the subject to his body and not solely on the degree of respiratory changes, as pronounced variations in respiratory function occurred without any complaints. In general, however, symptoms were found during the more pronounced respiratory changes.

Several mechanisms were involved in the production of symptoms. Most commonly a symptom resulted from the awareness of increased breathing. Although the breathing was already disproportionate to the bodily needs, the complaints indicated a feeling of difficulty in breathing or a need to breathe more deeply. Air hunger of this origin was just as pressing as that of subjects with metabolic or cardiac disease. The subject's interpretation of this symptom is closely linked to the real and symbolic importance of breathing to the organism. The subjects with asthma complained of dyspnea arising from the above mechanisms, and in addition, bronchial narrowing and the accumulation of mucus sometimes produced actual impedance to breathing, which intensified the complaint of difficulty in breathing. The occurrence of wheezing depended both upon the degree of bronchial narrowing and upon the secretion of bronchial mucus. Symptoms of constriction, tightness, or "lumps in the chest" are probably mediated through increased muscle tension and spasm in the intercostal muscles and diaphragm.

Relation of Respiratory Changes to Emotional States and Attitudes. The preceding observations show the intimate relationship between breathing and emotional states. It seems likely that this relationship arose from the purposeful adaptation of respiration to the physical needs of the body in response to various stressful situations. Respiratory changes now continue to be evoked by symbolic stimuli which are no longer met with the same physical activity. Thus an increase in rate and depth of breathing is associated with a reaction to stress with preparation for struggle or flight. On the other hand, there is a preliminary diminution in respiratory function when there is a tense expectation in preparation for action. Decreased breathing also occurs when the subject feels overwhelmed, depressed, or defeated. If the threat results in conflict between feeling and appropriate action, there is a reflected irregularity of respiration. Such concepts may be extended to the interpretation of the prolongation of expiration found in asthmatic attacks and shown in the tracings of many of the subjects who experience asthmatic attacks during emotional disturbances. In situations of stress in which decisive action is indicated, such subjects frequently show tentative, indecisive, evasive, or withdrawing behavior. These attitudes are reflected in the respirations which instead of being free and augmented are impeded and blocked.

SUMMARY

1. In a pneumographic study of 22 subjects, respiratory patterns were found to vary closely with the emotional state.

2. Increased rate or depth or both and sighing were found chiefly with anxiety but sometimes during anger and resentment. Decreased rate or depth or both were found when the subjects felt tense and on guard with feelings of anxiety or anger and when feeling sad or dejected.

3. Irregularity of respiration was commonly associated with anger, particularly when the feeling was suppressed. It was also associated with feelings of guilt and occurred during weeping.

4. A prolongation of expiration during periods of emotional disturbance was found in a higher proportion of subjects with asthma than in those with anxiety. In three asthmatic subjects this change was associated with wheezing and dyspnea and in one with dyspnea alone.

5. Discussions of attitudes and conflicts known to be associated with respiratory symptoms (dyspnea and chest discomfort) evoked such symptoms in more than half of the subjects, and the symptoms were related to changes in the respiratory pattern.

6. It is concluded that respiratory symptoms associated with emotional disturbances may arise from altered respiratory function in response to symbolic stimuli to action and often are related to conflict concerning such action.

REFERENCES

Alexander, F., and Saul, L. J. Respiration and personality, Psychosom Med, 2: 110, 1940.

Baker, D. M. Sighing respiration as a symptom, Lancet, 1:174, 1934.

Binger, C. The psycho-biology of breathing, Ann Intern Med, 11:195, 1937.

Cannon, W. B. Bodily Changes in Pain, Hunger, Fear and Rage. 2nd ed. New York, Appleton-Century-Crofts, 1929.

Christie, R. V. Some types of respiration in the neuroses, Quart J Med, 4:427, 1935.

Darwin, C. The Expression of the Emotions in Man and Animals, New York, Appleton-Century-Crofts, 1897.

Duncan, C. H., Stevenson, I. P., and Ripley, H. S. Life situations, emotions, and paroxysmal auricular arrhythmias, Psychosom Med, 12:23, 1950.

Faulkner, W. B., Jr. The effect of the emotions upon diaphragmatic function, Psychosom Med, 3:187, 1941.

Feleky, A. Influence of the emotions on respiration, J Exp Psychol, 1:218, 1916.

Finesinger, J. E. Effect of pleasant and unpleasant ideas on respiration in psychoneurotic patients, Arch Neurol Psychiat, 42:425, 1939.

——— and Mazick, S. G. The effect of a painful stimulus and its recall upon respiration in psychoneurotic patients, Psychosom Med, 2:333, 1940.

——— The spirogram in certain psychiatric disorders. Amer J Psychiat, 100: 159, 1943.

French, T. M., and Alexander, F. Psychogenic factors in bronchial asthma: Psychosomatic Medicine, Monograph IV. Washington, D.C., National Research Council, 1941.

Nielson, J. M., and Roth, P. Clinical spirography: Spirograms and their significance, Arch Intern Med, 43:132, 1929.

Stevenson, I. P., Duncan, C. H., Wolf, S., Ripley, H. S., and Wolff, H. G. Life situations, emotions, and extrasystoles, Psychosom Med, 11:257, 1949.

——— and Wolff, H. G. Life situations, emotions, and bronchial mucus, Psychosom Med, 11:223, 1949.

——— Duncan, C. H., and Ripley, H. S. Variations in the electrocardiogram with changes in the emotional state, Geriatrics, 6:164, 1951.

Treuting, T. F., and Ripley, H. S. Life situations, emotions and bronchial asthma, J Nerv Ment Dis, 108:380, 1948.

White, P. D., and Hahn, R. G. The symptom of sighing in cardiovascular diagnosis, with spirographic observations, Amer J Med Sci, 177:179, 1929.

Wolf, S. Sustained contraction of the diaphragm, the mechanism of a common type of dyspnea and precordial pain, J Clin Invest, 26:1201, 1947.

Ziegler, L. H., and Elliott, D. C. The effect of emotion on certain cases of asthma, Amer J Med Sci, 172:860, 1926.

7

The Conducting Airway and Associated Structures

The respiratory dead space is composed of two volumes. One is called the anatomic dead space and the other the physiologic dead space. The anatomic dead space is the volume of the conducting airway, including the mouth or nose down to the level of the respiratory bronchioles. The physiologic dead space includes the anatomic dead space and the "alveolar dead space" or the volume of air ventilating alveoli without blood flow, and the volume of air ventilating alveoli in excess of that required to saturate the blood with oxygen. The physiologic dead space will not be discussed in this chapter.

ANATOMIC DEAD SPACE

The anatomic dead space can be measured by several different methods. Commonly utilized are the Bohr equation and expired nitrogen or carbon dioxide curves which have been integrated with volume curves. In this study the latter method was used. It has been shown that, by using this method, the dead space volume can be increased by the injection of atropine and decreased with histamine. Increasing flow or volume tends to increase the anatomic dead space, and decreasing flow or volume tends to decrease the dead space.

Changes in the diameter of the airway during emotional reactions have been demonstrated by Faulkner, who reported bronchoscopic observations. He found that with feelings of resentment and hostility and perhaps helplessness, the airway lumen constricted by one-third while with feelings of security and elation dilation occurred. Dekker reported x-ray studies that showed a considerable narrowing of the cervical and thoracic trachea and the main bronchi during attacks of asthma.

Of equal importance to that of the individual anatomic dead space measurements is the measurement of the minute dead space. An increase in respiratory rate and/or anatomic dead space can cancel out an increase in minute ventilation, resulting in no change in the alveolar ventilation or actual hypoventilation. To the observer the subject appears to be hyperventilating because of the increase in respiratory rate and effort of breathing.

The anatomic dead space measurements used in this study were corrected when necessary by "dummy" dead space measurements as described in Chapter 5.

SUBJECT 1. This subject was an anxious, idealistic, 25-year-old white male—a divorced college student. During the separation and divorce from his wife, he was unable to continue his schooling and found work as a technician in the laboratory in which these studies were undertaken. At the time, he was experiencing considerable emotional upheaval because of his decision to return to college and being asked to terminate his employment. In this setting his reaction was that of avoiding his job responsibilities. He did not report to work except when requested by the experimenter, and hence was quite anxious about entering the laboratory.

During the above-described period his anatomic dead space was noted to be at very low levels. He was subsequently given an intramuscular injection of 1/100 g of atropine. Anatomic dead space measurements followed at 1- and 3-hr intervals postinjection. Initially, the dead space measurements were low and were not influenced by relaxation and sleep. One hour after injection, the dead space volume was doubled while the subject was dozing but remained at preinjection levels when he was alert. Three hours after injection, when the subject was relaxed, dead space values were doubled over the preinjection values while the subject was alert, but were almost tripled while he was dozing (Table 1).

The illustrated dead space changes occurred independently of tidal volume and the time required to expire the dead space or tidal volume. However, as dead space increased, the length of time required for one respiratory cycle decreased. This is also illustrated in Table 1.

COMMENT. The exact duration of inspiration was not measured during these experiments. Because the duration of the total respiratory cycle decreased as the dead space increased, there is the possibility that low dead space volumes were produced by an inspiratory pause allowing diffusion of gas up the airway. However, breaths with similar respiratory cycle durations before and after the injection of atropine show the same differential in dead space volume. The low dead space volumes are thought to be a result of a reduction in the diameter of the conducting airway.

The effects of emotion on dead space volume were seen to be partially offset by a parasympathetic blocking agent. However, the drug did not prove adequate, and only after dispelling the subject's anxiety was the dead space volume returned to normal levels. The increase in dead space volume

Table 1. Anatomic Dead Space Variations in a 25-Year-Old Male Experiencing a Life Crisis

	No of Obser-vations	V_D* ml	Range	V_T ml	Range	TT† sec	Range	V_tT‡ sec	Range	V_DT§ sec	Range
Pre-Atropine¶	23	72	59–96	680	455–1300	8.3	5.3–11.9	3.1	1.8–4.3	0.36	0.20–0.55
1 Hr after 1/100 gr atropine											
Dozing	41	116	87–130	644	338–1300	6.4	4.2–11.8	2.9	1.9–5.7	0.51	0.25–0.85
Alert	12	77	67–91	680	200–988	7.6	4.4–9.3	3.5	2.2–6.2	0.48	0.18–0.70
3 Hr after atropine											
Alert	9	112	107–129	542	411–658	6.8	5.0–9.3	2.6	2.0–3.0	0.52	0.45–0.65
Dozing	6	138	129–167	507	397–644	4.4	3.7–5.8	2.8	2.1–3.8	0.54	0.43–0.85

* Corrected.
† Length of time between each tidal volume.
‡ Time required to expire the tidal volume.
§ Time required to expire the anatomic dead space.
¶ $p = < 0.001$ compared with 1-hr post-atropine dozing and 3-hr post-atropine dozing and alert

was more pronounced during the period when the effects of the atropine should have been disappearing.

The same subject volunteered for four different headband experiments (see Chapter 10). His response to the headband was that of acute anxiety, nausea, urge to vomit, hypersalivation, tinnitus, restlessness, irritability, sweating, warm flushes, loss of awareness of his surroundings, a great desire to "get the damned thing off," hyperventilation, increased blood pressure, and a dull aching headache.

In contrast with most subjects, who showed no change or an increase in dead space volume during the pain, he decreased the volume of his dead space. This decrease was associated with an elevated tidal volume and a decreased duration of expiration. Low dead space volumes were found only when the pain was maximal. If at other times he was asked to breathe with the large fast tidal volumes, similar to those found during maximal pain, a marked increase in dead space volume would result. If, on the other hand, without the pain, slow, deep respirations were used, a low anatomic dead space would result. Figure 1 compares a fast deep breath and a slow

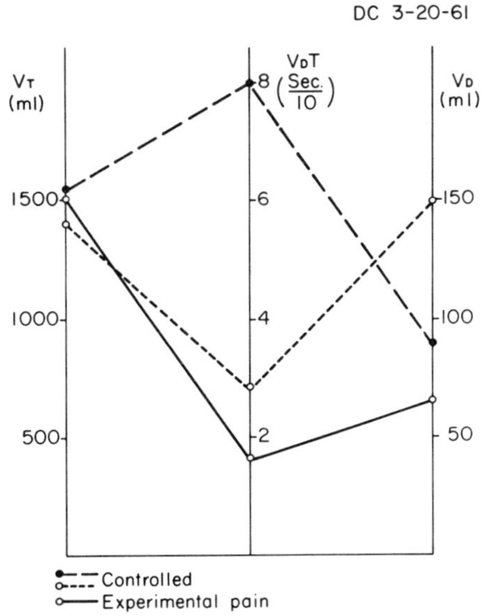

Fig. 1. Decreased anatomic dead space during experimental head stimulation in Subject 1. Also included were two tidal volumes taken prior to maximal response to pain. During these two tidal volumes, dead space expiratory time (V_DT) of 0.8 sec was associated with drop in anatomic dead space, and decrease in dead space expiratory time to 0.3 sec was associated with increase in anatomic dead space—despite identical tidal volumes. However, during height of headband stimulation, decrease in dead space expiratory time was associated with decrease in anatomic dead space. This is thought to represent decrease in diameter of major airways.

deep breath during controlled voluntary breathing with a breath during the height of the head pain. As shown, very slow deep breathing (as indicated by the V_DT or length of time required to expire the dead space volume) decreases the anatomic dead space, and fast breathing at the same tidal volume increases the dead space volume in the absence of head pain. During maximal head pain, dead space was at a minimum despite the fast breathing with identical tidal volumes.

The changes in anatomic dead space during head pain varied from the decrease in Subject 1 to two- and threefold increases in other subjects. Fig. 2 shows the changes in anatomic dead space produced by the pain in three subjects. Anatomic dead space may decrease, remain unchanged, or increase with similar changes in tidal volume and duration of the respiratory cycle.

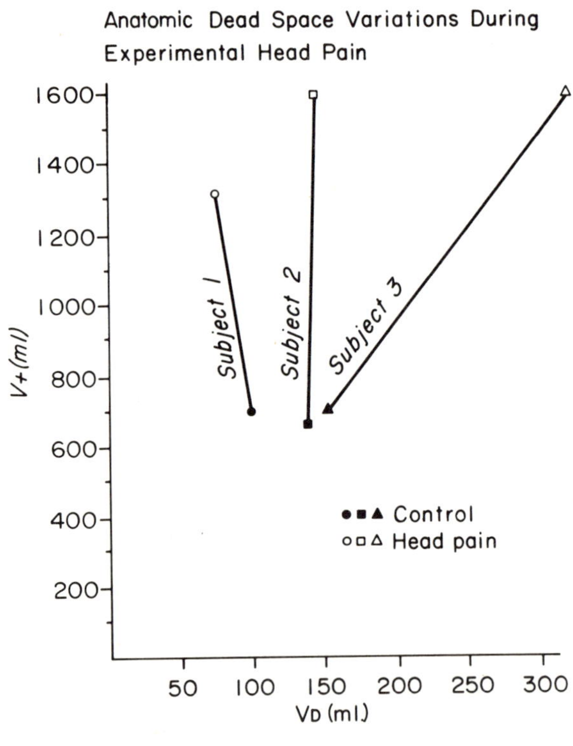

Fig. 2. Comparison of changes in anatomic dead space in three subjects in response to noxious stimulation of the head. Despite changes in tidal volume and increases in flow rate, dead space increased in some, did not change in one, and was reduced in the other.

MINUTE DEAD SPACE CHANGES

Changes in minute dead space volume ($\dot{V}_D$) assume vital importance in assessing changes in ventilation. As shown in Figure 3, an elevation in respiratory rate may lead to hypoventilation. To the observer this may resemble hyperventilation. However, the shallow breathing and increased minute dead space have produced a decrease in the alveolar ventilation. In some patients, the minute ventilation is seen to rise while the alveolar ventilation falls because of the increase in minute dead space. The same is true of slow breathing. A change from rapid to relatively slow respirations may be a change from hypoventilation to hyperventilation. During slow breathing the tidal volume and minute dead space may be such as to produce an increase in alveolar ventilation even though the minute ventilation may be unchanged.

Also, even though alveolar ventilation is increased or decreased, this

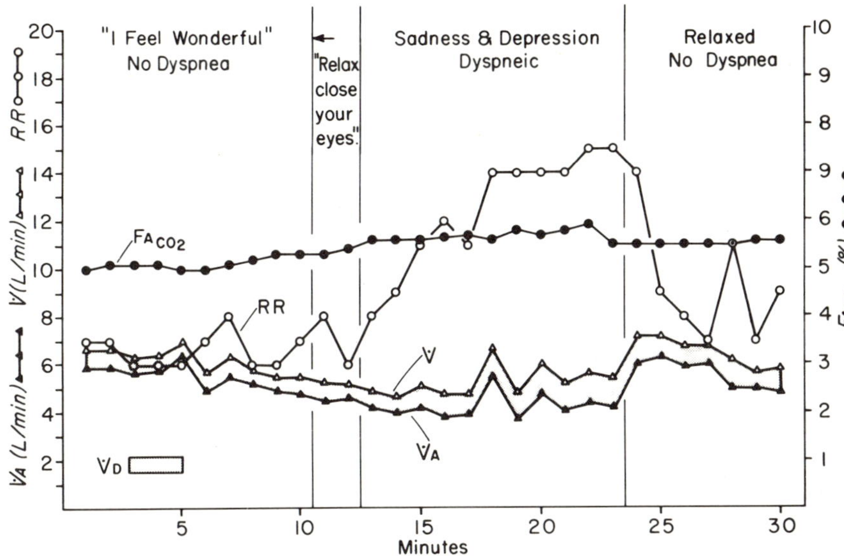

Fig. 3. Hypoventilation during suggestion of depression with increase in respiratory rate. Hypoventilation response was produced by both an increase in minute dead space and decrease in tidal volume. With some subjects hypoventilation occurs with increase in minute dead space secondary to increase in respiratory rate alone with no change or a slight increase in tidal volume. Measurement of respiratory rate alone with visual observation of chest movement may or may not give accurate indication of hyper- or hypoventilation.

does not automatically indicate hyperventilation or hypoventilation. Metabolic need may have increased or decreased out of proportion to ventilation and the $F_{A_{CO_2}}$ will rise or decrease as the patient is actually hypoventilating or hyperventilating, respectively, in relation to his needs.

COMMENT. When measuring changes in ventilation it is of utmost importance to have an accurate estimate of the alveolar ventilation and the $F_{A_{CO_2}}$; this is the only sure way of avoiding misinterpretation of the data.

WEEPING

The close association of the lacrimal glands with the upper airway anticipates that the function of these glands would be associated and integrated with changes in the airway. The following observations, although preliminary, support this contention.

Weeping is seen as a method of relieving suffering. During weeping behavior there are changes in the nasal mucous membranes and probably in bronchial mucus production as well. Unlike dyspnea, which provides destructive feedback (see Chapter 16), weeping is seen as providing emotional relief. It is always associated with helplessness but not with any specific emotion. As such, it may be associated with anger, anxiety, or depression when helplessness is a predominant component of the emotion. In four observations on three subjects this was found to be the case. In one, sobbing and weeping was associated with a panic state and helplessness; in two, with sadness and helplessness; and in one, with frustration and helplessness. The weeping depended on the subject's perception that his current situation might be impossible for him to solve but there was someone somewhere who could help him. Cultural values make weeping difficult in males even in the face of appropriate feelings of helplessness. They therefore have to use different methods of asking for help or may be unable to do so. All three of the subjects in whom weeping was studied were females.

SUBJECT 1. Subject 1 was a 31-year-old housewife who experienced feelings of sadness, loneliness, and helplessness when thinking of a recently deceased aunt (see Chapter 8). While thinking of her aunt she hypoventilated. Toward the end of one of four experimental periods, when feelings about the deceased aunt were suggested, she began weeping. The weeping was associated with an increase in ventilation and respiratory rate and a fall in the alveolar carbon dioxide concentration. After approximately 30 secs the weeping was terminated and respiratory variables fell to the previous hypoventilatory levels and were subsequently returned to eupneic levels by suggestion of pleasant topics.

SUBJECT 2. Subject 2 was a 43-year-old supermarket checker, who began sobbing during a reaction of panic and helplessness (see Chapter 8). The sobbing behavior necessitated her removal from the measuring apparatus. After sobbing for a period of 10 min she was able to control herself and she was again attached to the measuring instruments. At that point it was found that her preceding hyperventilation was partly relieved and she felt more at ease. There had been no attempt by the experimenter to comfort her during the sobbing. After subsequent reassurance by her ward physician her ventilation returned to eupneic levels.

SUBJECT 3. Subject 3 was a 50-year-old commercial artist, who experienced weeping on two occasions in response to severe frustration, sadness, and helplessness when thinking of her deceased father, and once when she felt depressed and helpless about her tenuous social and psychologic adjustment (see Chapter 8).

She had very strong feelings about weeping which were expressed as follows: [Do you feel like crying when you feel like that?] "I won't let myself. I feel like it, yes. I feel like breaking down and crying until I can't see straight." [What keeps you from crying?] "I feel like a heel when I cry." [Why?] "I don't know why. It's childish, sissy-like. I feel sort of like a man would feel if he cried."

During periods of depression and helplessness she usually did not weep, but on one occasion was observed to have tears streaming down her face. This was associated with hypoventilation.

When thinking of her deceased father she felt dyspneic, frustrated, helpless, and sad. She expressed herself as follows: "I feel a terrible loss, a terrible sadness. There's nothing I can do. Even thinking of happy things about him makes me sad. There's nothing I can do except eliminate him from my mind. Hardly a day passes when I don't think of him. I don't know where he is . . . [buried]. I don't know which one [cemetery] it is. I deliberately forget. I can't bring him back and I can't find anyone to replace him." She was obsessed with thoughts of joining him or bringing him back. This response of frustration and need for action was associated with hyperventilation and at times with weeping.

COMMENT. Weeping behavior appears to be an effective method of relieving suffering. If the subject is helpless and action-oriented, weeping appears to relieve both the ongoing psychologic and physiologic reaction. If the subject is helpless and nonaction-oriented, weeping has the same effect, but in the opposite direction.

The old adage, "let go, cry, and get it over with," may in many cases be sound advice. Apparently weeping behavior in some way provides a relatively nonpainful method of discharging emotion. As such it should be looked upon as an important protective device. The statement that men should not cry is culturally acceptable, but denies men a method of providing relief from suffering which may not be replaceable by other methods.

The effectiveness of weeping in relieving suffering is thought to depend upon its association with washing painful or uncomfortable material from the eyes. In this way, weeping becomes associated with relief of discomfort and becomes generalized to discomfort of any kind rather than just that experienced in the eyes.

THE NOSE*

These data represent a view of studies on reactions of the nasal mucous membrane occurring in man during a variety of experimentally induced and naturally occurring stressful life situations. The various methods of investigation used have been detailed elsewhere. The choice of technique employed depended on the nature of the experimental situation and the question asked.

Anxiety and Nasal Hyperfunction. The following observations on nasal function were made during the course of an interview productive of anxiety, conflict, and other strong feelings in the subject. The threat to the subject's security depended for its force on the communication and understanding of symbols which, because of past conditioning experiences, had acquired special meaning for him.

A 40-year-old itinerant salesman had noted recurrent nasal obstruction and rhinorrhea since his marriage 14 years ago. Both his parents were Russian-Jewish immigrants. His father was a humorless, domineering baker who made liberal use of corporal punishment. His mother was a tearful, unhappy individual who, from the date of her marriage, was almost continuously pregnant until she had had 11 children. The patient was the oldest. He quit school in the seventh grade at the age of 14, and began working as a traveling salesman in defiance of his father's orders to continue his education. He left home and saw little of his family thereafter. Two of his younger brothers later became lawyers. The patient was always concerned only with his own pleasures and gratifications and never developed warm emotional ties to others.

While this subject's nasal structures were under observation he began a discussion of his current preoccupations. Prior to the interview his nasal mucous membranes appeared pale red in color and there was a slight amount of secretion and swelling, with very slight obstruction to breathing. During the discussion which concerned his wife, who had been asked to accompany him on the visit to the hospital so that she, too, might be questioned, he became anxious and tremulous and was "on the verge of tears." At this time the membranes became intensely hyperemic. Secretion was copious, the turbinates were considerably swollen, and obstruction to breathing was pronounced. Following the interview, as the patient became relaxed, the hyperfunctioning mucous membranes returned to the control levels.

* This section is adapted from an article originally published in *Trans Amer Acad Ophthal Otolaryng*, 59:439, 1955, by Holmes, T. H.

COMMENTS. Observations of nasal function have been made during the application of a wide variety of stimuli. It has been found that the inhalation of the fumes of ammonium carbonate and of allergens such as mixed ragweed pollen, experimentally induced head pain, and exposure to cold air produce a reaction in the nasal mucous membranes which is indistinguishable from that documented in the above experiment.

Thus it appears that the nasal mucous membranes react to symbols or threats of danger with a pattern of function which is identical to that which occurs in response to a direct assault by noxious physical or chemical agents acting either directly on the mucous membranes or other parts of the body.

As a protective reaction pattern, nasal hyperfunction contributes to the preservation of nasal tissue integrity by shutting out, neutralizing, and washing away noxious agents. Such a response is both appropriate and relatively effective against chemical fumes but inappropriate and relatively ineffective in response to assaults upon other parts of the body or to symbols which threaten security.

SIMULTANEOUS OBSERVATION OF NASAL AND GASTRIC FUNCTION DURING ANXIETY. The following observations made on an adult male subject with a large gastric fistula document the fact that stressful situations provoking nasal reactions may induce concomitant alterations in other physiologic systems. This case is also illustrative of variations in function of the same system at different times. The specificity of the reactions appears to depend on the way in which the individual defines his relationship to the stimulus situation and what, if anything, he feels like doing about it.

At the time of one observation, the subject's wife was about to visit the hospital because of troublesome varicose veins. His concern about hospitals and sickness and his dependence upon his wife for the proper conduct of the home engendered conflict, with feelings of anxiety and resentment. Hyperemia and engorgement were noted in both the gastric and nasal mucosae.

Another observation was made during a serious threat to the subject's security when he became convinced that certain newspaper publicity concerning his gastric fistula had caused him to be identified by his acquaintances in the community in which he lived. In consequence, he became anxious, resentful, and humiliated at what he considered public exposure. Again both the gastric and nasal mucosae were unusually red and swollen.

ANXIETY AND TISSUE DAMAGE. During a period of good spirits and relative freedom from nasal disturbance, a 36-year-old white male was engaged in vigorous discussion of fundamental personal conflicts. At the outset of the interview the nasal structures were of relatively normal appearance. Immediately after this observation, a biopsy was made of the left lower turbinate under local 10 percent cocaine anesthesia. Microscopic examination of the tissue revealed essentially normal mucosal structure with a moderate round cell infiltration. During the next hour, as the subject discussed his lack of success in his job, his inadequate sexual adjustment and inability to assume his responsibilities as a husband and father, and his difficulties with his father-in-law, he became anxious and restless and was on the verge of tears. In addition to anxiety, his feelings included resentment, humiliation, and guilt. At this point, 1 hr after the first biopsy, examination revealed the mucous membrane in the right nasal cavity to be a deep violaceous red color with maximal swelling, secretion, and obstruction. A second biopsy specimen was then obtained from the right lower turbinate. Microscopic examination revealed hyperreacting mucous glands, prominent dilated vascular and lymphatic channels, and edema of the stroma.

COMMENT. From this experiment it is evident that threats of danger evolving from stressful life situations may become important etiologic forces in the genesis of illness. Often the discomfort and tissue damage evoked by symbols are indistinguishable from those produced by noxious physical and chemical agents or infectious microorganisms. Therefore, it appears relevant to an understanding of the natural history of many nasal disorders to consider the effects on the nasal mucous membranes of the interaction of multiple noxious stimuli applied simultaneously.

SUMMATIVE OR ADDITIVE EFFECTS: ANXIETY-PROVOKING STIMULI INTRODUCED DURING EXPOSURE OF HAY FEVER PATIENT TO POLLEN. The subject of these observations was a 57-year-old Negro housewife, born in the British West Indies of mixed Negro and white stock. She complained of "hay fever" of five years duration and had a strongly positive ragweed skin-test reaction.

The experiment was performed during the hay fever season at a time when the subject was feeling calm, secure, and relaxed. She was free of hay fever symptoms, and her nasal mucous membranes were moderately red, with small amounts of secretion and swelling evident. She was then exposed in the experimental pollen room for 109 min. Nasal hyperfunction, characterized primarily by a mild increase in secretion, was first observed 30 min later. At the same time mild symptoms of rhinitis occurred, which included two transient "twinges of burning pain" in the nostrils, awareness of a small amount of accumulated secretion in the nasal chambers, and two episodes (lasting 1 min each) of mild tearing and photophobia which accompanied the burning nasal pain. These symptoms then completely subsided within 8 min of their onset, and aside from some obstruction to breathing in the nasal cavities, the patient remained comfortable for a period of 10 min.

At this point an interview was begun which the patient quickly directed toward the unsatisfactory relationship which existed between her husband and her second daughter. As she discussed this situation of conflict she became tense and anxious, and her voice became whining and petulant as she expressed her feelings of resentment, frustration, and humiliation evolving from her memories of her husband's behavior. Examination of her nose during this period of the interview revealed a marked increase in the degree of nasal hyperfunction. At the same time, symptoms of rhinitis recurred with increased intensity and included awareness of free accumulation of secretion in both nasal cavities with increased postnasal drip, complete obstruction to breathing, paroxysms of sneezing, persistent tearing and photophobia, and a "full feeling" in the head and face.

After this problem had been discussed for 33 min, the subject was diverted to neutral topics and felt much reassured. Gradually over the next 28 min she regained her feelings of well-being; despite the fact that she was still being exposed to pollen in the pollen room, nasal hyperfunction subsided, symptoms disappeared, and she remained comfortable for the duration of the experiment.

NEURAL MECHANISMS: NASAL FUNCTION FOLLOWING UNILATERAL STELLATE GANGLION BLOCK. Following suitable control observations on nasal function, 6 cc of 2 percent procaine was injected into the left stellate ganglion of a 58-year-old Negro male who suffered from seasonal hay fever. Accompanying the other objective signs of the unilateral Horner's syndrome were hyperemia, swelling, hypersecretion, and moderate obstruction to breathing in the left nasal cavity.

COMMENT. This observation suggests that impulses mediated by cholinergic fibers in the parasympathetic nerve supply to the nasal mucous membranes are responsible for the production of nasal hyperfunction engendered by discussions of life situations provoking conflict. This inference is in agreement with the work of other investigators.

NEURAL MECHANISMS: EFFECT OF SUSTAINED NOXIOUS STIMULATION ON THE HYPERFUNCTIONING NASAL MUCOSA. At the point of maximal nasal hyperfunction, 20 min after the stellate block described above, 2 mg of mixed ragweed pollen were introduced into each nasal chamber. The response of additional hyperemia, swelling, hypersecretion, and obstruction in the left side was intense and dramatic, and the symptoms produced in the left nasal cavity were those of "hay fever." In the right nasal chamber, however, the hyperfunction was delayed in its appearance and of brief duration, and it was not of sufficient magnitude to produce symptoms.

COMMENT. This experiment indicates that during the phase of nasal hyperfunction induced by stellate ganglion block, the functionally altered mucous membrane reacts promptly and vigorously to contact with pollen, culminating in frank manifestations of hay fever rhinitis. On the other hand, the introduction of pollen onto the functionally intact mucous membrane in the absence of pre-existing hyperfunction, even in a known "hay fever" sufferer, induced only a transient hyperfunction which fell well within the physiologic budget of the nasal tissues and was well tolerated. It is suggested that the mechanisms involved in this experiment are applicable, at least in part, to the summative effects of pollen and anxiety demonstrated previously.

DISCUSSION

Isolated observations indicate that the anatomic dead space is not a static measurement and is influenced by emotional stimulation. This is also found to be true of the minute dead space which may increase to the point of cancelling out an increase in minute ventilation. Because the alveolar ventilation, not the minute ventilation, gives a direct reflection of the amount of functional air available to the individual, this volume is emphasized in the following chapters. In this way possible errors owing to dead space changes can be eliminated.

The dead space air represents one of many variables which have psychophysiologic relevance and pertinence to the conducting airway and to the production of symptoms and disease. Stevenson and Wolff reported increased mucus secretion in the bronchial tree during conflict, anxiety, and resentment which are probably associated with similar changes in the nasal mucous membranes. It is probable that depressive reactions lead to decreased mucus secretion in the bronchi just as they do in the nose and vagina. The role the respiratory cilia may play in the above reactions is unexplored.

In patients with impaired bronchial drainage the changes in mucus secretion mentioned above can set the stage for respiratory infections. In addition, however, the dramatic emotionally induced increase in sputum production noted by Stevenson can be exceedingly difficult to manage even with good bronchial drainage, and it represents a negative social value. In some patients, the increased sputum production forces them into social isolation and seriously limits their productivity as well as being very uncomfortable. Stevenson and Wolff also noted increases in bronchial mucus secretion in asthmatics which could be treated with psychotherapy and thereby avert serious physiologic difficulty.

The lacrimal glands were seen as participating in the reactions of the upper airway. Rather than having specific associations with specific emotions, lacrimal gland overactivity was associated with the feeling of helplessness which could be present with anger, anxiety, or mild depression. The tears thus produced are partly discharged on the face and partly into the nose by the lacrimal ducts. Their production was seen to be highly culturally determined. Of the many patients which were studied in preparation of this monograph, women were the only ones who allowed themselves to cry in their attempts to combat discomfort. Crying was seen as being effective in producing relief from emotions and their physiologic counterparts.

It has been demonstrated repeatedly that the alterations in nasal function accompanying conflictual settings are often of sufficient magnitude to produce troublesome nasal symptoms and pathologic tissue changes. Also, from a study of the histories of patients exhibiting common nasal disorders and from observations on individuals followed at frequent intervals over long periods of time, it has been possible to establish a correlation between a setting of conflict and anxiety productive of nasal hyperfunction and an exacerbation of nasal disease. Further, as conflicts evolving from difficulties in interpersonal and social adjustments often remain unresolved for long periods of time, the accompanying state of anxiety and nasal hyperfunction may become both intense and sustained. In such a setting the nasal tissues become unable to tolerate the additional alterations in nasal function engendered by new noxious threats or assaults on bodily integrity. Thus nasal hyperfunction that appears as a part of an individual's response to a threatening life situation engendering conflict and anxiety may constitute a major etiologic factor in the genesis of nasal dysfunction. When combined with other environmental stimuli capable of producing nasal hyperfunction, it becomes relevant to the genesis of many common acute and chronic disorders of the nasal and paranasal spaces.

REFERENCES

Association for Research in Nervous and Mental Diseases: Life Stress and Bodily Disease. Baltimore, The Williams & Wilkins Co., 1950.

Chorobski, J., and Penfield, W. Cerebral vasodilator nerves and their pathway from the medulla oblongata, with observations on the pial and intracerebral vascular plexus, Arch Neurol Psychiat, 28: 1257, 1932.

Comroe, J. H., Forster, R. E. Dubois, A. B., Briscoe, W. A., and Carlsen, E. The Lung, 2nd ed. Chicago, Year Book Medical Publishers, 1962.

Darwin, C. Expression of Emotions in Man and Animal. New York, Philosophical Library, 1955.

Dekker, E., and Groen, J. Asthmatic wheezing (compression of the trachea and major bronchi as a cause), Lancet, 272:1064, 1957.

Faulkner, W. B. Influence of suggestion on size of bronchial lumen: Bronchoscopic study and report of one case, Northwest Med, 40:367, 1941.

Fowler, E. P., Jr. Unilateral vasomotor rhinitis due to interference with the cervical sympathetic system, Arch Otolaryng, 37:710, 1943.

Fowler, W. S. Lung function studies: II. The respiratory dead space. Amer J Physiol, 154:405, 1948.

Gardner, W. J., Stowell, A., and Dutlinger, R. Resection of the greater superficial petrosal nerve in the treatment of unilateral headache, J Neurosurg, 4:105, 1947.

Grace, W. J., and Graham, D. T. Relationship of specific attitudes and emotions to certain bodily diseases, Psychosom Med, 14:243, 1952.

Holmes, T. H., Goodell, H., Wolf, S., and Wolff, H. G. The Nose: An Experimental Study of Reactions Within the Nose in Human Subjects During Varying Life Experiences. Springfield, Ill., Charles C Thomas, Publisher, 1950.

——— Goodell, H., Wolff, G., and Wolf, S. Evidence on the genesis of certain common nasal disorders, Amer J Med Sci, 218:16, 1949.

——— Treuting, T., and Wolff, H. G. Life situations, emotions and nasal disease: Evidence on summative effects exhibited in patients with "hay fever," A Res Nerv Ment Dis Proc (1949), 29:545, 1950.

McAuliffe, G. W., Goodell, H., and Wolff, H. G. Experimental studies on headache: Pain from the nasal and paranasal structures, A Res Nerv Ment Dis Proc 23:185, 1943.

Severinghaus, J. W., and Stupfel, M. Respiratory dead space increase following atropine in man, and atropine, vagal or ganglionic blockade and hypothermia in dogs, J Appl Physiol, 8:81, 1955.

Stevenson, I. P., and Wolff, H. G. Life situations, emotions and bronchial mucus, Psychosom Med, 11:223, 1949.

Wolf, S., and Wolff, H. G. Human Gastric Function. New York, Oxford University Press, 1947.

Wolff, H. G. Stress and Disease. Springfield, Ill., Charles C Thomas, Publisher, 1953.

——— Wolf, S., Grace, W. J., Holmes, T. H., Stevenson, I., Straub, L., Goodell, H., and Seton, P. L. Changes in form and function of mucous membranes occurring as part of protective reaction patterns in man during periods of life stress and emotional conflict, Trans Asso Amer Physicians, 61:313, 1948.

Young, A. C. Dead space at rest and during exercise, J Appl Physiol, 8:91, 1955.

8

Ventilation and Metabolism

This chapter consists of data collected from 22 subjects. Subjects were considered eligible for study if they could communicate well and were experiencing emotional changes. There were no other considerations for selection. The subjects were either patients or employees of a tuberculosis hospital; 19 had tuberculosis or a diffuse obstructive pulmonary syndrome, or both, and 3 had normal lungs. Serial psychologic and physiologic observations were made on a daily or weekly basis over periods of time varying from 2 to 100 weeks. The number of observations on each subject varied from 5 to 44 with a mean of 15. There were an equal number of males and females whose ages ranged from 15 to 68 with a mean of 36 years.

Days on which psychologic changes occurred were compared with relaxed or "normal" days. Once outstanding naturally occurring life situations were identified they were subsequently suggested to the subjects. The suggestion was used without hypnosis. After a 10- to 15-min control period in which the subject kept his eyes closed and was instructed to relax completely, he was asked to concentrate on the currently stressful life event. Statistical analysis utilized Student's *t* test for paired samples.

GROUPED DATA

Twenty of the 22 subjects in this group were found to respond to short-term naturally occurring adverse life situations and/or suggestion of such situations with hyperventilation and one or more of the following: anger,

This chapter is adapted from an article originally published in *Psychosom Med*, 26:645, 1964, by Dudley, D. L., Martin, C. J., and Holmes, T. H.

anxiety, irritability, restlessness, desire to act, hostility, tension, or panic (Table 1). The increase in respiratory rate, alveolar ventilation, and oxygen

Table 1. HYPERVENTILATION IN RESPONSE TO SUGGESTED AND NATURALLY OCCURRING STIMULI (20 SUBJECTS)

	RR	$\dot{V}_A$ (L/MIN)	F_{ACO_2} (%)	$\dot{V}_{O_2}$ (ML/MIN)*
Control	15	4.1	5.4	203
Response	19†	6.6‡	4.8‡	251†

* 4 subjects.
† $p = <0.02$.
‡ $p = <0.001$.

consumption, and the decrease in the fractional concentration of alveolar carbon dioxide were statistically significant. During the hyperventilation period these subjects expressed their desire to take action with both verbal and nonverbal behavior. Eight of the subjects reported varying degrees of shortness of breath during the hyperventilation.

Eight of the 22 subjects were found to respond to short-term adverse life situations or suggestions of such situations at some time or another with hypoventilation and one or more of the following: despair, withdrawal, apathy, sadness, or hopelessness (Table 2). The decrease in alveolar ven-

Table 2. HYPOVENTILATION IN RESPONSE TO SUGGESTED AND NATURALLY OCCURRING STIMULI (8 SUBJECTS)

	RR	$\dot{V}_A$ (L/MIN)	F_{ACO_2} (%)	$\dot{V}_{O_2}$ (ML/MIN)*
Control	13	4.5	5.7	271
Response	12	3.6†	6.1‡	248

* 2 subjects.
† $p = 0.01$.
‡ $p = 0.05$.

tilation and increase in the fractional concentration of alveolar carbon dioxide were statistically significant. Oxygen consumption was reduced. These subjects were generally physically limp during the reaction period. Several of the subjects reported shortness of breath during the hypoventilation. Five of these subjects also displayed the hyperventilation reaction on one or more occasions.

Seven of the 22 subjects responded to long-term naturally occurring adverse life events with sustained changes in behavior and emotion. With anger or anxiety and related states, carbon dioxide production was found to be elevated as well as the alveolar ventilation, so that the fractional concentration of alveolar carbon dioxide remained unchanged. With despair, sadness, or hopelessness and related states, carbon dioxide production was found to be decreased as well as the alveolar ventilation, so that once again the fractional concentration of alveolar carbon dioxide remained unchanged. As it is the change in carbon dioxide production that was of interest, the six subjects in the anger/anxiety group were placed with the one subject in the grief/despair/hopelessness group (Table 3). Significant

Table 3. Physiologic Adjustment to Slowly Occurring or Long-Term Changes in Psychologic Orientation (7 Subjects)

	RR	$\dot{V}_A$ (L/MIN)	F_{ACO_2} (%)	$\dot{V}_{CO_2}$ (ML/MIN)
Control	14	4.7	5.1	237
Response	17	6.7*	5.3	357*

* $p = <0.02$.

changes were found in the alveolar ventilation and carbon dioxide production when relaxed control days were compared with the days of sustained behavioral and emotional change. Two of these subjects reported shortness of breath during the reaction period.

In order to validate physiologic similarities between sleep and depressive emotion, five subjects were asked to sleep after initial relaxation. They were requested to "close your eyes, relax, and try to sleep." These five subjects were usually able to sleep on request with relative ease. As shown in Table 4, a significant decrease in alveolar ventilation and increase in alveolar

Table 4. Hypoventilation in Response to Suggested Sleep (5 Subjects)

	RR	$\dot{V}_A$ (L/MIN)	F_{ACO_2} (%)
Control	14	4.9	5.1
Response	14	3.5*	5.7†

* $p = <0.02$.
† $p = <0.01$.

carbon dioxide concentration resulted from the suggestion of sleep—which is similar to the response to depressive emotion shown in Table 2.

The increase in ventilation and carbon dioxide production during stimulation by long-term adverse life events appears to be similar to the response to exercise lasting periods of minutes. Two previous investigators in this laboratory utilized 3-min periods of exercise in the study of chronic pulmonary disease. The response to exercise in eight of these subjects is shown in Table 5; the data are similar to those shown in Table 3. Other studies

Table 5. Actual Exercise (8 Subjects)

	RR	$\dot{V}_A$ (L/MIN)	F_{ACO_2} (%)	$\dot{V}_{CO_2}$ (ML/MIN)
Control	16	6.5	5.2	338
Response	21*	12.9†	5.5*	710†

* $p = < 0.05$.
† $p = < 0.001$.

done in our laboratory show that with suggestion of exercise, data similar to those shown in Table 1 are produced (see Table 6).

Table 6. Suggested Exercise (11 Subjects)

	RR	$\dot{V}_A$ (L/MIN)	F_{ACO_2} (%)	$\dot{V}_{O_2}$ (ML/MIN)
Relaxed	13	4.3	5.8	271
Exercise	21*	12.7†	4.0‡	377†
Relaxed	12	4.3	5.5	269

* $p = 0.01$.
† $p = < 0.01$.
‡ $p = < 0.001$.

COMMENT. From the above information behavior was divided into two categories. When action or desire for action formed a major component of a psychologic reaction the subject was called action-oriented. When inaction or desire for inaction formed the major component of a psychologic reaction, the subject was called nonaction-oriented.

ILLUSTRATIVE CASES

SUBJECT 1. Subject 1 was a 31-year-old white married, once widowed housewife and mother of four children. She had a long history of major illness dating back 18 years. When this study was undertaken her diagnoses were active pulmonary tuberculosis, chronic bronchitis, and a hysterical adjustment pattern.

When first seen in the laboratory, she appeared withdrawn and passive, seemed to have given up trying to solve her many problems and said, "I just don't feel like doing anything." At this time she was easily able to sleep on request during the experiments. When asked to sleep, she would close her eyes and immediately began to hypoventilate as illustrated in Figure 1. During the thirteenth measuring period, she hyperventilated when requested to sleep and appeared tense and upset. After the recording she said that she had been thinking of her husband and her problems during the experimental session. Upon further questioning it was found that she had been feeling resentful toward her husband for a number of years because of his irresponsible behavior. When thinking of her husband she expressed her feelings as follows, "I feel insecure. I feel anxious. I feel mad and unhappy, like I would like to do something and change things. I would like to run away and go home with the children. If things do not work out this time, I'll get a divorce. Nothing I do pleases him,

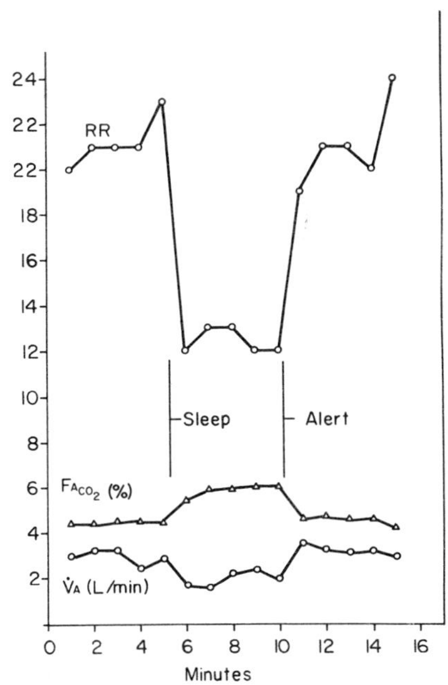

Fig. 1. Physiologic response of Subject 1 to suggested sleep. Sleep response was no longer produced with ease after subject had changed from her initial withdrawn passive behavior, to relative activation.

and I have tried everything." Whenever she was asked to think of her husband she became short of breath, tense, and restless, and clenched her fists.

The hyperventilation reaction was reproduced a total of ten times when she was asked to think of her husband and twice when she spontaneously thought of him. In order to terminate the hyperventilation she was asked to think of her children, a subject which usually evoked feelings of pleasure. The hyperventilation response of this subject while thinking of her husband is illustrated in Figure 2. The only consistent change in the cardiovascular measurements was that of an elevation in pulse rate.

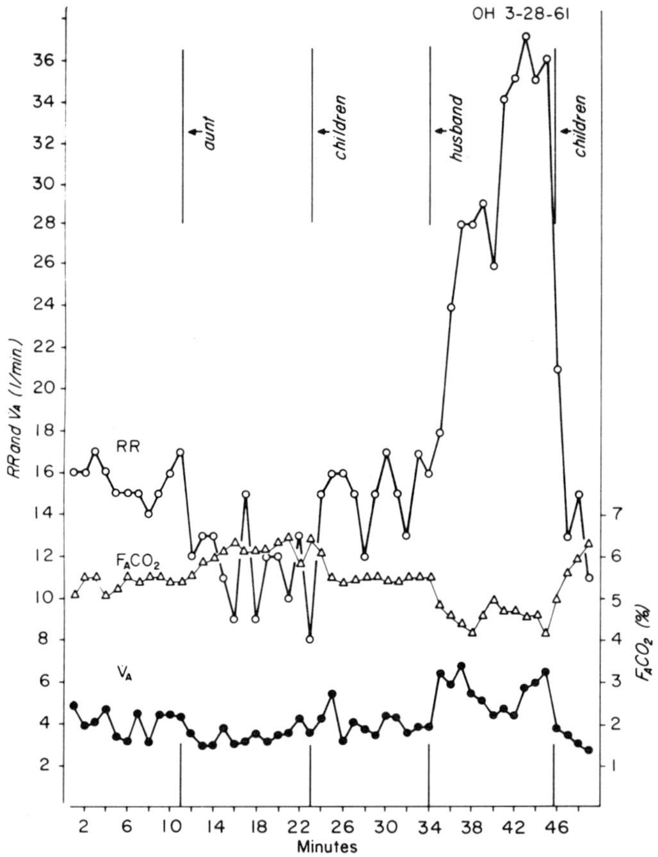

Fig. 2. Physiologic response of Subject 1 to suggestions of her deceased aunt and her husband. After patient had dissipated some of her feelings about these two people, reactions illustrated were not so easily produced. Physiologic response to thinking of her aunt was similar to that noted during suggestion of sleep. Physiologic response to thinking of her husband was similar to that noted during suggestion of exercise (which will be illustrated in succeeding chapters). Her children, always a source of relaxation and contentment, provided stimulus to return her to a relatively pleasant, relaxed condition.

Over the two-month period that suggestions of her husband were used as a stimulus, she gradually became more alert and aggressive. Associated with this increased self-assertiveness was an increase in the control values for ventilation and a reduction in the ventilatory response to suggestion of her husband. This two-month period was punctuated by the death of an aunt who had been her only confidante. For many years, the subject had been dependent upon her aunt for counseling and guidance during periods of emotional turmoil. For the period immediately following news of her aunt's death, the subject experienced feelings of sadness and loneliness when thinking of her relative. These feelings were illustrated by the following statements, "I feel lost. I feel sad. I feel like crying. I feel all alone. She was the one person I could confide in." While thinking of her aunt, she hypoventilated with irregularity in depth, frequency, and flow. This was similar to her reaction to the suggestion of sleep, with the exception of the irregularities in respiration (see Fig. 2). An increase in pulse rate also occurred during suggestion of her aunt. The reaction to thinking of her aunt was induced by suggestion on three occasions. It was noted that the hypoventilation reaction to thinking of her aunt was no longer present after the subject recovered from her acute sense of loss. Figures 3 and 4 illustrate further the ease with which these responses could be produced and terminated in this suggestible subject. Figure 4 also directly compares the physiologic response to the suggestion of sleep to the physiologic response to thinking of her aunt.

As she changed from her original withdrawn and passive outlook to more

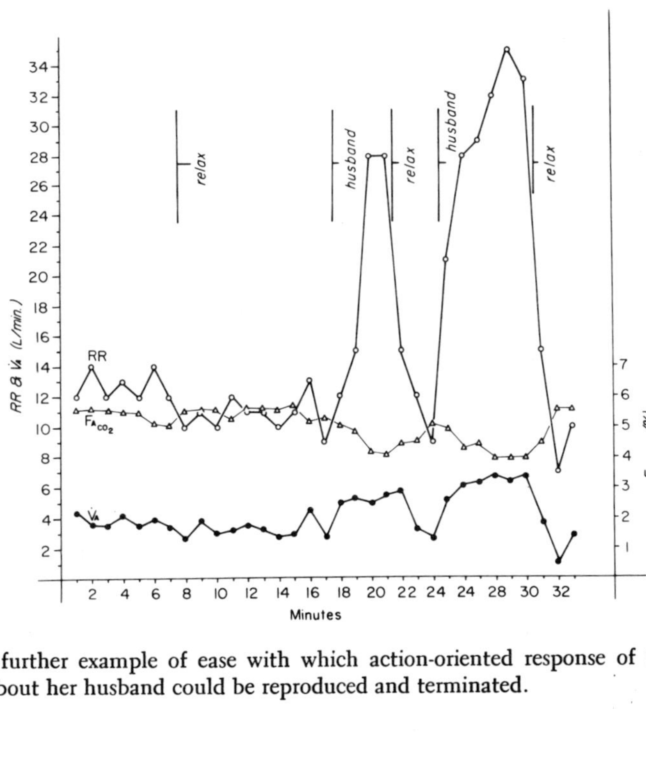

Fig. 3. A further example of ease with which action-oriented response of Subject 1 to thinking about her husband could be reproduced and terminated.

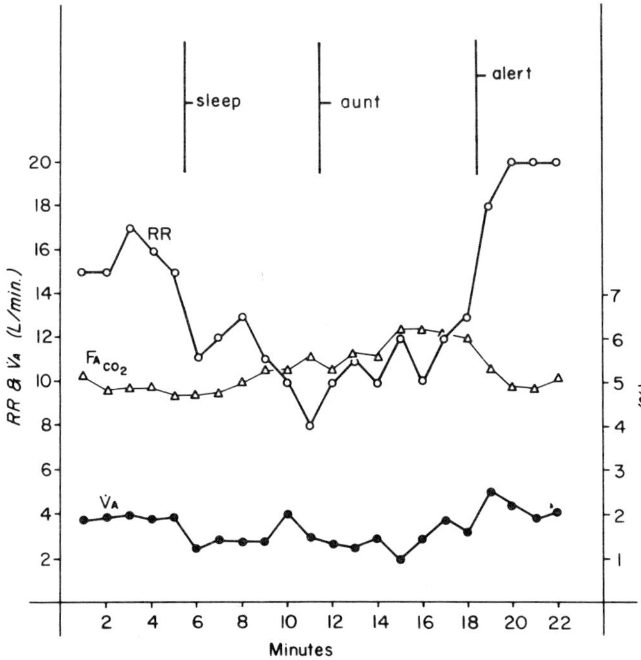

Fig. 4. A further example of ease with which nonaction-oriented response of Subject 1 to thinking about her deceased aunt could be reproduced. Also illustrated is the similarity in ventilation between suggestion of sleep and suggestion of the aunt.

assertive and outgoing behavior, she increased ventilation, carbon dioxide production, blood pressure, and pulse rate. The respiratory and cardiovascular values for her first five consecutive days in the study, as compared to measurements made during five consecutive days eight weeks later, are shown in Table 7. During the last five-day period she was more outgoing and communicative and was no longer able to sleep easily on request. After this last period of measurements she was discharged from the hospital.

She was subsequently recalled one month after discharge for further studies. When she came into the laboratory, it was noted that she seemed alert and much more assured than at any time previously. At this time she was measured for a period of more than 90 min. Instead of waiting for the investigator to terminate the experiment, which had always been the course of events in the past, she terminated the experiment herself and said that she did not have time for any more measurements as she wanted to visit some of the patients on the wards. At this time she became hostile toward the experiments for the first time and asked, "What does all this have to do with my tuberculosis?" The physiologic measurements for this action oriented period are also illustrated in Table 7. The measurements for this period are in contrast to the same measurements during the previous periods and show an elevation of ventilation, carbon dioxide production, and blood pressure.

Table 7. DATA ON SUBJECT 1

	RR	RANGE	$\dot{V}_A$	RANGE	$F_{A_{CO_2}}$	RANGE	$\dot{V}_{CO_2}$	RANGE	BP	RANGE	PR	RANGE
Control (all 28 days)	16±3		3.7±0.6		5.3±0.4		197±32		104±9/71±7		86±7	
First 5 days	17	14–21	3.3	2.8–3.7	5.2	4.2–5.8	175	126–209	92/64	88–100/58–70	82	72–94
Last 5 days	18	15–24	4.0	3.8–4.3	5.0	4.5–5.4	199	175–232	111/77	106–112/73–82	97	88–106
Recalled	20		4.8		5.6		269		128/83		82	

COMMENT. In this subject the effect of both long-term and short-term naturally occurring adverse life stimuli upon respiration can be seen. During short-term psychologic stimulation (whether naturally occurring or suggested) the subject is seen to increase or decrease alveolar ventilation, and decrease or increase the fractional concentration of alveolar carbon dioxide in a typical hyperventilation or hypoventilation reaction. When, however, a change in psychologic orientation occurs over a long period of time (in this case over eight weeks), there is no fall in the fractional concentration of alveolar carbon dioxide even though the alveolar ventilation is increased. This represents an increase in carbon dioxide production and thereby an increase in metabolism as this subject became more action oriented. Changes in blood pressure and pulse rate are seen to occur concurrently with the respiratory and psychologic changes.

SUBJECT 2. Subject 2 was a 58-year-old white male divorced lawyer and father of three children. An admission diagnosis was made of irreversible diffuse obstructive pulmonary syndrome and hypoxia, and a mixed psychoneurosis with anxiety and depressive features. Throughout his stay in the hospital he experienced panic states which were manifested by agitation and shortness of breath. They lasted several minutes and were usually relieved by a subcutaneous injection of sterile saline.

He was measured a total of 18 times during which he complained constantly and stamped his feet on the floor. On the nineteenth time he was placed in a smaller, darker, enclosed laboratory to be measured, and was seated in an easy chair from which he was unable to extricate himself without help. His response was, "Oh, Jesus–I don't think I can stand it." After being measured for 1 min he had to stop; he said, "I can't do it–I just can't. I've got to get out of here." At this time he appeared restless and agitated. He was told that the measurements would have to be carried out in the small laboratory until the regular laboratory was again available. He then left.

On the day of the next test, he walked to the laboratory, became very short of breath and gasped for air. Before he could be measured he had to leave the room several times in order to get his breath. He said, "I can't do it. I can't stay in this room." At this time he was very tense and restless. After several trips in and out of the laboratory, he agreed to be measured provided he could be placed in a chair from which he could get out easily. After the measurement he was too short of breath to walk back to his ward and had to be taken by wheelchair.

The change in ventilation during this period was well outside of two standard deviations from the mean. The mean values for the 27 days of measurement were: RR 19 ± 3.6; V_A 5.8 L ± 2.8 L; $F_{A_{CO_2}}$ 4.3 percent ± 0.4 percent. Values for the above illustrated reaction were: RR 34; $\dot{V}_A$ 14.7 L; $F_{A_{CO_2}}$ 4.0 percent. Cardiovascular measurements made during another similar anxiety attack with severe shortness of breath were as follows: preattack–BP 130/90; PR 112; ST 25.0; attack–BP 160/100, PR 134, ST 26.0; 18 min after intramuscular placebo medication–BP 132/88, PR 116, ST 26.8.

After the incident described above there was a dramatic change in this subject's relationship to the investigator. He felt that the experiment was no longer voluntary and that his stay in the hospital and his friendship with the investigator depended upon his performance in the laboratory and the whims of the experimenter. He ceased to complain about the experiments and indicated that he was "more than willing to cooperate all that I can." After his changed behavior he said, "You noticed quite a change in me? Are the records better?" During this period of forced cooperation, which lasted three weeks, the subject was noted to have increased alveolar ventilation but showed no change in the fractional concentration of alveolar carbon dioxide (Fig. 5). His general outlook was noted to have changed from one of helplessness and nonaction-orientation to one of cautious optimism and action-orientation.

COMMENT. This man was inadvertently placed in an untenable position in which he felt trapped and overwhelmed. His reaction was one of agitation, helplessness, restlessness, lack of cooperation, and direct action. In this setting he hyperventilated. Considering the striking elevation of alveolar ventilation, the change in the fractional concentration of alveolar carbon dioxide is not impressive. This finding suggests an increase in carbon dioxide production and hence an increase in metabolism.

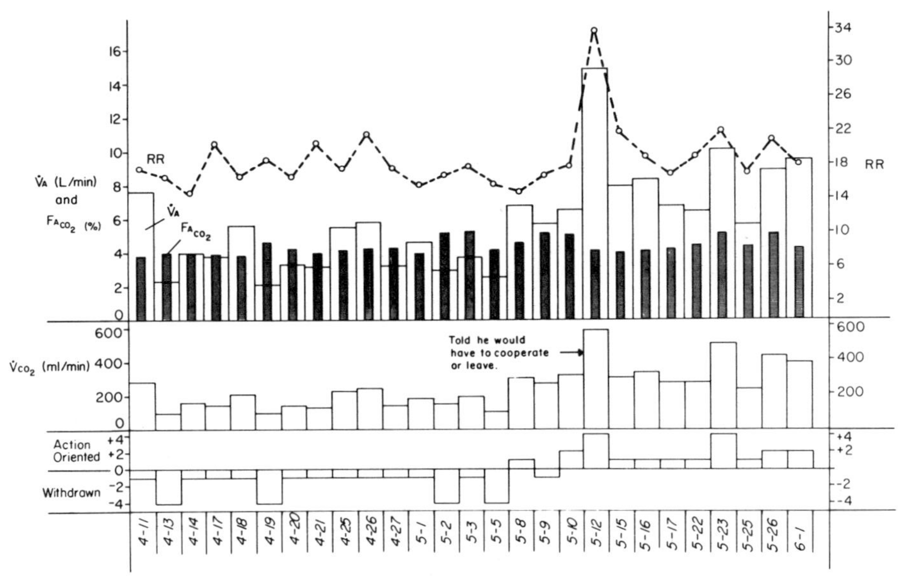

Fig. 5. Physiologic response of Subject 2 to sustained change in behavior and affect. During period of withdrawal or nonaction-orientation he was found to have relatively low alveolar ventilation and carbon dioxide production. During subsequent period of action-orientation, alveolar ventilation and carbon dioxide production were high. There were no significant changes in fractional concentration of alveolar carbon dioxide. This was seen as a result of adjustment of metabolic rate of changes in ventilation which occurred over relatively long period of time.

Subsequent studies indicated that the situation mentioned above was one of the factors responsible for a change in general outlook. The change in outlook was correlated with simultaneous changes in ventilation and metabolism. Low ventilation and low carbon dioxide production were shown to be consistent with nonaction-orientation, while high ventilation and high carbon dioxide production were shown to be consistent with action-orientation.

SUBJECT 3. Subject 3 was a 50-year-old white female, three-times-divorced commercial artist who had been hospitalized previously three times for the treatment of pulmonary tuberculosis and irreversible diffuse obstructive pulmonary syndrome, once for the treatment of severe abdominal pain, once for medical and social evaluation, and once for experimental study purposes.

When initially brought to the laboratory, she was short of breath, tense, and restless, and had an uncontrollable tremor of her hands. She later described this period as being "the lowest mentally" in her life. She said, "I was afraid. Like everything was over. Nothing picked me up." During this time she complained of numerous pains with special significance being placed on severe stomach pain. After being in the hospital for a short time, it was found that she had a rather large peptic ulcer (> 3 cm). Treatment of the ulcer and subsequent relief from the pain were correlated with alleviation of the shortness

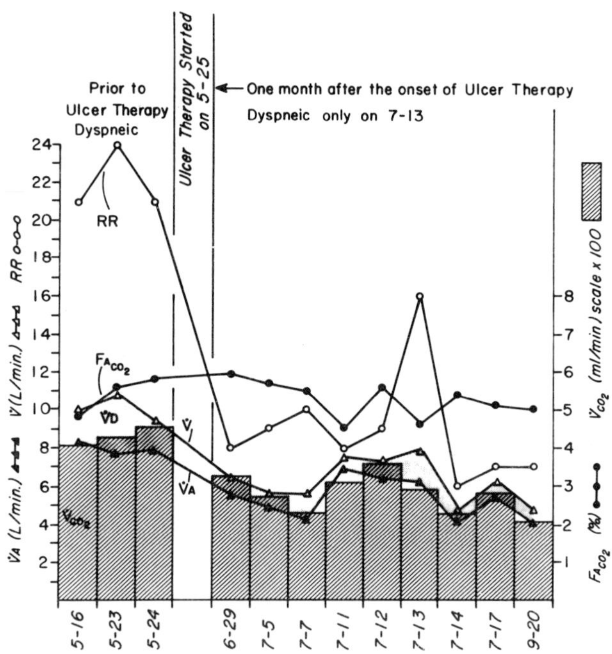

Fig. 6. Relief of dyspnea and respiratory hyperfunction following alleviation of ulcer symptoms in Subject 3.

of breath, a 20-lb weight gain, and a marked change of mood. She then said that she "felt enthused" and "as well as possible physically." The alteration in behavior coincided with a drop in the alveolar ventilation and carbon dioxide production (Fig. 6).

During her stay in the hospital she frequently displayed hostility toward individuals who played a directive role in her life or who she thought had slighted her in some way. She developed a particularly strong dislike of two female patients. When thinking of these two people she became tense, hyperventilated, and developed a gasping shortness of breath and a pounding of her heart. Her feelings toward these two females were expressed as follows, "I'm sorry to say I felt contempt—almost hatred. I've always felt that way about people of that caliber. I would like to get the two of them together and beat the holy 'H' out of them." [Would you do it?] "Oh, no! I'm not the kind of person who goes around fighting people. I feel a mixture of fear and hatred." The hyperventilation response to such anger is illustrated in Fig. 7. She displayed hostility and hyperventilation to five other adverse life stimuli.

She complained of being continually depressed and was preoccupied with thoughts of suicide. As illustrated above, however, the depression was frequently broken by periods of irritability and anger. During periods of severe depression she felt as though she was "just barely getting enough air into my lungs to keep going." In order to reproduce this shortness of breath and depression in the laboratory it was sufficient to ask her to think of how she felt when she was depressed, tired, and at the end of her rope. The depression was described by the subject as follows, "The most lonely feeling in the world. I feel like breaking

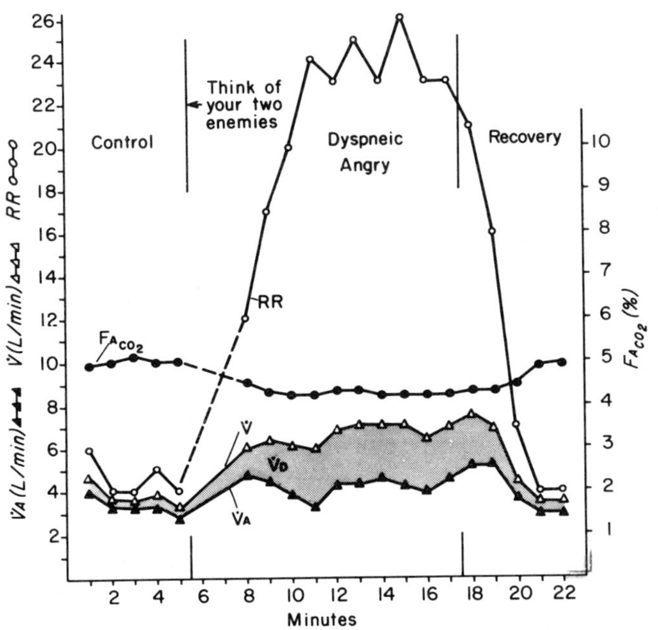

Fig. 7. Dyspnea in association with anger and hyperventilation in Subject 3.

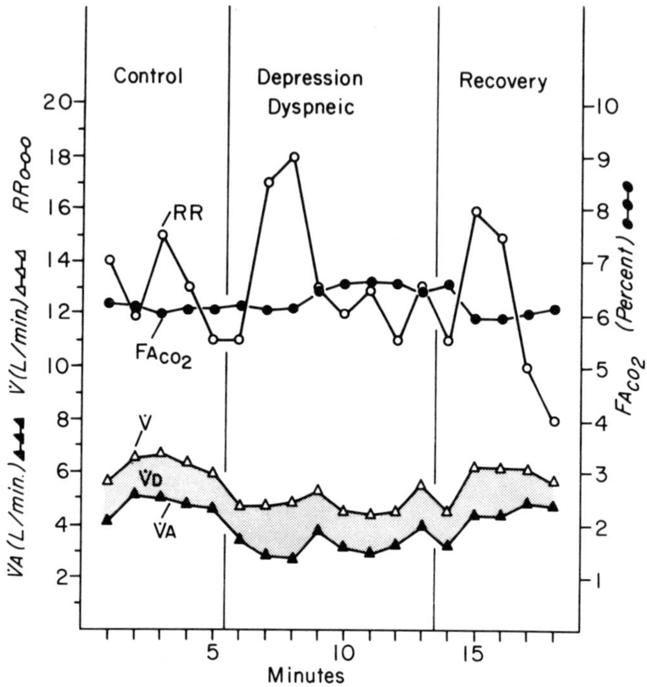

Fig. 8. Dyspnea in association with depression and hypoventilation in Subject 3.

down and crying until I can't see straight. What in the world is the use of keeping on in this rat race. I don't feel like actually doing anything. I don't feel well and I'm so tired." The subject's hypoventilation reaction to the above suggestion was duplicated on eight occasions. The reaction is illustrated in Figure 8. When asked to relax and sleep, her level of ventilation was similar to that of being told to think of depression.

COMMENT. Behavior on the part of individuals around the subject called forth a reaction of hostility which never found adequate expression in action. When the subject was subsequently asked to think about these people or events, a reaction of hyperventilation and action-orientation resulted. With suggestion of depression, she readily hypoventilated and became nonaction-oriented. It should be noted that she experienced shortness of breath with hyperventilation, hypoventilation, anger, and depression.

SUBJECT 4. Subject 4 was a 43-year-old white female, married, childless, a supermarket checker, who seldom had been ill previous to contracting pulmonary tuberculosis. She was admitted to the sanatorium for the treatment of advanced active pulmonary tuberculosis and tuberculous largyngitis. She was an aggressive woman who tried to dominate everyone with whom she came into contact. She experienced considerable difficulty in adjusting to the confinement of the tuberculosis hospital. She frequently became upset and dealt with problems with anger and action. On the twenty-eighth and last day that she was measured she came into the laboratory appearing tense and agitated and repeated over and over, "My back's against the wall. I can't take any more. If I meet one of those nurses I'll smash her. I feel like smashing things." She was measured for a period of 15 min shortly after entering the laboratory and was found to be hyperventilating. During the measurement she was tense, shaking, and clenching her fists. At this time her blood pressure was 150/108 (which is outside of 3 S.D. from the mean of control values) and the fingertip skin temperature was 31.4° C. After the first 15 min of measurement she broke down sobbing and said, "I didn't want to do this. I'll be all right in a minute." After the sobbing episode the hyperventilation subsided somewhat. Following the preliminary recordings she talked to her ward physician for 30 min, during which she constantly referred to being in a corner with her back against the wall. After the talk, she said, "I feel relaxed and tired. This is the one place I can relax." During this period of measurement, ventilation was noted to be in the low normal range for her. Also at this time she developed a fluctuating blood pressure and a throbbing headache. She said that her breathing had been labored during the hyperventilation period and that she had experienced chest pain and a "knot in the stomach." Toward the end of the observation her fingertip skin temperature was 25.6° C and her blood pressure varied from 120/90 to 150/100. The increase in alveolar ventilation during the attack was outside of two standard deviations from the mean of the 28 days measured. The above incident is illustrated in Figure 9.

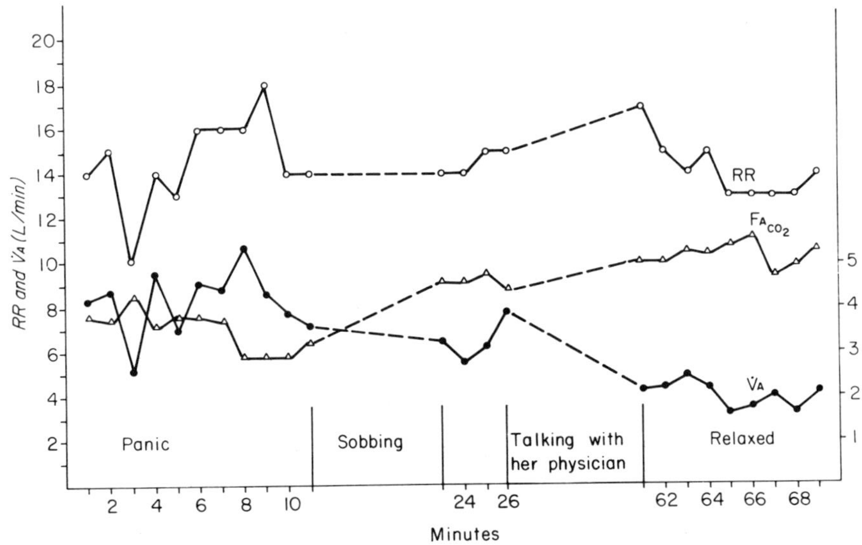

Fig. 9. Respiratory hyperventilation in Subject 4 during period of panic. Patient was able partially to relieve her feelings by sobbing, during which there was no effort to comfort her. After talking to her physician and working out the immediate problem, her ventilation returned to normal values and she felt relaxed and comfortable.

On another day she appeared aggressive and admitted feeling worried, tense, and angry. However, she did not feel panicked by the situation she found herself in and believed that the investigator could solve her problems if she confided in him. She was mad at her doctor because he broke up her pool game and made her get some laboratory tests done. In addition, she had previously tried to find out from the doctor approximately how long she would be in the hospital. When he would not tell her she responded, "The only way to get out of this place is to get pregnant," and left in a huff. After her disagreements with her physician, one of the patients told her to "Straighten up your shoulders." She told the patient, "Why don't you . . . ," and walked away.

In addition to the above she was "worried" about her conduct on the ward the preceding night. At 12:40 A.M. one of the nurses came into her room and asked her to turn out her light and go to bed. She was working on a ceramic plate at the time and threw the plate at the nurse, missing her but striking the door. She then chased the nurse down the hall. The nurse escaped to the treatment room where she locked herself in for protection. The subject then "told off" several "curious" patients and retired to her room.

When she entered the laboratory she was concerned about possible repercussions from her activities over the past 24 hr and was angry at her physician. She said, "Boy, am I mad," but admitted to being worried also. Initially she was found to be hyperventilating. Her blood pressure was 120/80, pulse rate

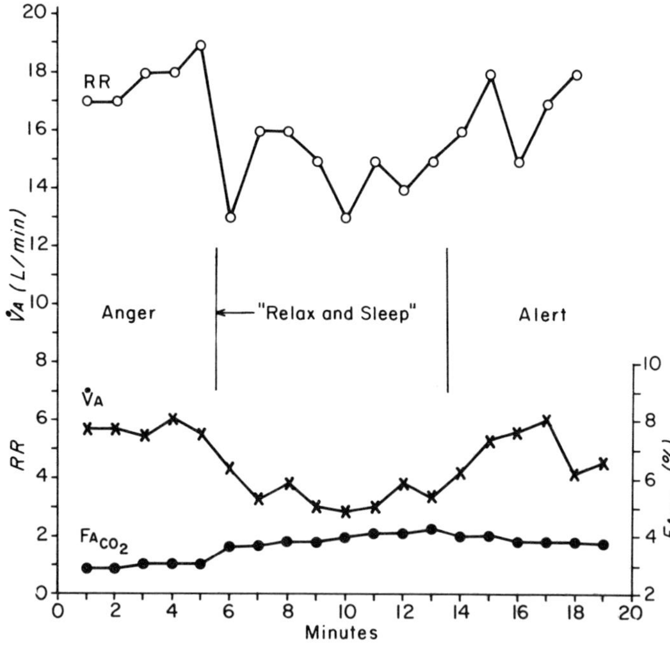

Fig. 10. Interruption of period of mixed emotions with anger predominating in Subject 4 with suggestion of relaxation and sleep. In general, such mild suggestion techniques worked remarkably well in most subjects.

92, and skin temperature 22.8°C. After she was asked to relax, her ventilation dropped but blood pressure and pulse rate remained unchanged. Skin temperature rose to 31.4° C. Subsequently, when asked to remain alert, ventilation increased but blood pressure and skin temperature remained unchanged. Pulse rate dropped to 82. This period of mixed emotional response is illustrated in Figure 10.

Although this subject was never measured during a period of depression, her response to the suggestion of sleep was similar to other subjects' response to suggested depression.

COMMENT. The data above illustrate several periods of anxiety and anger in a highly aggressive woman who openly expressed her feelings and often acted out her impulses. She commonly created disturbances on the ward and was feared by a number of patients and ward personnel.

SUBJECT 5. Subject 5 was a 25-year-old white male tuberculous patient with severe emotional problems and known asthma since the age of seven. At the time of the study he had a severe irreversible component to his diffuse obstructive pulmonary syndrome. He contracted anterior poliomyelitis at the age of three months, and spent most of his life in hospitals until the age of 16 years. At one time his divorced mother left him in the hospital for nine years (age 7–16) without visiting him.

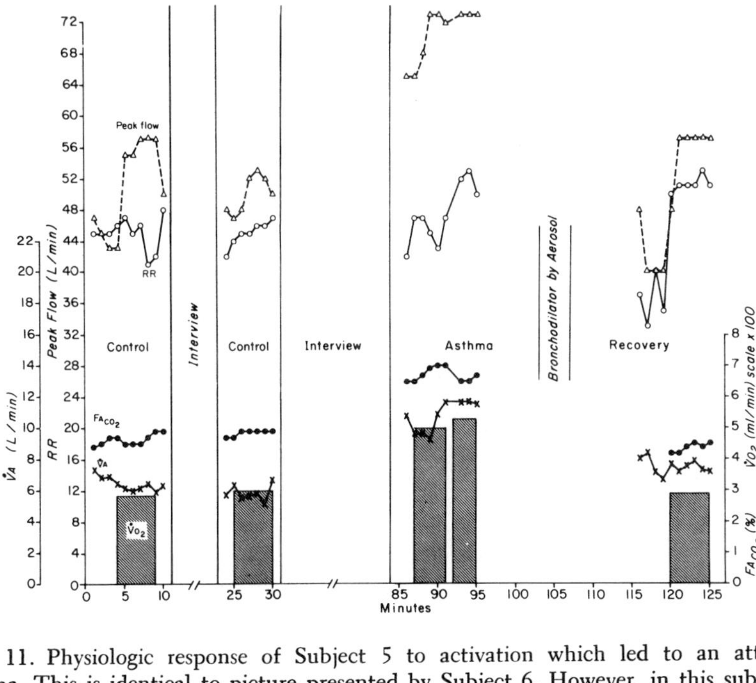

Fig. 11. Physiologic response of Subject 5 to activation which led to an attack of asthma. This is identical to picture presented by Subject 6. However, in this subject increased resistance and impaired flow rates were partially reversible.

He was unable to walk until after a surgical operation for correction of polio-induced foot deformities at the age of seven. After this first of nine operations he developed a severe attack of asthma which lasted for several days. His asthma got progressively worse until at the time of this study he had attacks almost daily.

Measurements of respiratory and cardiovascular variables were made during four naturally occurring attacks of asthma and one hypnotically induced attack. During an attack he was observed to sweat freely, tremble, wheeze, and become cyanotic. He appeared irritable and petulant and complained of shortness of breath. He said, "I want what I want and I want it now." Only two of the attacks were amenable to termination by suggestion and talking of neutral and pleasant topics. The other attacks were terminated by a bronchodilator administered by aerosol. Placebo aerosols were not effective. As illustrated in Figure 11, asthmatic reactions in this subject were correlated with respiratory hyperfunction. This hyperfunction ceased abruptly at the termination of an attack. After an attack he appeared relaxed and pleasant and stated, "I want to go to sleep and just rest." Cardiovascular measurements taken prior to an attack were: BP 134/100; PR 119; ST 28.0° C. During the attack: BP 160/102; PR 144; ST 30.6° C. Seven minutes after a bronchodilator: BP 134/100; PR 140; ST 28.8° C.

COMMENT. The data on this subject suggest an intimate relationship between emotional and physiologic change. The attacks of asthma occurred both spontaneously and secondary to psychologic stimulation. During an attack the physiologic change led to increased irritability, anger, and restlessness, thus accentuating the symptoms. During asthma this subject is breathing at the limit of his ability. Even though he increases his ventilation and flow to the maximum that he is capable of, it is not sufficient, and there is an increase in the fractional concentration of alveolar carbon dioxide and the development of cyanosis, as ventilation does not compensate adequately for the increase in metabolism. Thus ventilation cannot "keep up" with metabolism.

SUBJECT 6. Subject 6 was a bitter, anxious, 66-year-old white married male, with tuberculosis and severe irreversible DOPS. His hospital course was marked by periods of panic during which he was cyanotic and incapacitated by dyspnea. Many of these attacks appeared to be related to his strong feelings of hostility concerning his wife's long-term hospitalization in a mental institution and in his inability to deal with her or the institution. The panic could be interrupted by suggestion of topics associated with relaxation and pleasant memories. This was particularly so with suggestion of the good times he used to have with his three sons before they deserted him and married.

Figure 12 illustrates the rise in ventilation during panic in this subject. The increase in $F_{A_{CO_2}}$ along with the observable cyanosis indicate an increase in oxygen consumption and carbon dioxide output which could not be compensated for by his failing respiratory system. The levels of ventilation shown during the panic day are of a magnitude which approach his maximal breathing capacity.

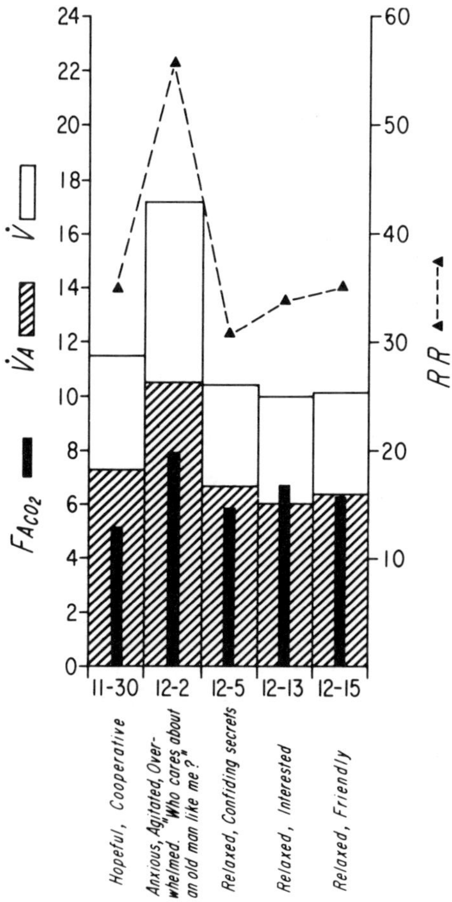

Fig. 12. Comparison of relatively relaxed days with day characterized by anxiety and agitation in Subject 6. During anxious day both alveolar ventilation and fractional concentration of alveolar carbon dioxide increased because of his inability to increase ventilation and thereby match changes in oxygen consumption and carbon dioxide production. Fixed pulmonary deficit thereby dictates amount of emotional expression that the lungs can participate in.

COMMENT. This subject illustrates the devastating effect of an emotionally induced increase in metabolism in a patient with a fixed pulmonary defect. Unlike the asthmatic it is not transitory, but represents a fixed ceiling on the man's ability to respond with ventilatory changes at any time. The panic and fear induced by this defect in a relatively primitive patient who already has difficulty adjusting is overwhelming. It takes an exceedingly understanding and well-informed physician to deal with this kind of adjustment problem.

DISCUSSION

In a group of 22 subjects, action-oriented behavior has been correlated with hyperventilation in 20 subjects in response to short-term adverse life situations. Eight of the 22 subjects were found to hypoventilate in response to short-term adverse life situations to which they reacted with nonaction-orientation. Seven of the 22 subjects were found to react to long-term adverse life stimuli with sustained changes in psychologic orientation and increased or decreased ventilation without a corresponding change in the fractional concentration of alveolar carbon dioxide. These data illustrated lowered carbon dioxide production during nonaction-orientation and increased carbon dioxide production during action-orientation.

Respiratory changes occurring during action-orientation were seen to be similar to those occurring during real or suggested exercise, and respiratory changes occurring during nonaction-orientation were found to be similar to those occurring during real or suggested sleep.

The significance of these changes in metabolism and ventilation to the healthy individual is that of matching body physiology and psychologic intent in terms of activity levels. The patient with compromised ventilation and borderline blood gas values may get into serious difficulty by reacting with either of the above patterns. A subject whose ventilation is already being severely taxed may not be able to increase ventilation to meet psychologic and physiologic demands when reacting to a stimulus with the action-oriented pattern. Thus he may become hypoxic and hypercarbic as a result of the increased metabolic load and the failure of ventilation to compensate by increasing the supply of air. The nonaction-oriented pattern is less well understood, but patients appear to decrease ventilation in excess of the change in metabolism and the net result is, again, a relative ventilatory inadequacy so that the subject becomes hypoxic and hypercarbic because of the discrepancy between the supply and demand of oxygen. An additional factor in this kind of response is that it may lead to difficulty in breathing which in turn produces anxiety and the patient then begins to react with the action-oriented pattern. Once the patient is dyspneic, whether from an initial action-oriented pattern or from the nonaction-oriented pattern, his anxiety is increased and he becomes more dyspneic and more hypoxic and hypercarbic. These factors may react in a vicious circle, the end result of which is increasing ventilatory inadequacy.

The reason for the lag of oxygen consumption and carbon dioxide production behind ventilatory changes is unknown, but this lag accounts for the symptoms of the classic hyperventilation syndrome in which the Pa_{CO_2}

falls to symptom-producing levels. A chronic idiopathic hypoventilation syndrome has been described, but there are no studies that indicate that depression is a primary cause. An acute hypoventilation syndrome has not been described, but from the data presented it appears to exist and is manifested by dyspnea and probably other symptoms as well.

REFERENCES

Anderson, R. W. Psychic influences in pulmonary ventilation. Medical Thesis, University of Washington School of Medicine, 1960.

——— Psychic influences in pulmonary ventilation. Unpublished data, 1962.

Dudley, D. L. The psychophysiology of pulmonary ventilation. Medical Thesis, University of Washington School of Medicine, 1964.

——— Holmes, T. H., Martin, C. J., and Ripley, H. S. Changes in respiration associated with hypnotically induced emotion, pain and exercise, Psychosom Med, 26:46, 1964.

——— Martin, C. J., and Holmes, T. H. Psychophysiologic studies of pulmonary ventilation, Psychosom Med, 26:645, 1964.

Gleeson, F. G. The relationship of mood, dyspnea and pulmonary function studies in respiratory cripples, Medical Thesis, University of Washington School of Medicine, 1958.

Rodman, T., and Close, H. P. The primary hypoventilation syndrome, Amer J Med, 26:808, 1959.

Stevenson, I., and Ripley, H. S. Variations in respiration and in respiratory symptoms during changes in emotion, Psychosom Med, 14:476, 1952.

9

Catecholamine Excretion and Reversible Obstructive Disease

Cranial parasympathetic nervous system impulses to the respiratory tree probably play an important role in the genesis of many cases of bronchial asthma and other psychophysiologic respiratory mucous membrane reactions. Little is known, however, about the function of the sympathetic nervous system during the asthmatic reaction or its possible contribution to host susceptibility or resistance to the disorder.

The initial phase of the study was designed to observe the excretory products of sympathetic nervous system function in naturally occurring asthma. Two asthmatic patients were observed daily in their homes over a period of a month and catecholamine excretion in fractionated 24-hr urine samples was correlated with the patient's behavior before, during, and after asthmatic attacks. The second phase of the study was designed to examine under laboratory conditions some of the relationships observed during the longitudinal study. With use of a standardized interview as the stimulus, the behavioral response of 17 asthmatic subjects was observed and correlated with catecholamine excretion.

The timed urine samples were refrigerated until processed, or frozen if a lapse of several days occurred before processing. The quantity of metadrenalin (MA) and normetadrenaline (NMA) was determined by acid hydrolysis of the urine, passage through Dowex 50-W resin, separation of the metabolites by bidimensional paper chromatography, elution, and the photometric quantitation of the visualized spot. The excretion titers were expressed in micrograms per hr. All samples were checked for creatinine excretion (see Chapter 5). Statistical analysis utilized Student's t test for paired samples.

This chapter is adapted from an article originally published in *J Psychosom Res*, 10:255, 1966, by Masuda, M., Notske, R. N., and Holmes, T. H.

THE LONGITUDINAL STUDY

SUBJECT 1. Subject 1 was a 43-year-old white housewife and mother of two daughters. At age 23, 20 years prior to the study, she had had her first asthma attack simultaneously with an "infection." During the next 20 years she averaged two to three attacks a year, usually in association with an upper respiratory infection. During the last eight years the symptoms increased in frequency and intensity. The diagnosis of an irreversible progressive diffuse obstructive pulmonary syndrome was made four years prior to the study.

Information abstracted from entries made in a diary each day and during the interviews, revealed a persistent depressive element characterized by feelings of helplessness commingled with hopelessness. During the first two weeks of observation her complaints were: "Hard to breathe," "If I could only get my breath," or "Getting tired of breathing." The depression in the second half of the study was more intense and the complaints included: "Down in the dumps," "Down and discouraged," "Very discouraged," "Nothing I do helps." Accompanying the increased depression was an irregular menstrual period, an upper respiratory infection with increased sputum, and intermittent ankle swelling.

The subject reported a few "good" days, with a minimum of respiratory complaints. These were followed either that night or the next day by a series of "bad" days with increased discomfort. After an enjoyable "non-short-of-breath day" at a family picnic, this subject returned home exhausted and thereafter proceeded downhill and ultimately into the hospital.

Data for Subject 1 are seen in Figure 1. The first three samples represent

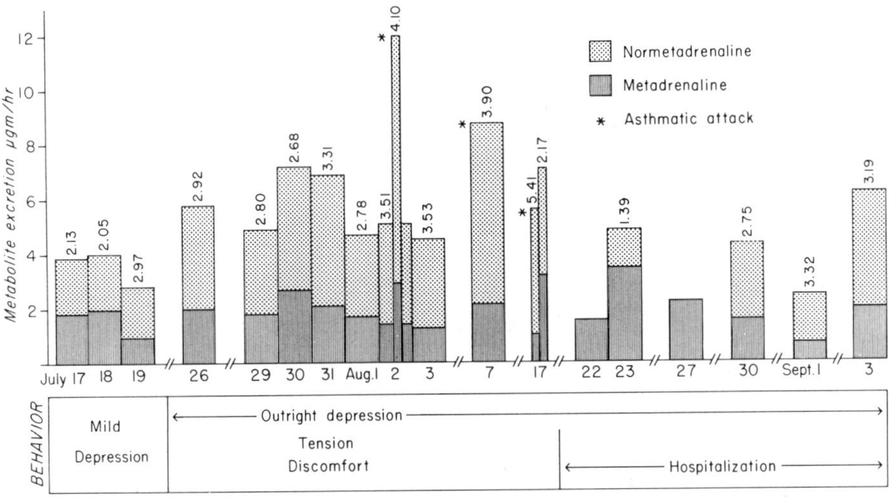

Fig. 1. Behavioral and biochemical data for Subject 1. Wide columns represent 24-hr urine collection periods and narrow columns represent fractional (1- to 4½-hr) collections. Collections marked with asterisk encompassed period of asthmatic attack. Numbers above each column are NMA/MA ratio for that collection.

catecholamine excretion during the two-week period of mild depression. In the subsequent weeks of depression, three asthmatic attacks were observed. Analysis of the accompanying urine samples revealed a high NMA to MA ratio indicating a disproportionate secretion of noradrenaline to adrenaline during the asthmatic attack. The absolute level of NMA was elevated in two attacks but not in the third.

SUBJECT 2. Subject 2 was a 46-year-old white housewife and mother of a 3-year-old girl. Her first asthma attack came 19 months after her first husband's death, when she sold her small store and married a bachelor 14 years her senior, who lived with his two sisters and 95-year-old mother. Soon after the marriage she became pregnant for the first time (age 43) and this was accompanied by frequent exacerbations of her disease.

The daily diary and the interview revealed a pattern of oscillation between "good" and "bad" days, similar to that of the first subject. On the "good" days the subject was energetic and active and had few complaints. The "bad" days that promptly ensued were characterized by "weakness and exhaustion," "let-down," an increase in bodily complaints, and, finally, asthma.

The three attacks observed were associated with the following events: (1) news of her husband's being in an automobile accident, (2) news of the approaching termination of this study, and (3) news of the death of her father. Two of the three asthmatic attacks were preceded by an afternoon of hard work in the yard.

Data for Subject 2 are shown in Figure 2. The most striking catecholamine

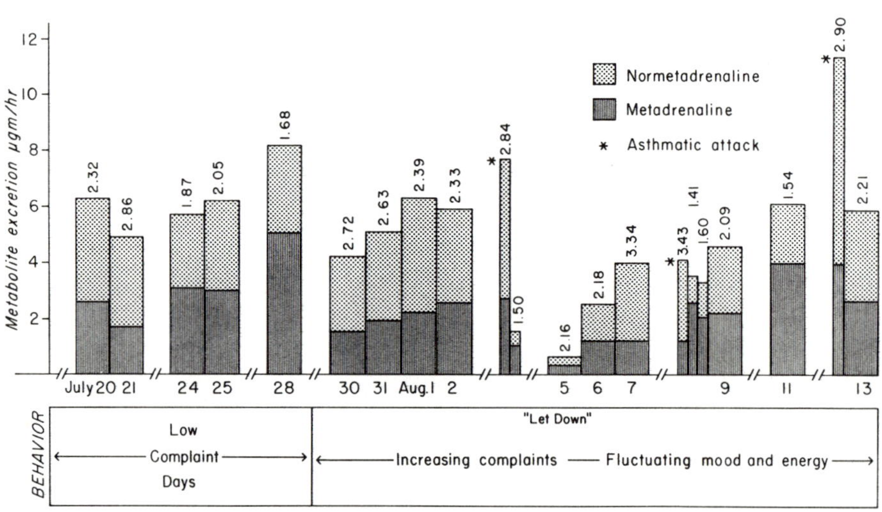

Fig. 2. Behavioral and biochemical data for Subject 2. Wide columns represent 24-hr urine collection periods and narrow columns represent fractional (1- to 4½-hr) collections. Collections marked with asterisk encompassed period of asthmatic attack. Numbers above each column are NMA/MA ratio for that collection. Consistently high NMA/MA ratios are seen during the period around asthmatic attacks (see Fig. 1).

change is noted on the day (August 5) which was characterized as a "letdown" day when she was exhausted from the previous day's activity. The asthma, as with the first subject, was associated with the highest NMA to MA ratios but not necessarily with high absolute catecholamine excretion levels.

Table 1. Catecholamine Metabolite Excretions in Two Asthmatic Subjects

	Metadrenaline μg/hr		Normetadrenaline μg/hr		NMA/MA	
	Non-attack	Attack	Non-attack	Attack	Non-attack	Attack
Subject 1	1.94	2.05	5.00	8.72	2.77	4.48
Subject 2	2.29	2.59	4.69	7.68	2.19	3.06

Mean of nonattack samples (N = 15 for Subject 1; 18 for Subject 2).
Mean of attack samples (N = 3 for Subjects 1 and 2).
Lines connect titers that are significantly different at <0.05 level.

The average excretions of MA and NMA for these two subjects are shown in Table 1. During the asthmatic periods, both subjects showed significant changes in the execretion of NMA, but not in the excretion of MA. This disproportionate response during the attack is also reflected in a corresponding increase in the NMA to MA ratio, with Subject 1 showing a significantly higher ratio during an attack than Subject 2. Subject 1 was the more seriously ill and incapacitated of the two.

THE SHORT-TERM STUDY

This portion of the investigation was designed to evaluate more precisely the pattern of catecholamine excretion identified in the study of naturally occurring asthma.

Seven of the 19 subjects exhibited a respiratory reaction during the interview: four progressed from no ausculatory wheezing to distinct wheezing; three changed from occasional wheezing to constant generalized wheezing. In all seven, the most intense wheezing occurred during that part of the interview dealing with the subject's attitudes, emotions, and behavior during a typical asthmatic attack. This reaction usually occurred between one-third to two-thirds of the way through the interview. At this time the reacting group was judged to be more involved in the interview than the nonreacting group. Topics were discussed at greater length and affect of greater intensity was communicated. In the seven reacting subjects the intensity of affect and wheezing diminished during the discussion of neutral topics toward the end of the interview. The other ten subjects discussed the same topics in the same order but did not develop any wheezing.

All 17 asthmatic subjects exhibited varying degrees of dependency, depression, and dissatisfaction in interpersonal and social relationships. Conflict—with feelings of helplessness, being mistreated, or misunderstood—commonly engendered a state of frustration culminating in onset of asthmatic symptoms. Verbal statements conforming to the asthma attitude defined by Grace and Graham—i.e., "feeling left out in the cold, alone, or shut out"—were readily identified in only four reactors and three nonreactors.

Table 2. Catecholamine Metabolite Excretion in Asthmatic Subjects and College Students

		Metadrenaline μg/hr		Normetadrenaline μg/hr		NMA/MA	
	N	Control	Interview or Experimental	Control	Interview or Experimental	Control	Interview or Experimental
Asthmatic nonreactor	10	3.68	4.25	6.61	7.35	1.76	2.07
Asthmatic reactor	7	2.45	2.55	4.63	6.55	1.73	2.93
College students	24	4.52	4.99	6.14	6.62	1.40	1.36

Lines connect means that are significantly different at <0.05 level.

Table 2 compares the mean urinary excretion of MA and NMA in those who developed wheezing and those who did not. Also included in Table 2 for comparison are metabolite excretion data from another study in which college students were used. These latter subjects had, in the experimental period, undergone a series of challenging events including partial sensory isolation, electric shock, exposure to white noise, and mathematical testing. Control collections were made just prior to the experimental session.

The data in Table 2 indicate that the asthmatic nonreactors showed no significant changes in catecholamine metabolite excretion between the control and interview periods. The asthmatic reactors, however, showed a significant increase in excretion of NMA during the interview as compared with the control period, but no change in MA. The reactors had a significantly reduced excretion of MA compared with that of the nonreactors during the interview situation. This disproportionate excretion was reflected in a higher NMA/MA ratio in the reactor group, though not to the level of significance. It was also noted that in the control period titers of MA and NMA had a tendency to be lower in the reactor group.

A comparison of the metabolite excretions of the college students with that of the asthmatic nonreactors showed no significant differences, although there was a tendency toward a lower MA excretion in the latter. The asthmatic reactors, however, showed significantly lower excretion levels of MA as compared with the college students in both the control and the experimental periods, while the NMA excretion showed no difference between the two groups. These differences were reflected in a significantly higher NMA/MA ratio in the reactors as compared to the college students.

DISCUSSION

The relationship of bronchial asthma to psychodynamic, psychopathologic, personality, constitutional, emotional, and behavioral factors has been studied and formulated by numerous investigators who have used diverse techniques and theoretical points of view.

There is general consensus among workers in the field that psychophysiologic mechanisms are important to the natural history of asthma. The present study of alterations in the function of the sympathetic nervous system as indicated by urinary metabolites excreted during asthmatic behavior is a further attempt to define bodily mechanisms which contribute to the genesis of the disorder.

Adrenaline and noradrenaline are secreted by the adrenal medulla and the adrenergic neurons, respectively. The metabolism of these substances has been clarified in recent years with the discovery of O-methylation which converts adrenaline to metadrenaline, and noradrenaline to normetadrenaline. The derivatives are excreted in the free and conjugated forms. It has been hypothesized that noradrenaline is formed and stored in the nerve endings in at least two forms of binding, ostensibly in equilibrium. The loosely bound noradrenaline that is released in response to neural activity mediates the end organ response. It is this secreted noradrenaline which is physiologically active that is metabolized to normetadrenaline by the body tissues or released into circulation. The metabolism of adrenaline secreted by the adrenal medulla appears to be less complicated as its hormonal action at the tissue level is dependent on its release into the circulation. The measures of metadrenaline and normetadrenaline can be regarded as an index of the circulating and/or physiologically active catecholamines, adrenaline and noradrenaline.

The longitudinal study revealed that the level of normetadrenaline increased during an asthmatic attack. However, the striking change was the relative disproportion of the catecholamine excretion. The normetadrenaline to metadrenaline ratio during the attack was the highest in the series. This observation was confirmed in the short-term study. The reactors who responded during the interview with wheezing also showed increased levels of normetadrenaline, no change in metadrenaline levels, and an increase in the normetadrenaline to metadrenaline ratio. This was also evident in the comparison of the metabolite excretion levels in asthmatics with that of college students. The students showed no change in normetadrenaline/metadrenaline ratio in response to the experimental situation, while the asthmatics showed an apparent graded preferential secretion of noradrenaline.

The low excretion of metadrenaline in the asthmatics was demonstrated in the data from the longitudinal studies as well as in the reactor group of asthmatics. In addition to the lower metadrenaline excretion level, it is also clear that the precipitation of acute attacks—whether by naturally occurring circumstances or by standardized interview—does not result in elevation of these levels. It would seem, therefore, that the adrenal medulla functions at a lower level in asthmatics and fails to respond in the setting productive of asthmatic behavior.

Knauff, Fruhmann and Verbeck found that the asthmatic attack was accompanied by increased amounts of urinary noradrenaline but not of adrenaline (increasing the noradrenaline/adrenaline ratio from 5.7 to 8.8). They also found that the (nonattack) asthmatic in remission had a higher noradrenaline/adrenaline ratio than did control nonasthmatic individuals (5.7 as against 3.3). However, their results indicated that the asthmatic's adrenaline and noradrenaline levels were significantly higher than controls.

Concerning the relevance of the data in this study to the genesis of bronchial asthma, the following formulation is offered. Asthma can be viewed as an epiphenomenon or by-product of adaptive behavior evoked in part by difficulties in social and interpersonal relationships. Although this mode of problem solving usually lacks relevance and pertinence to the stimulus situation, it is, nevertheless, a well-integrated pattern of behavior. Grace and Graham's definition of the essence of this behavior—"feeling left out in the cold"—provides a universe of discourse compatible with many of the divergent psychological theories concerning this disorder and with most of the physiological and constitutional data. Many of the functional changes involving the respiratory tree as it participates in the behavior of "feeling left out in the cold" result from parasympathetic stimulation of smooth muscle and mucous membrane, and are similar to changes that occur when human subjects are actually exposed to cold atmosphere.

Change in function of other bodily systems is also commonly observed. Some of these include decrease in skin temperature, increase in heart rate and blood pressure, and hyperpnea, with increase in alveolar ventilation and oxygen consumption. The fact that some of these physiological changes are mediated via sympathetic nerves is compatible with data from this study which indicate increased excretion of noradrenaline. Although sympathetic neural activity may be increased during asthmatic behavior, the sympathetic humoral activity of the adrenal medulla remains low and unchanged. The absence of medullary stimulation from this biologically inappropriate adaptive behavior deprives the body of one of its important protective resources, adrenaline. The failure of the adrenal medulla to secrete adrenaline may be construed as one of the mechanisms by which resistance to asthma is lowered or susceptibility increased.

SUMMARY

Two asthmatic subjects were followed daily to ascertain their attitudes, emotions, and clinical status. Coincident to this was a collection of 24-hr urine samples with fractional collections during attacks. A cyclic phenomena of "good" days followed by a series of "bad" days culminating in an asthmatic attack was seen as a behavioral feature of the longitudinal studies.

In short-term studies 17 asthmatic patients were interviewed in such a manner as to allow their reliving the attitudes, emotions, and events which had surrounded their individual asthmatic attacks. Seven of the 17 subjects showed an increase in wheezing during the interview.

The subjects who developed wheezing were differentiated from those who did not by their lower excretion levels of metadrenaline during the interview, which reflected a less responsive adrenal medulla. In addition, the asthmatic had initial or daily levels of metadrenaline which were lower than those seen in a group of healthy college students. During an asthmatic attack, whether naturally occurring or induced, there was an increase in the normetadrenaline/metadrenaline ratio that indicated the disproportionate increase in activity of the sympathetic nervous system as differentiated from adrenal medullary output. Normetadrenaline levels were not different among groups. These results indicate that the adrenal medulla is hypoactive and hyporesponsive during an asthmatic attack.

REFERENCES

Abramson, H. A. Pseudoallergenic schizophrenia, Ann Allerg, 17:576, 1959.

Adams, W., David, F., and Hansen, L. New method for determination of creatinine in urine by ion exchange separation and ultraviolet spectrophotometry, Analyt Chem, 24:854, 1962.

Alexander, F. Emotional factors in respiratory disturbances, in Psychosomatic Medicine. New York, W. W. Norton, 1950.

——— and French, T. M. Studies in Psychosomatic Medicine. New York, Ronald Press, 1948.

Axelrod, J., Senoh, S., and Witkop, B. O-methylation of catecholamines in vivo, J Biol Chem, 233:697, 1958.

Bacon, C. The role of aggression in the asthmatic attack, Psychoanal Quart, 25: 309, 1956.

Bastiaans, J., and Groen, J. Psychogenesis and psychotherapy of bronchial asthma, in Modern Trends in Psychosomatic Medicine. O'Neill, D., ed. London, Butterworth, 1955.

Beale, H. D., Fowler, W. S., and Comroe, J. H., Jr. Pulmonary function studies in 20 asthmatic patients in the symptom free interval, J Allerg, 23:1, 1952.

Burgin, L. B. Emotion as an allergen, Pediat Clin N Amer, 6:657, 1959.

Bursten, B. Psychological state and sputum eosinophilia, Psychosom Med, 24: 529, 1964.

Dekker, E., Barendreet, J. T., and Devries, K. Allergy and neurosis in asthma, in Advances in Psychosomatic Medicine, Vol. 1., Jores A., and Stokvis, B., eds. Basel/New York: S. Karger, 1960.

——— Felser, H. A., and Groen, J. Conditioning as a cause of asthmatic attacks, J Psychosom Res, 2:97, 1957.

——— and Groen, J. Asthmatic wheezing, Lancet, 272:1064, 1957.

——— and Groen, J. Reproducible psychogenic attacks of asthma, J Psychosom Res, 1:58, 1956.

Deutsch, F. Basic psychoanalytic principles in psychosomatic disorders, Acta Psychother, 1:102, 1953.

Dudley, D. L., Martin, C. J., and Holmes, T. H. Psychophysiologic studies of pulmonary ventilation, Psychosom Med, 26:645, 1964.

Dunbar, F. Emotions and Bodily Changes. New York, Columbia University Press, 1954.

——— Psychoanalytic notes relating to syndromes of asthma and hay fever, Psychoanal Quart, 7:25, 1938.

Funkenstein, D. H. Variations in response to standard amounts of chemical agents during alterations in feeling states in relation to occurrence of asthma, Res Publ Ass Nerv Ment Dis, 29:566, 1950.

Grace, W. J., and Graham, D. T. Relationship of specific attitudes and emotions to certain bodily diseases, Psychosom Med, 14:243, 1952.

Graham, D. T. Some research on psychophysiologic specificity and its relation to psychosomatic disease, in Physiological Correlates in Psychological Disorders. Roessler, R., and Greenfield, N., S., eds. Madison, University of Wisconsin Press, 1962.

Herxheimer, H., and Prior, F. N. Further observations on induced asthma and bronchial hyposensitization, Int Arch Allerg, 3:189, 1953.

Holmes, T. H., Goodell, H., Wolf, S., and Wolff, H. G. The Nose: An Experimental Study of Reaction Within the Nose in Human Subjects During Varying Life Experiences. Springfield, Ill., Charles C Thomas, Publisher, 1950.

Kerney, E. L. The history of asthma from Hippocrates to Meltzer, J Allerg, 35: 215, 1964.

Knapp, P. H. Models and methods: A psychodynamic predictive approach to bronchial asthma, J Nerv Ment Dis, 135:440, 1956.

——— and Nemetz, S. J. Acute bronchial asthma, Psychosom Med, 22:42, 1960.

——— and Nemetz, S. J. Personality variations in bronchial asthma, Psychosom Med, 19:443, 1957.

——— and Nemetz, S. J. Sources of tension in bronchial asthma, Psychosom Med, 19:466, 1957.

Knauff, H. G., Fruhmann, G., and Verbeck, G. Die Ausscheidung von adrenaline und noradrenalin bei asthma bronchiale und bei lumenemphysem, Klin Wschr, 40:411, 1962.

Kopin, I. J., and Gordon, E. K. Metabolism of norepinephrine-H^3 released by tyramine and reserpine, J Pharmacol Exp Therap, 138:351, 1962.

LaBrosse, E. Axelrod, J., and Kety, S. O-methylation, the principle route of metabolism of epinephrine in man, Science, 128:593, 1958.

Lowell, F. C., Schiller, I. W., and Lynch, M. T. Estimation of daily changes in the severity of bronchial asthma, J Allerg, 26:113, 1955.

Masuda, M. Differing adaptive metabolic behaviors, J Psychosom Res, 10:239, 1966.

——— and Bakker, C. B. Personality catecholamine metabolites and psychophysiological response to diazepam, J Psychiat Res, 4:221, 1966.

McIlroy, M. B., and Marshall, R. The mechanical properties of the lungs in asthma, Clin Sci, 15:345, 1956.

Neely, F. L. Experimental asthma: Therapy with histaminase, J. Lab Clin Med, 27:319, 1941.

Notske, R. N. Catecholamines and asthmatic behavior. M.D. Thesis, University of Washington School of Medicine, Seattle, 1965.

Oberndorf, C. F. The psychogenic factors in asthma, NY J Med, 35:41, 1935.

Rees, L. An etiological study of premenstrual asthma, J Psychosom Res, 7:191, 1963.

Rees, L. Physical and emotional factors in bronchial asthma, J Psychosom Res, 1:98, 1956.

Stein, M. Etiology and mechanisms in the development of asthma, in Psychosomatic Medicine, Nodine, J. H., and Moyer, J. H., eds. Philadelphia, Lea & Febiger, 1962.

Stevenson, I. P., and Ripley, H. S. Variations in respiration and respiratory symptoms during changes in emotion, Psychosom Med, 14:476, 1952.

——— and Wolff, H. G. Life situations, emotions, and mucus, Psychosom Med, 11:223, 1949.

Trendelenburg, U. Modification of the effect of tyramine by various agents and procedures, J Pharmacol Exp Therap, 134:8, 1961.

Treuting, T. F., and Ripley, H. S. Life situations and bronchial asthma, J Nerv Ment Dis, 108:380, 1948.

Van Arsdel, P. P., Jr., and Motulsky, A. G. Frequency and hereditability of asthma and allergic rhinitis in college students, Acta Genet, 9:101, 1959.

Von Euler, U. S. Autonomic neuroeffector transmission, in Handbook of Physiology: Section 1, Neurophysiology, Magoun, R. W. ed. Baltimore, Waverly Press, Vol. 1, p. 215, 1959.

——— Franksson, C., and Hellstrom, J. Adrenaline and noradrenaline output in urine after unilateral and bilateral adrenalectomy in man, Acta Physiol Scand, 31:1, 1954.

Webb, P. Air temperature in respiratory tracts of resting subjects in cold, J Appl Physiol, 4:378, 1951.

Whelan, R. F., and Young, M. I. The effect of adrenaline and noradrenaline infusions on respiration in man, Brit J Pharmacol, 8:98, 1953.

Wolff, H. G. Stress and Disease. Springfield, Ill, Charles C Thomas, Publisher, 1953.

Section III

Experimentally Induced Change

This section contains reports of experiments in which either artificial stimulation (noxious head stimulation) or hypnotic and nonhypnotic suggestion of naturally occurring situations or artificial situations were utilized to induce psychologic and physiologic change. These experiments followed chronologically the observations described in Chapter 8. They were intended to elaborate on the findings based on naturally occurring life change. It was believed that similar findings resulting from the use of different stimulus techniques would increase confidence in the design and conduct of future experiments, which would lead to some assurance that the laboratory results represented real-world events and would be useful in a clinical setting.

10

Noxious Head Stimulation: General Observations and Case Reports

In this study, experimental stimulation of the head was utilized to elicit psychologic and physiologic change. Subjects were studied before, during, and after stimulation with a metal headband with 14 adjustable rubber-tipped screws around the edges. This device produced a pressure headache and physical and mental discomfort when the adjustable screws were fixed tightly against the circumference of the head. The objective was to produce a significant change in behavior from that of the control state; therefore time and magnitude of pressure were held as variables rather than constants. The end point was determined by the subject and was defined as that point at which he could no longer tolerate the experience. Following application of the pressure device to the head the screws were tightened at intervals of 5 to 8 min, until the end point was achieved. Time required to reach the level of intolerance and termination of the noxious stimulus ranged between 11 and 39 min.

A total of 50 experiments involved 26 volunteer subjects. The number carried out on each subject varied from one to six. There were 3 females and 23 males in the experimental group; their ages varied from 21 to 50, with a mean of 26. Twenty-one subjects had normal lungs and five had tuberculosis. All but two of the 21 subjects with normal lungs were medical students. These two were laboratory technicians. The five tuberculosis subjects were patients who were participating in a parallel study. The only criterion for selection of subjects was that they be available and willing to take part in the experiments.

This chapter is adapted from an article originally published in *J Psychosom Res*, 9:209, 1965, by Dudley, D. L., Masuda, M., Martin, C. J., and Holmes, T. H.

Table 1. Experimental Head Pain
(26 Subjects)

	RR	$\dot{V}_A$ (L/MIN)	F_{ACO_2} (%)	$\dot{V}_{O_2}$* (ML/MIN)	Blood Pressure Systolic	Blood Pressure Diastolic	Heart rate	Skin Temperature (°C)†
Control	12	5.5	5.6	301	128	80	81	29.7
period	±6	±0.8	±0.6	±43	±14	±12	±17	±3.2
Pain	14	11.0‡	4.3‡	386‡	158‡	102‡	87§	28.3§
period	±6	±4.3	±0.8	±75	±25	±17	±13	±2.8
Recovery	13	4.9	5.2	281	129	85	77	29.9
period	±7	±1.1	±0.6	±39	±10	±10	±16	±2.3

* 15 subjects.
† 25 subjects.
‡ $p < 0.001$.
§ $p < 0.05$.
(Differences are between control and pain periods.)

The respiratory and cardiovascular data shown in the tables in this chapter were based on 5 min measurement periods, even though continuous measurements were made before, during, and after stimulation. The choice of 5 min was made for convenience and because after being stimulated for a period of 15 to 20 min the subjects responded maximally for approximately 5 min. Mean changes and their interrelation with catecholamine excretion will be discussed in Chapter 11. Thus in the tables variations in measurements which occurred between the control period and subsequent period of maximal response are not represented. Data analysis utilized Student's t test for paired samples and the standard deviation from the mean.

OBSERVATIONS

Hyperventilation with Action-Orientation

The reasons given for participating in the experiments varied from feelings of obligation to the department or the experimenters, to those of six medical students who believed it was a requirement. Most expressed interest in what might happen during the experiments and were apprehensive about participating. All subjects felt "trapped" into participating and most would have considered withdrawing if it had not meant appearing "weak," "unable to take it," or that they were flouting the authority of the faculty members who requested that they participate.

The 26 subjects reacted to the stimulus with action-orientation (anger, anxiety, resentment, and a strong desire to end the experiment) directed at the headband and/or the experimenter and action-oriented behavioral responses (hypermobility and irritability) of varying degrees of intensity. The physiologic changes associated with the stimulus were those of hyperventilation, increased oxygen consumption, increased blood pressure and pulse rate, and decreased skin temperature. These changes are shown in Table 1. There were no statistically significant changes in respiratory rate. The mean length of time that the stimulus was tolerated was 24 min, with a range of 11 to 39 min. The verbal responses of the subjects when asked what they felt like doing at the point of maximum discomfort are shown in Table 2. As shown, most subjects felt like taking action of some form.

Exceptions to the Majority Reaction

Inspection of the individual protocols revealed that the behavior of three subjects in response to the stimulus was markedly different from the ma-

Table 2. Answers to the Question "What Did You Feel Like Doing at the Height of the Pain?"

Subject	Statement	Med. Stud.	Lab. Tech.	Tb. Subj.
1	I wished it were off. I would do anything just to terminate the pain.	X		
2	I wanted to ask you to stop. I wished it would hurry up and get over. I felt like getting out of the situation somehow.	X		
3	I got a little nervous toward the last. It didn't bother me much. It hurt all right, but it didn't aggravate me in any way. I can grin and bear that headband. I didn't feel like doing anything.			X
4	There was nothing I could do. The pain didn't bother me.			X
5	I didn't feel like doing anything about it. It just felt like a band of pain. It didn't particularly bother me.			X
6	I felt like taking the damned thing off. I kept thinking if you don't take the damned thing off I'm going to.			X
7	I wanted to take it off.			X
8	I just wanted to get out. I felt like grasping the damned clamp and throwing it off.	X		
9	I felt like waving my hands and saying let's chuck it. God Almighty I've got to get this thing over with.	X		
10	I felt like getting the . . . off, throwing the mouthpiece off and getting up. I was about ready to take the damned thing off.	X		
11	I wished the experiment were over and I were out of here. I just wished it were over with.	X		
12	I felt like taking it off. I felt like telling you to take it off.	X		
13	I wanted to get the darned thing off at any cost. I just wanted to get away. I wanted to get away at any cost.	X		
14	To hell with this . . .! Let me out of here. Enough! Enough! Enough!	X		
15	Just couldn't stand it for even another thirty seconds. [Too traumatized to communicate his feelings.]		X	
16	I felt like getting it off. I felt just like getting out.	X		
17	I felt like moving around. I felt like taking off the clamp.	X		
18	I wanted to make my escape actively. I felt like taking it off. I had a restless sensation to escape.	X		

19	I thought I had better do something about it.	X	
20	Either I wanted to get up and stamp my feet and move around or just call off the experiment. I felt that if it wasn't taken off I would have to quit.	X	
21	I just wanted to get out. I wanted to do something and couldn't.	X	
22	I would have liked to have taken it off if I thought I could have. I couldn't take much more and nearly said so. The thought flashed through my mind to tear the thing off.	X	
23	I wanted to take it off. I had to restrain from reaching up and unscrewing it. I said to myself that that was going to be it.	X	
24	I just felt like getting it off. I wanted to have the band taken off as soon as possible.	X	
25	I didn't feel like doing anything; I just wanted to get it off.		X
26	I wanted to rip that crown off my head, and then break up the place. I felt I was going to jump through the ceiling–rip that thing off–run around the room and then go to sleep.	X	

jority (Subjects 3, 4, and 5; Table 2). Although they admitted awareness of noxious sensations, they denied being "disturbed" or "upset" by the discomfort. However, each appeared to be tense, restless, and irritable, and asked to have the experiment discontinued when these reactions were marked. In contrast to the rest of the subjects they denied wanting to do anything to terminate the stimulus. As shown in Table 3, these subjects had

Table 3. DENIAL OF HEAD PAIN (3 SUBJECTS)

	RR	$\dot{V}_A$ (L/MIN)	F_{ACO_2} (%)	$\dot{V}_{O_2}$ (ML/MIN)*	Blood Pressure Systolic	Blood Pressure Diastolic	Heart Rate	Skin Temperature (°C)
Control period	20	7.0	5.0	281	119	88	92	28.6
Pain period	18	7.2	5.2	285	145	103	94	29.3
Recovery period	22	7.5	5.2	314	127	93	91	27.2

* One subject.

minimal changes in ventilation during the stimulus period. Oxygen consumption and VMA (3-methoxy 4-hydroxymandelic acid) measurements done on one of the subjects also showed little change (Fig. 4b). However, the blood pressure elevation was of a magnitude reached in many of the subjects who responded to the stimulus with overt emotional change. Two of the three subjects were the only subjects in the study with pulmonary disability (decreased exercise tolerance), and all three had had active pulmonary tuberculosis in the past. Two were females, age 46 and 50 (the oldest subjects in the study), and the third was a male, age 25. Two of these subjects will be presented in the case studies to follow.

In order to convey the essence of the emotions and behavior experienced during the experiments the observations on typical experiments are reported in detail.

Individual Case Reports

SUBJECT 1. Subject 1 was a 24-year-old white male, married medical student. During the course of the experiments he was working in the laboratory as a research fellow. Prior to the beginning of the first experiment the subject felt confident of his ability to manage the pain and maintained this attitude throughout the experiment. At the first adjustment and tightening of the headband the subject felt alert and tense, but experienced minimal discomfort. After 8 min the headband was tightened a second time and the subject experienced transitory head pain and an increasing feeling of general physical and mental discomfort.

At 15 min the band was tightened a third time. The pain was no longer transitory and the subject experienced a diffuse steady dull pain over the entire head region. During this period the subject felt tense and restless and kept thinking, "I wish it were off. What did I do it for?" Over the next 5 min the pain and feelings of restlessness steadily increased and the subject found it impossible to think of anything but the head pain and the urge to terminate it. From 17 to 20 min, the subject was aware of breathing fast and hard and felt numbness and tingling in his hands and arms. There was an increase in the systolic and diastolic blood pressure and pulse rate. He broke out in a cold sweat and was observed to have twitching of the facial muscles. He experienced feelings of helplessness, resentment, and agitation.

At 20 min he felt that he could no longer tolerate the pain, and the headband was removed.

After removal of the band the discomfort vanished and the subject was profoundly relieved. At this point he felt as though he had just finished some difficult, demanding physical task. The physiologic and biochemical data on this experiment are illustrated in Figure 1. Note the increase in VMA levels during the stimulus period.

Two days later the same subject was tested again. On this day he felt blue and tense. He lacked confidence in his ability to take the pain and forced himself to participate from fear of ridicule.

After the headband was placed and tightened he felt an overwhelming desire to sleep and his eyes felt too heavy to keep open. At 10 min the pain was of a low intensity which was easily ignored and the subject felt restless. After 17 min the band was tightened a second time, and it produced a severe,

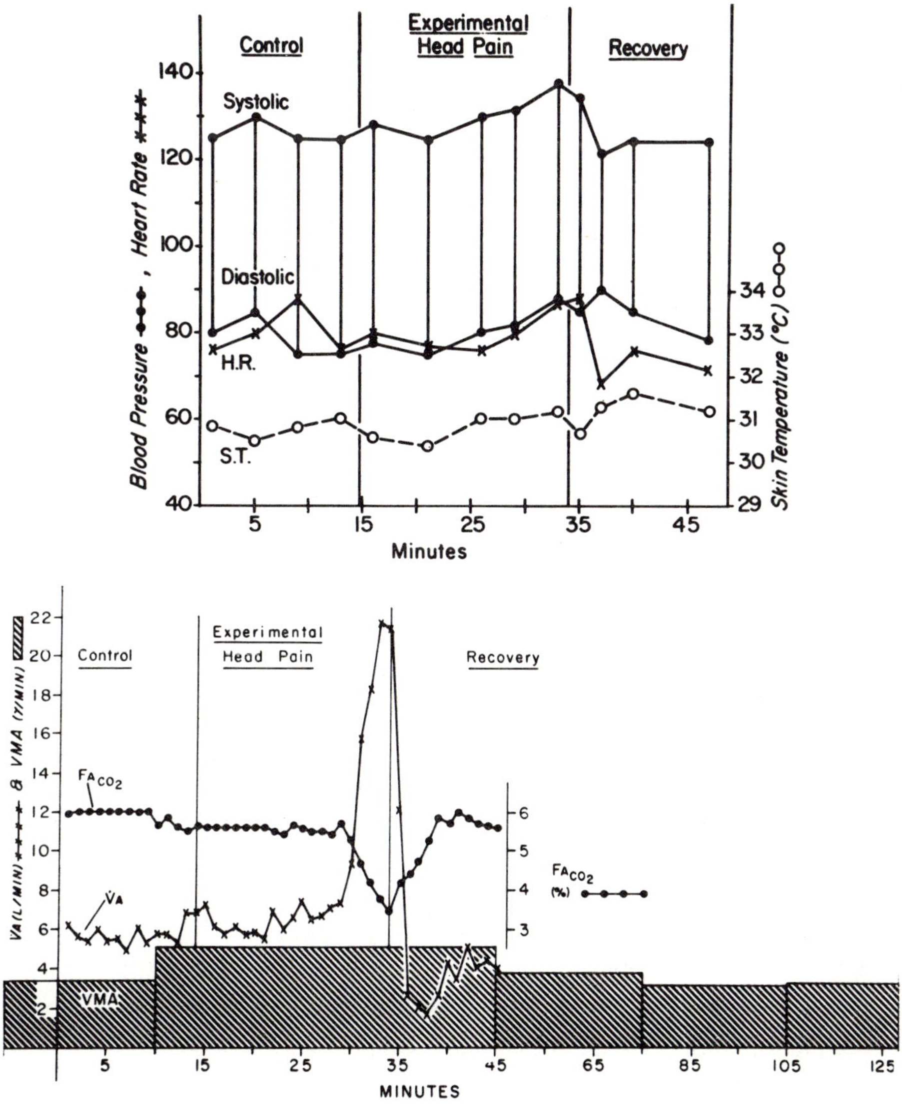

Fig. 1. Top. Cardiovascular response of Subject 1 to experimental head stimulation on day when he felt confident and sure of his ability to withstand stimulus situation. Bottom. Respiratory response of Subject 1 to experimental head stimulation on day when he felt confident and sure of his ability to withstand stimulus situation. Note elevation of VMA excretion.

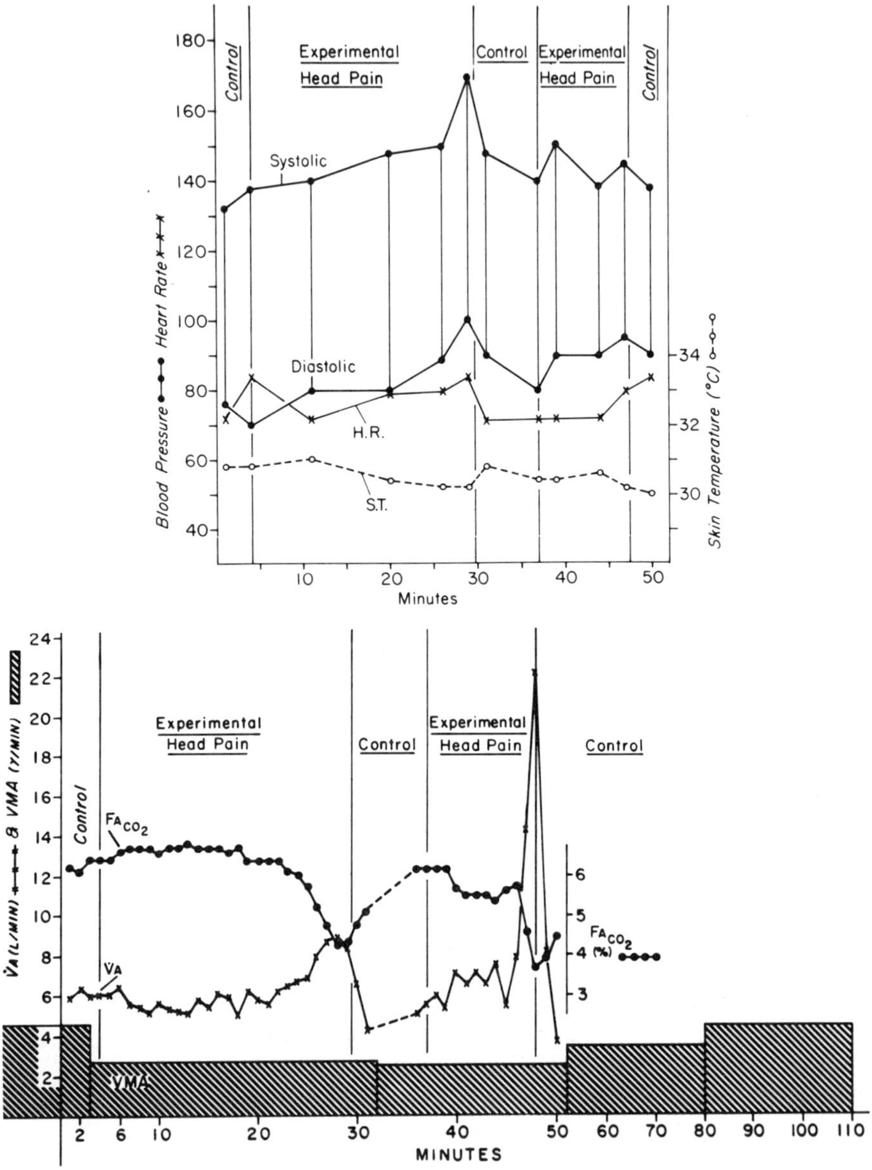

Fig. 2. Top. Cardiovascular response of Subject 1 to experimental head stimulation on day when he felt depressed and unsure of his ability to withstand stimulus. Bottom. Respiratory response of Subject 1 to experimental head stimulation on day when he felt depressed and unsure of his ability to withstand stimulus situation. Note decrease in VMA excretion.

dull, steady pain over the entire head superior to the band. The subject could no longer sit still and he kept thinking, "What in the hell am I doing this for?" and felt resentful and anxious. He was warm, sweating, and exceedingly uncomfortable. After 25 min he felt that he had had all he could take and the band was removed. At this point one of the experimenters wondered out loud if this subject had withstood as much pain as the other subjects. As a result the subject believed that he had to "prove myself" and he volunteered to have the experiment repeated even though he felt "miserable and depressed."

After collection of a urine sample the band was placed on the subject's head and tightened. Three minutes later the band was tightened again. At this time the subject again became very restless, resentful, and anxious. The pain quickly reached a peak and the band had to be removed after 12 min.

After the experiment the subject felt exceedingly relieved and very tired—much more so than during the previous experiment. Data on this experiment are shown in Figure 2. Note the decrease in VMA excretion.

SUBJECT 2. Subject 2 was a 25-year-old white male, married medical student who reacted to the pain in a manner very similar to that of Subject 1. The pain was constant and dull and extended over the entire upper half of the head. He felt restless and could not concentrate. He felt that his respiratory rate and blood pressure increased. He said that he felt "like getting out of the stituation somehow." The data on this subject are included here in order to illustrate changes in oxygen consumption and one of the greater increases in blood pressure and decreases in skin temperature noted during head pain (Figure 3).

SUBJECT 3. Subject 3 was a 25-year-old, divorced laborer who was admitted to the hospital with far-advanced pulmonary tuberculosis, bronchial asthma, and chronic obstructive pulmonary disease. He had contracted polio as an infant and crippling foot deformities had resulted. He was unable to walk until after the first of several surgical operations for correction of the deformities (at the age of seven). After this first of nine operations, he developed a severe attack of asthma which lasted for several days. He had never been free from attacks since that time. He had much pain associated with the corrective operations and subsequent physical therapy and lived at the hospital until he was 16 years of age. In this setting he dealt with pain by developing drowsiness or emotional detachment.

Two experiments with the headband were done. During the first head pain experience he felt an intense desire to sleep. He claimed that the pain had not aggravated him in any way, although toward the end of the experiment he said he felt a "little nervous." He did not feel like doing anything, even though he admitted that the band hurt. Respiratory rate and minute ventilation were reduced during the pain, blood pressure and skin temperature were increased, and there was minimal or no change in pulse rate or alveolar ventilation.

During the second pain experiment this subject also showed decreased respiratory rate and minute ventilation, but minimal to no change in the fractional concentration of alveolar carbon dioxide, alveolar ventilation, oxygen consumption, catecholamine excretion, blood pressure, and pulse rate over control values. Skin temperature changes were variable. These measurements are illustrated in Figure 4. The small change in alveolar ventilation shown is due to the fact that during the control period the dead space air occupied 38 per-

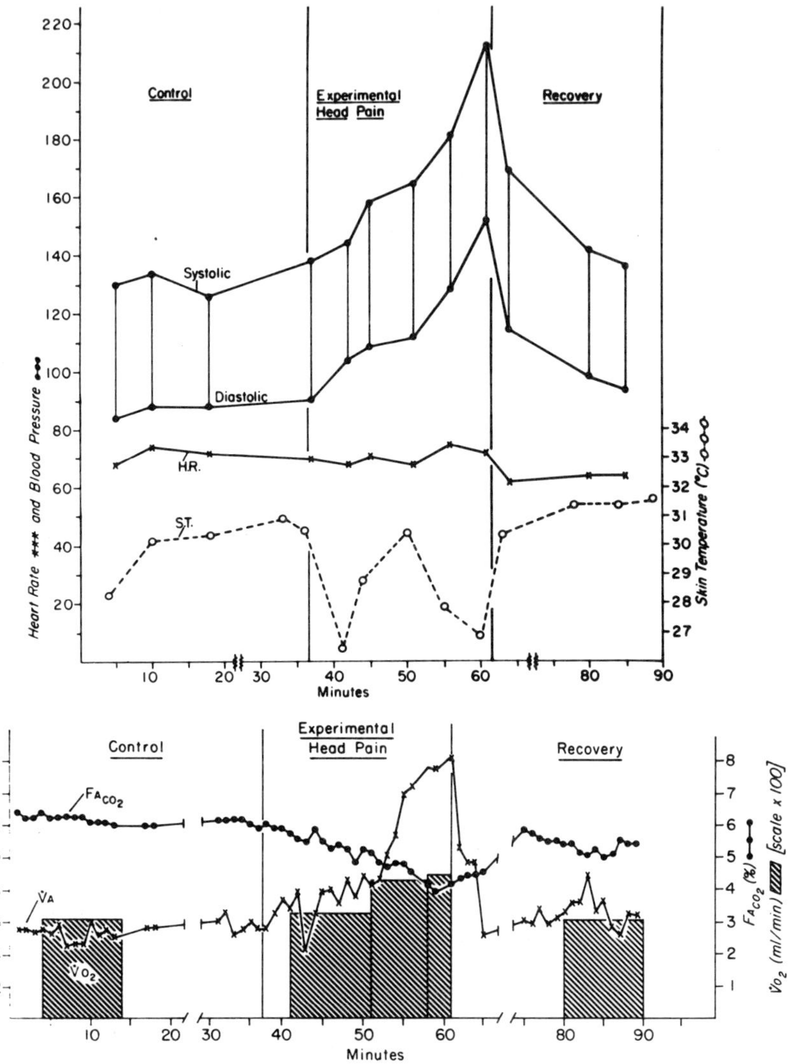

Fig. 3. Top. Cardiovascular response of Subject 2 to actual head stimulation. Bottom. Respiratory response of Subject 2 to actual head stimulation. Note increase in oxygen consumption which corresponds to period of increased muscular activity.

cent of the total ventilation and during the last minutes of the pain experiment, the dead space represented approximately 26 percent of the total ventilation. Thus, although there was a decrease in minute ventilation of approximately 1.5 L, because of the drop in dead space the alveolar ventilation remained essentially unchanged. Unlike Subjects 1 and 2, he showed no change in VMA execretion.

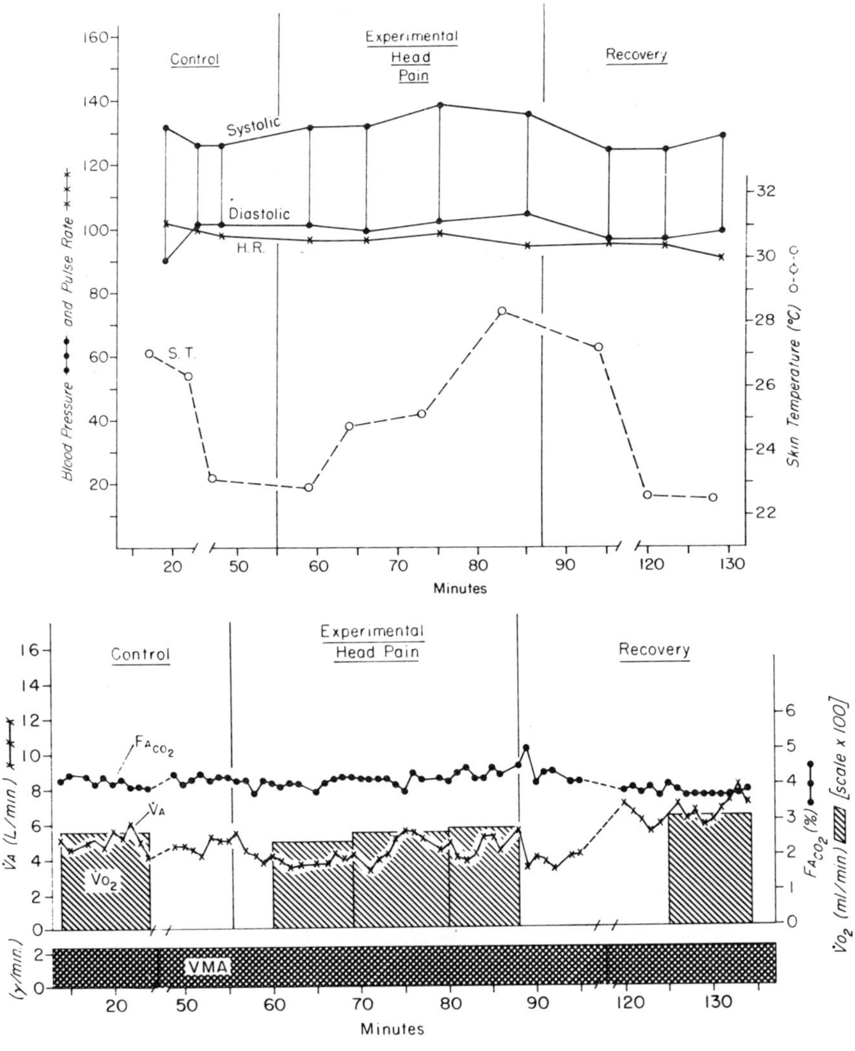

Fig. 4. Top. Cardiovascular response of Subject 3 to actual head stimulation. Bottom. Respiratory response of Subject 3 to actual head stimulation. Despite almost complete lack of respiratory system activation and lack of change in VMA, this subject showed marked changes in skin temperature and mild changes in blood pressure.

In contrast to the first pain experiment, he did not feel drowsy. He said that the pain made him feel "depressed" and stated "I just felt–something like being down in the dumps." He did not feel like doing anything about the pain as he felt that there was nothing that could be done. He admitted to getting a little irritated at the height of the pain, but insisted that "it didn't bother me a bit."

SUBJECT 4. Subject 4 was a 50-year-old white female, three-times-divorced commercial artist who was undergoing treatment for peptic ulcer. She had been hospitalized three times for tuberculosis and had experienced considerable shortness of breath on exertion and with emotional upsets.

Prior to the headband experiment she described her breathing as good and said that her spirits were high. During the experiment she admitted to feeling an intense pressure on her head, caused by the band, but denied that it was ever severe enough to lead to termination of the experiment. Instead, she terminated the experiment because of a severe, sharp, superficial pain in her stomach which came in waves and was much more severe than the pressure on her head. During the stimulus period she felt warm, sweated profusely, experienced nausea, wanted to vomit, was short of breath and "panicky," and developed

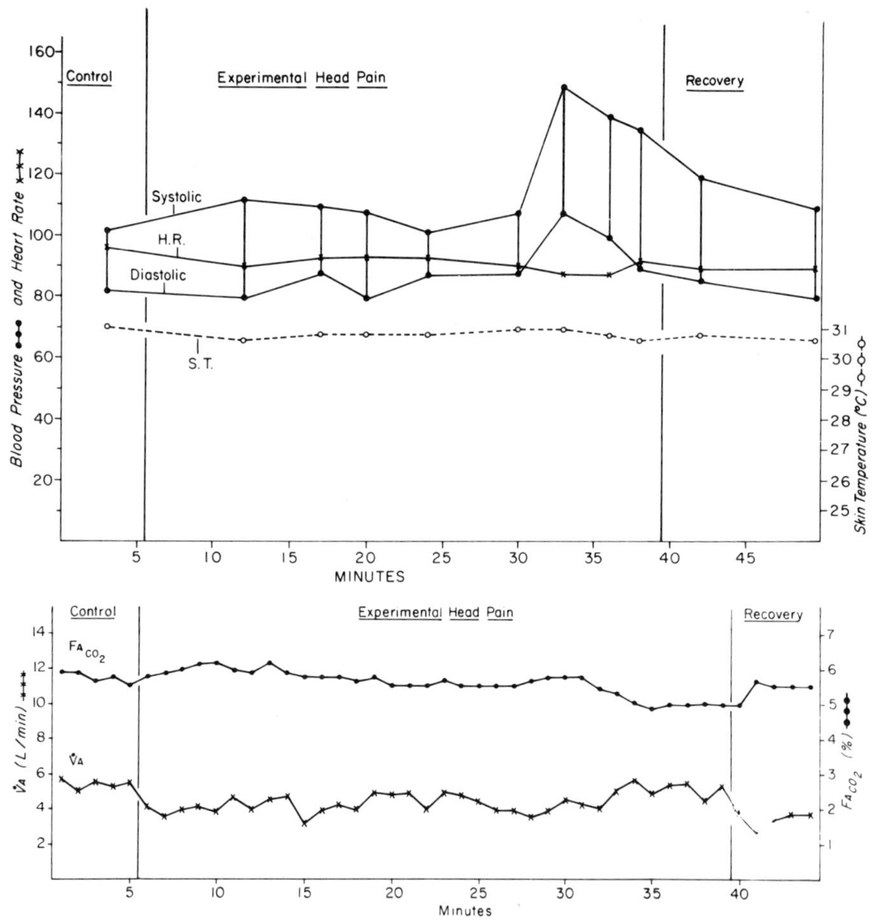

Fig. 5. Top. Cardiovascular response of Subject 4 to actual head stimulation. Bottom. Respiratory response of Subject 4 to actual head stimulation.

obvious distention of her abdomen. She remarked that "there was nothing I could do about it."

For 25 min after the stimulus these symptoms continued with a gradual decrease in severity. During the poststimulation period she reported that the pain and nausea were identical to that which occurred when "painful people bother me."

When she left the laboratory 50 min after stimulation, she was almost fully recovered. However, her stomach remained swollen. At this time she indicated that anyone who could not take the headband was a "sissy" and she hoped that she had not ruined the experiment by terminating after 34 min. She persisted in her contention that the head pain was not the stimulus which caused her to terminate the experiment, but that the severe stomach pain was responsible.

As shown in Figure 5 there was a mild hyperventilation response with an increase in blood pressure and essentially no change in pulse rate or skin temperature.

DISCUSSION

Pain is a sensation which foretells of tissue injury and thereby warns the organism to remove the stimulus producing the pain or to escape. This statement also applies to noxious sensations in general, provided action is possible and is an acceptable form of response. For this reason it was thought that the headband used in this experiment should produce a relatively pure, action-oriented response in the experimental setting described. It is recognized that the pain produced by the headband constituted only a part of the stimulation experienced by the subjects. Therefore, the experimental setting has been termed a "noxious situation" and includes factors in addition to the pain (e.g., anxiety about the experiment and anger at the experimenter for placing the subject in a situation from which he could not gracefully escape) which contributed to the total psychologic and physiologic response.

In the largely young male population utilized, the response to the noxious situation was almost always that of action-orientation exemplified by the emotional, behavioral, and physiologic changes described. The biological usefulness of this response is that of placing the body in an optimal position to respond by physical exertion. In an appropriate setting this response would be advantageous. However, in the setting in which it occurred, it is lacking in relevance and pertinence.

Examination of individual protocols revealed three subjects who had nontypical reactions. Two of these subjects were middle-aged women and one was a 25-year-old male. All three had had active tuberculosis in the past. They were observably upset during the experiments, as evidenced by restlessness and irritability. However, they would not admit that the stimulus bothered them and denied wanting to terminate the experiment. Despite their denial of desiring to terminate the experiment, they all indicated that they had had enough of the experiment when their irritability and restlessness reached a high level. After the experiment was over they persisted in saying that the stimulus had not bothered them and they only ended the experiment because "I had had enough" or because of "the stomach pain." They showed minimal to no respiratory hyperfunction and an increase in blood pressure. Their responses appeared to be a mixture of action-orientation and nonaction-orientation.

Subject 3 provides an example of how the action orientation of behavior can be modified to produce the variant response found in these three subjects. This 25-year-old male had experienced painful medical procedures for the correction of polio-induced foot deformities from age 3 months to 16 years. From age 7 to 16 his divorced mother left him in a children's hospital without visiting him. In this setting he learned that dealing with pain by action was largely ineffective and he thereby responded with detachment, depression, and drowsiness. Also, pain became equated with desirable medical procedures and thereby was something to accept. As a result of these past conditioning experiences he responded to the headache with a mixture of action-orientation and nonaction-orientation. This reaction was characterized by depression, drowsiness, irritability, hyperactivity, increased blood pressure, and a lack of respiratory hyperfunction.

The data on VMA show that VMA excretion does not correlate with changes in the cardiovascular and respiratory parameters. This is well illustrated by Subject 1. Although this subject reacted to the stimulus with resentment, anxiety, and physiologic hyperfunction during the second pain experiment, as he had during the first, the psychologic setting of the experiment was different in that he did not feel confident of his abilities to withstand the stimulus as he had during the first experiment. This change in psychologic outlook was followed by a fall in VMA excretion, whereas VMA excretion had increased during the first experiment.

Catecholamine excretion during noxious head stimulation will be discussed in Chapter 11.

SUMMARY

1. Twenty-six subjects were studied before, during, and after stimulation with a metal headband.

2. The predominant response was that of emotional, behavioral, and physiologic activation.

3. Changes in VMA were not associated with changes in respiratory and cardiac physiology.

4. The variations in physiologic changes associated with the stimulus are seen as different methods of preparing the subject to undertake physical activity.

REFERENCES

Wolff, H. G. Headache and Other Head Pain, 2nd ed. New York, Oxford University Press, 1963.

11

Noxious Head Stimulation: Integration of the Physiologic Response

The autonomic nervous system has long been monitored as an indicator of the state of "arousal" or "activation" of the organism. This oversimplification of a complex psychological and physiological state is an extension of the function of the sympathetic nervous system as envisioned by Cannon. The sympathetic response was conceived as being a mass discharge through the system, preparing the organism by mobilizing its "energies" in the face of an external challenge. The role of the autonomic system in environmental exchanges has been extended to include a particularistic relationship between physiological and psychological events.

In this investigation, the pattern of physiologic response to a specific challenge (noxious head stimulation) was studied further. The stimulus—as noted in Chapter 10—results in a spectrum or amalgamation of changes including headache, pain, anger, frustration, anxiety, or withdrawal.

The subjects were 28 young male medical students, studied before and during stimulation with a metal headband having 14 adjustable rubber-tipped screws around the edges (see Chapter 10).

Twenty-one subjects (Group 1) had physiological, catecholamine, and behavioral variables measured during the stimulus. In the remaining seven subjects (Group 2), only the catecholamine metabolite excretion was measured. This latter group also had catecholamine excretion measurements done at similar time periods when the subjects were engaged in their regular daily routine. The mean values for the entire stimulus period were utilized in the totals to be described.

This chapter is adapted from an article originally published in *J Psychosom Res*, 12:205, 1968, by Masuda, M., and Dudley, D. L.

OBSERVATIONS

Group 1

Figure 1 is a graphic representation of the mean changes in the cardiovascular and respiratory variables during the prestimulus and stimulus pe-

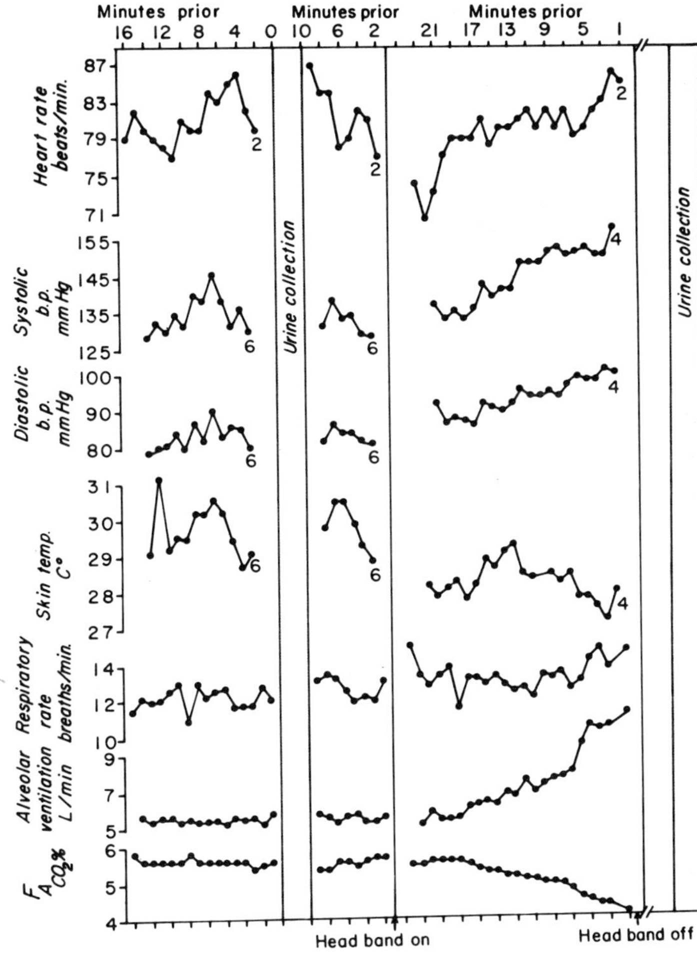

Fig. 1. Mean measurements of cardiovascular and respiratory variables during prestimulus and stimulus periods. Numbers on figure indicate that values represent 2-, 4-, or 6-min moving averages. Respiratory rate, alveolar ventilation, and fractional concentration of alveolar carbon dioxide were measured continuously. Values given are means for all 21 male medical students in Group 1.

riods. The cardiovascular variables are represented as curves of moving averages. It is readily evident that there were parallel increases during the noxious stimulation period in the diastolic and systolic blood pressures, the heart rate, and alveolar ventilation. The $F_{A_{CO_2}}$ curve shows an inverse downward trend. These relationships were corroborated by using Spearman's rank order correlation coefficients between the moving averages of these variables during the stimulation. In addition, skin temperature showed a negative correlation to the respiratory rate and the latter a negative correlation to the $F_{A_{CO_2}}$.

The mean titers during the headband stimulation are compared with those during the prestimulation period in three categories of physiological variables (Table 1). Significant increases were seen in respiratory rate, alveolar ventilation, and oxygen consumption, with a concomitant decrease

Table 1. MEAN MEASURES OF VARIABLES ACCORDING TO URINE COLLECTION PERIODS

VARIABLE	PRE-STIMULUS	STIMULUS	PERCENT CHANGE*	SIGNIFICANCE (P)†
Respiratory				
Respiratory rate, breaths/min (RR)	12.2	13.3	+11	<0.01
Alveolar ventilation, liters/min ($\dot{V}_A$)	5.51	7.16	+30	<0.01
Alveolar carbon dioxide, % ($F_{A_{CO_2}}$)	5.63	5.20	−6	<0.01
Oxygen consumption, cc/min ($\dot{V}_{O_2}$)	301	354	+12	<0.01
Cardiovascular				
Heart rate, beat/min (HR)	82.4	82.1	+0.4	NS
Systolic blood pressure, mm Hg (SBP)	130	142	+9	<0.01
Diastolic blood pressure, mm Hg (DBP)	81	91	+12	<0.01
Skin temperature, C° (ST)	29.6	28.4	−4	<0.01
Urinary				
Urine flow, cc/min (U)	.98	1.15	+29	<0.05
Creatinine, mgm/min (CR)	1.31	1.36	+14	NS
3-methoxy-4-hydroxymandelic acid, μg/min (VMA)	2.38	2.78	+19	<0.05
Normetadrenaline, μg/hr (NMA)	5.51	6.12	+23	NS
Metadrenaline, μg/hr (MA)	5.70	6.62	+28	NS

* Percent change as mean of individual percent changes.
† Wilcoxon signed rank test (paired replicates).

in alveolar carbon dioxide concentration. In the cardiovascular variables, increases in systolic and diastolic pressures were accompanied by a drop in skin temperature, but with no significant change in the mean heart rate. There were increases in the urinary variables of flow rate and VMA, but no changes in the NMA, MA, and creatinine. Thus the distinctive mean changes which occurred in the respiratory and cardiovascular variables during the experimental period were less evident than those in the urinary variables.

In a further analysis of the data, the incremental changes which occurred in the variables between the control and the experimental period ($Vx_{1\text{-}2}$ vs $V_{Y_{1\text{-}2}}$) were correlated. The significant correlations (Spearman's rho) are shown in Table 2. There is a sharp contrast to the data of Figure 1.

Table 2. Significant (Spearman's Rho) Intercorrelations of Variables Using Incremental Changes on Stimulation

	1	2	3	4	5	6	7	8	9	10	11	12	13
	HR	SBP	DBP	ST	RR	$\dot{V}_A$	F_{ACO_2}	$\dot{V}_{O_2}$	U	CR	VMA	NMA	MA
1						.534				−.564	−.592		
2			.836									−.548	
3													
4													
5													
6													
7													
8													
9											674	.527	.564
10											.547		
11													
12													884

$r_s = 0.05 = 0.521.$

Within the respiratory and cardiovascular groups of variables, the only intracategory change which was positively correlated was that of systolic and diastolic blood pressures. Within the urinary category, the urine flow change was positively correlated to the catecholamine metabolites. The VMA excretion change showed a positive correlation to creatinine and the changes in NMA and MA excretions were highly and positively correlated.

The number of significant intercorrelations between variables of the three different categories are also few in number. Heart rate changes showed a positive correlation with the alveolar ventilation and a negative correlation with the changes in creatinine and VMA excretions. There was a negative correlation between systolic blood pressure change and the change in the excretion of normetadrenaline which is unexplained.

The changes from prestimulus to stimulus titers in the spectrum of variables of each individual revealed considerable difference in patterns. The number of individuals showing changes in each of the variables are shown in Table 3. Significance in the cardiovascular and respiratory variables was judged by the Wilcoxon rank sum method applied to the individuals' titers. In the case of the urinary variables which involved single determinations on each collection period for each individual, there is no

Table 3. NUMBERS OF INDIVIDUALS SHOWING CHANGES IN VARIABLES FROM PRESTIMULUS TO STIMULUS PERIODS

CHANGE	HR	SBP	DBP	ST	RR	$\dot{V}_A$	F_{ACO_2}	$\dot{V}_{O_2}$	U	CR	VMA	NMA	MA
Increase	3	16	15	1	5	15	0	8	15	9	14	14	14
No change	12	5	6	9	15	6	7	6	0	0	3	0	0
Decrease	6	0	0	11	1	0	14	0	6	12	4	7	7

statistical device for the determination of significant changes. In Table 3 these responses are noted as simple positive or negative changes from the initial titer.

It is evident that comparable numbers of individuals were responding to stimuli with increases in systolic and diastolic blood pressures and alveolar ventilation. Comparable numbers of individuals showed reductions in skin temperature and F_{ACO_2}. These changes were in the expected direction (Fig. 1; Table 1). However, the same individuals who showed increases in one variable were not necessarily the same individuals who showed increases in another.

Evidence for the above-noted observation is shown in Figure 2, which presents four diagrams of selected individual patterns of responses. Each individual's pattern is represented as a circle of response changes with each category of system variables as a halved trisection of the circle. The horizontal midline demarcates two semicircles or areas that above the line represent physiological activation and/or increase in titer and below the line represent physiological inhibition and/or decrease in titer. The radial lines indicate the variables, the direction of change, and the percent change from the initial level of each of the variables. The initial level is represented as the heavy inner circle. The outer circle represents a 100 percent change from the initial value, and the fainter middle circle indicates a 50 percent change utilized as an index of the magnitude of the response change. A significant change (as previously defined) is marked with an asterisk. A reduction in skin temperature and decrease in F_{ACO_2} are here represented as an activation process.

In Figure 2, two of the four response patterns, A and D, represent the

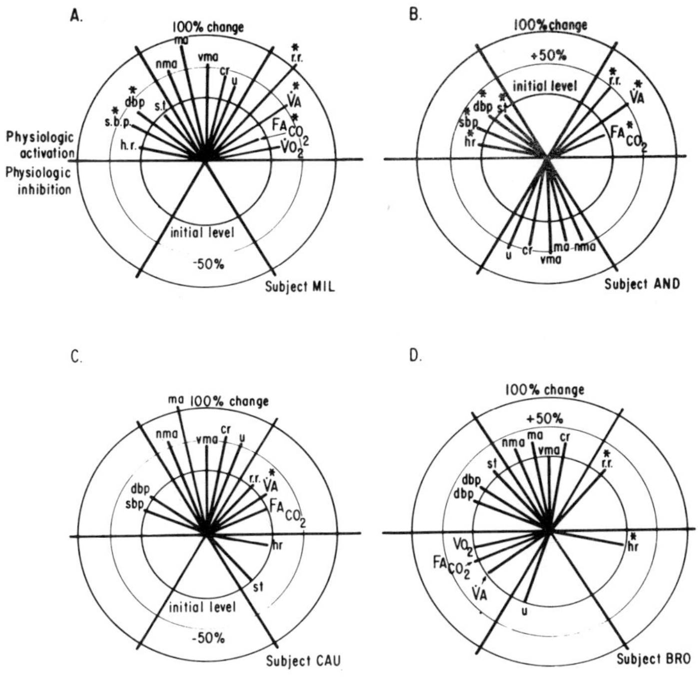

Fig. 2. Selected patterns of physiological responses to noxious head stimulation. Each individual's pattern is represented as a circle of change with each system represented as halved trisection of the circle. Initial level is represented as heavy inner circle. Plus and minus signs represent change in positive or negative direction. As illustrated, there is no one consistent pattern of response that characterized all subjects. However, most patterns represent various degrees of activation. Significant changes are marked with asterisk. Subject D represents the least degree of activation encountered and Subject A the most.

extremes of the activation and nonactivation concept. Response patterns B and C represent intermediate and mixed patterns. In response pattern A all variables were in the direction of activation. In the cardiovascular and respiratory systems, five of the seven variables were significantly changed and the oxygen consumption increase was 22 percent—almost double the mean oxygen consumption change (Table 1). The catecholamine metabolites showed increments in titers greater than 50 percent of the initial levels and more than double the mean percent changes (Table 1). The creatinine increase was also double the mean percent change (Table 1). The increase in urine flow of 28 percent was similar to the mean significant change of 29 percent (Table 1).

Response pattern D, by contrast, showed a significant increase only in respiratory rate, while displaying a significant decrease in heart rate. The urinary variables did not show changes that were impressive as assessed by the interindividual mean changes. In response pattern B, all cardiovascular and respiratory variables showed significant increases—but the urinary variables showed uniform reductions of 33 to 61 percent. Response pattern C, on the other hand, showed a significant change only in alveolar ventilation,

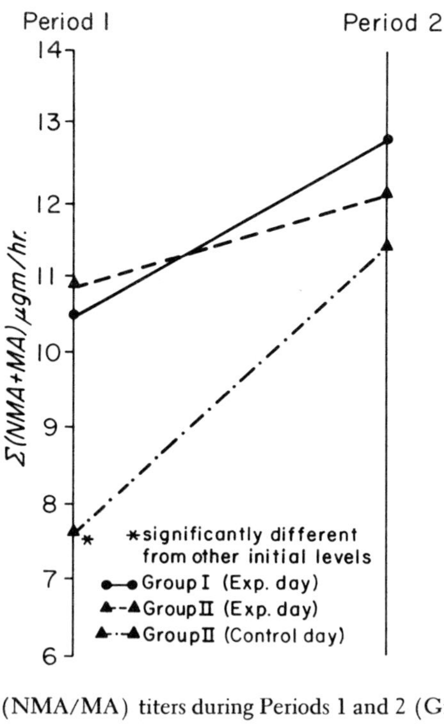

Fig. 3. Mean (NMA/MA) titers during Periods 1 and 2 (Groups I and II).

while most urinary variables showed increases of greater than 50 percent of control levels. The majority of the individual response patterns were of mixed types B and C, and were further complicated by nonuniformity of variables within the three system categories.

Group 2

In the seven medical students for whom head stimulation days and control days were compared, only the urinary NMA and MA were measured. In view of the preceding findings from Group 1 (Table 2) and previous findings from this laboratory of consistent and highly significant correlations of NMA and MA, these two urinary titers were summed as total 3-methoxycatecholamine metabolites Σ(NMA + MA). The data for these seven subjects on the experimental day and on a subsequent control day are shown in Figure 3. Also included for comparison is the Σ(NMA + MA) data from the 21 subjects of Group 1. The slight parallel rise in titer during the experimental head stimulation periods for both groups is not significant. On control day there was a significantly higher level in titer in period 2, the explanation for which is unknown. However, the most pertinent fact is that the levels for Group 2 period 1 on control day were significantly lower than the prestimulation levels on experimental days in both groups.

DISCUSSION

The response of subjects to the headband stimulation was generally one of heightened activation characterized by affects of anger and anxiety, and overt behavioral responses of restlessness and tension. An essential feature of the psychological response was the intense desire to act in a manner which would decrease or remove the stimulus.

These affective and behavioral changes were accompanied by physiological responses during the head stimulation period in the respiratory and cardiovascular systems. The concept of overall "activation" to the noxious head stimulus is supported by the time course of these physiological responses, which show distinct trends and a significant difference in the mean titers.

However, these distinct activation responses were not accompanied by mean increases in titers of NMA and MA, the 3-methoxycatecholamine metabolites. In view of the prime role of the sympathetic nervous system in psychophysiological responses, the lack of significant change in catecholamine metabolites is puzzling. Lack of uniformity in the direction of responses could possibly account for the absence of mean changes. If so, this might be evidenced as a difference in the variances of the mean prestimulus and stimulus titers of the catecholamines. No such difference of variance was found.

A second consideration which may account for the lack of catecholamine metabolite response in the face of distinct physiological, emotional, and behavioral change is the possible fallibility of the urinary NMA and MA as indices which reflect acute blood pressure changes. Previously the insensitivity of the VMA measure was explained on the basis of: (1) the efficiency of neuroeffector transmission; (2) the nonlinear and nonparallel curves relating physiological change to transmitter overflow; and (3) the probable production of the bulk of VMA at an intraneuronal catecholamine binding site. It had been anticipated that NMA and MA, being primary and differentiated metabolites, would reflect sympathetic activity changes. From a consideration of the data of Kopin and Gordon, it was evident that there was a decreasing order of sensitivity in the use of catecholamines and their metabolites as indices of acute change in the release of the neurotransmitter from the adrenergic neurone. This apparent increase in sensitivity of the NMA titer over the VMA titer was not sufficient to detect increased sympathetic activation. Thus the duration and the intensity of physiological activity are of importance in the consideration of the likelihood of these activities being reflected in the urinary metabolites.

A third and final factor which might result in an absence of urinary catecholamine response to the headband might be a result of the level of the initial titers in the prestimulus period. In Figure 3 it is evident that the control day prestimulus titers (period 1) were significantly lower than the prestimulus titers on the experimental day. This suggests that on experimental days the subjects came to the stimulus situation in a state of diffuse sympathetic activation such that imposition of the noxious stimulation did not elicit a further significant catecholamine secretion. The threat of the headband was sufficient to produce a state of overall sympathetic "arousal." The imposition of the headband changed this unknown generalized threat to a specific intense noxious challenge which the individuals met with individual patterns of physiological, emotional, and behavioral changes. The consistent increases in blood pressure are presumed to be a result of the channeling of the diffuse sympathetic discharge into specific cardiovascular channels.

Concomitant with the absence of changes in catecholamine metabolite excretion with noxious head stimulation was an increase in urine flow rate and no change in creatinine excretion. The studies of Schottstaedt et al. demonstrated that his behavioral Pattern A—"tension, increased demand, alert, ready, and confident"—was associated with decreased urine volumes and decreased creatinine excretions. Pattern B, also definable as an action oriented attitude, was characterized as "excitement, anxiety, apprehension, lack of confidence," while Pattern B^1, a variant, was characterized as "anger, aggressiveness, irritation." In both of these Pattern B states, urine flow and creatinine excretions were increased. It appears that the noxious stimulus used in this study led to an action-oriented attitude, but with such varying degrees of affect as to nullify significant trends. A further analysis of the urine flow and creatinine excretion changes with noxious stimulation in individuals did not show a predominance of any of the patterns described by Schottstaedt et al. Only one showed Pattern A; six showed Patterns B and B^1; and five showed no change in both variables. The other response patterns were mixed.

The cardiovascular system had responded to the stimulus with significant changes in systolic and diastolic blood pressure and in skin temperature. However, in the intercorrelations of the variable changes from prestimulus to stimulus, only the blood pressures were correlated to each other. This suggests that as a group and within individuals, the blood pressure changes were generally parallel. The skin temperature changes and heart rate changes were not related to pressure changes within individuals. The lack of covariance of cardiovascular variables has been reported by other investigators. Similarly, the intercorrelations of the mean respiratory titers seen during the head stimulation are nonexistent when one compares the incremental change in one variable with the change in another.

With regard to the intercorrelations of the changes in the urinary variables, there was a strong correlation between changes in NMA and MA titers—indicating the parallel secretory changes of NA and A. Urine flow changes were here correlated with the catecholamine metabolite excretions. The correlation of creatinine and VMA excretions is not unexpected in view of the evidence which relates VMA excretion to creatinine and body weight, and to intraneuronal metabolic degradation of continually synthesized and catabolized noradrenaline that is not physiologically active.

Intercorrelations of variable changes among the three categories of physiological variables were also notable for their scarcity (Table 3). This lack of intercategory correlations reveals that the individual pattern of response is far from uniform between systems. This is indicative not only of individuality of responses but also of the importance of prestimulus levels in the direction of individual responses.

The positive correlations found between measurements within physiological categories are taken as a consistency within particular systems which relates to a generalized pattern of coping behavior. The lack of consistency in patterns within and between physiological systems is indicative of the individual's ability to fragment physiological behaviors according to his individual style of adaptation.

Psychophysiological investigations have shown that there are many factors which can influence the direction and magnitude of autonomic and somatic variables—not the least of these is individual idiosyncrasy. A particularly favored response channel to certain stimuli has been termed "symptom specificity." An individual tends to retain his hierarchy of variable response patterns over time, and further, these patterns are reproducible by using a variety of stimuli.

The present study has demonstrated individualistic patterns of responses. The individual's pattern of response changes from prestimulus to stimulus and can be visualized as differences in the manner in which he copes with the stimulus. It is compounded of two phases: the preparatory or prestimulus coping behavior and the subsequent responsivity during the actual stimulation. Both behaviors are meaningful in the adaptive behavior process.

The fragmentation of behavioral responses may be analogous to the protective reaction pattern described by Wolff in relating disease processes to physiological changes. The selection of a particular localized reaction is a fragmentation of the many reactions possible within any particular system and follows the "principle of parsimony" which states that an individual will utilize a minimum of responses as a means of adaptation to an external challenge. This concept is extended here beyond consideration of disease processes to encompass the response patterns in those physiological systems which participate in an adaptive reaction. The fragmented response patterns are an end result of the individual's past experience and represent —whether appropriate or not—a workable, useful physiological behavior, often specifically channelled and individually adapted.

SUMMARY

1. Twenty-eight male medical students were subjected to experimental intense noxious stimulation of the head. Three categories of physiological responses were measured before and during the experimental period.

2. Significant mean differences were found between the prestimulus and stimulus periods in the respiratory variables of alveolar ventilation, oxygen consumption, alveolar carbon dioxide concentration, and respiratory rate. In the cardiovascular responses, mean differences were found in systolic and diastolic blood pressures and skin temperature, but not in heart rate. No mean differences were found in the creatinine excretion rate and

the catecholamine metabolite excretion rates of normetadrenaline (NMA) and metadrenaline (MA).

3. The absence of mean catecholamine metabolite changes with the noxious stimulation, despite behavioral, emotional, and physiological activation, is attributed to elevated prestimulus levels and/or insensitivity of these urinary metabolites.

4. The lack of intercorrelations in the changes within and between categories of physiological responses is attributed to individual response patterns and interpreted as indicating the ability of the individual to "fragment" and "channelize" functions in terms of his own protective or adaptive, metabolic, and behavioral needs.

REFERENCES

Axelrod, J. The uptake and release of catecholamines and the effect of drugs, in Progress in Brain Research, Vol. 8, Biogenic Amines, Himwich, H. E., and Himwich, W. A., eds. New York, Elsevier Publishing Co., 1964, p. 81-89.

Brodie, B. B. Recent views on mechanisms for lowering sympathetic tone, Circulation, 28:970, 1963.

Brown, G. L., and Gillespie, J. S. Output of sympathin from the spleen, Nature, 178:980, 1956.

Cannon, W. B. Bodily Changes in Pain, Hunger, Fear, and Rage, 2nd ed. Boston, Charles T. Branford Co., 1953.

Celander, O. The range of control exercised by the sympathicoadrenal system, Acta Physiol Scand, 34 (Suppl. 116), 1954.

Dudley, D. L., Holmes, T. H., Martin, C. J., and Ripley, H. S. Changes in respiration associated with hypnotically induced emotion, pain, and exercise, Psychosom Med, 26:46, 1964.

——— Masuda, M., Martin, C. J., and Holmes, T. H. Psychophysiological studies of experimentally induced action oriented behavoir, J Psychosom Res, 9:209, 1965.

Folkow, B. Impulse frequency in sympathetic vasomotor fibers correlated to the release and elimination of the transmitter, Acta Physiol Scand, 25:49, 1952.

Kopin, I. J., and Gordon, E. K. Metabolism of norepinephrine-H^3 released by tyramine and reserpine, J Pharmacol Exp Therap, 138:351, 1962.

Lacey, J. I. Psychophysiological approaches to the evaluation of psychotherapeutic process and outcome, in Research in Psychotherapy, Rubinstein, E. A., and Parloff, M. B., eds. Washington, D.C., American Psychological Ass. Inc., 1959, p. 160-208.

Malmo, R. B., Shagass, C., and Davis, F. H. Specificity of bodily reactions under stress: A physiological study of somatic mechanisms in psychiatric patients. Res Publ Ass Res Nerv Ment Dis, 29:231, 1950.

Masuda, M. Differing adaptive metabolic behaviors, J Psychosom Res, 10:239, 1966.

——— and Bakker, C. B. Personality, catecholamine metabolites, and psychophysiological response to diazepam, J Psychiat Res, 4:221, 1966.

McDonald, R. K., and Weise, V. K. The excretion of 3-methoxy-4-hydroxymandelic acid in normal and in chronic schizophrenic male subjects, J Psychiat Res, 1:173, 1963.

Nelson, G., Masuda, M., and Holmes, T. H. Correlation of behavior and catecholamine metabolite excretion, Psychosom Med, 27:216, 1966.

Schottstaedt, W. W., Grace, W. J., and Wolff, H. G. Life situations, behavior, attitudes, emotions, and renal excretion of fluid and electrolytes: I. Method of study, J Psychosom Res, 1:75, 1956.

——— Grace, W. J., and Wolff, H. G. Life situations, behavior, attitudes, emotions, and renal excretion of fluid and electrolytes: II. Retention of water and sodium; diuresis of water, J Psychosom Res, 1:147, 1956.

——— Grace, W. J., and Wolff, H. G. Life situations, behavior, attitudes, emotions, and renal excretion of fluid and electrolytes: III. Diuresis of fluid and electrolytes, J Psychosom Res, 1:203, 1956.

——— Grace, W. J., and Wolff, H. G. Life situations, behavior, attitudes, emotions, and renal excretion of fluid and electrolytes: IV. Situations associated with retention of water, sodium, and potassium, J Psychosom Res, 1:287, 1956.

——— Grace, W. J., and Wolff, H. G. Life situations, behavior, attitudes, emotions, and renal excretion of fluid and electrolytes: V. Variations in the excretion of endogenous creatinine, J Psychosom Res, 1:292, 1956.

Von Euler, U. S. Autonomic neuroeffector transmission, in Handbook of Physiology: Neurophysiology. Washington, D.C., Amer Physiol Soc, 1959, Sect. 1, Vol I, Chapter 7, p. 215-237.

Wenger, M. A. Some problems in psychophysiological research, in Physiological Correlates of Psychological Disorder, Roessler, R., and Greenfield, N. S., eds. Madison, Univ. of Wisconsin Press, 1962, p. 97-114.

Weiner, H. Some psychological factors related to cardiovascular responses: A logical and empirical analysis, in Physiological Correlates of Psychological Disorder, Roessler, R., and Greenfield, N. S., eds. Madison, Univ. of Wisconsin Press, 1962, p. 115-141.

Wolff, H. G. Headache and Other Head Pain, 2nd ed. New York, Oxford University Press, 1963.

——— Stress and Disease. Springfield, Ill., Charles C Thomas, Publisher, 1953.

12

Hypnotic Suggestion of Emotion, Pain, and Exercise

Hypnosis was used as a means of validating observations made with naturally occurring stimuli, suggestion of such stimuli, and head pain. A total of 21 experiments was carried out on 11 volunteer male subjects aged 21 to 28. Ten were normal male medical students and one a patient with tuberculosis. Ten were studied before, during, and after stimulation with a metal headband (see Chapters 10 and 11), and 11 were studied before, during, and after hypnotic suggestion of relaxation, depression, anxiety and/or anger, head pain, and exercise in that order. The suggestion of anxiety and/or anger, exercise, and head pain was terminated with the suggestion of relaxation. Only one of the subjects had been previously hypnotized.

All subjects were interviewed several days prior to the experiments to allay their fears about the procedures. At the same time, information was obtained about specific situations which were accompanied by strong emotions of anxiety, anger, and depression, and about experiences with active participation in physical exercise. The hypnotic suggestion was based upon data gained in these interviews and was confined to these previous experiences. Emotion was defined as a state having both psychic and physiologic components. The ideation in anxiety was apprehension; in anger, indignation and wrath; and in depression, dejection and hopelessness. Prior to the suggestion period, hypnosis was induced by eye fixation on a light and suggestion of relaxation and drowsiness. During the induction period, the subjects were continually told that they were growing more and more relaxed and that their eyelids were growing heavy. When it became difficult for them to keep their eyelids open they were told that they should close their eyes and they would then become more deeply relaxed. At that point

This chapter is adapted from an article originally published in *Psychosom Med*, 26:46, 1964, by Dudley, D. L., Holmes, T. H., Martin, C. J., and Ripley, H. S.

the subject's arm relaxation was evaluated by lifting the arm as a measure of the depth of relaxation. After induction, life situations and the headband experience were suggested to the subjects.

During the experiments, the depth of the trance and the response to suggestion were indicated by the subjects' pained facial expressions, clenching of fists, pounding on the arms of the chairs, and verbal expressions of experiencing discomfort. They experienced vivid imagery and memories during hypnosis and had posthypnotic amnesia for traumatic events. At the termination of the experiments all subjects were told, "When you awaken you will be relaxed and have a sense of well-being." This suggestion was effective in all cases. During and after hypnosis the subjects were questioned about their feelings, and observations were made of their overt behavioral responses.

At the end of each experiment the subjects were questioned further about their sensations and emotional reactions during the experimental procedures. The psychological and physiological data were then recorded by two investigators who worked independently.

In general, attention could be restricted under hypnosis so that life situations in which there had been active exercise and those accompanied by relatively pure emotion could be revived. However, in a number of instances the intended uncomplicated single emotion was not produced. Instead, mixed or overlapping emotions, such as anxiety and depression or anger and depression, occurred in association with relived experiences. Data analysis was done with Student's *t* test for paired samples.

Table 1. Comparison of Respiratory Variables During Suggested Emotions (10 Subjects)

	RR	$\dot{V}_A$ (L/MIN)	F_{ACO_2} (%)	$\dot{V}_{O_2}$ (ML/MIN)
Relaxed before hypnosis*	14	5.5	5.8	308
Relaxed during hypnosis	13	5.1	5.7	277
Depression	13	4.6	5.8	284
Anger and/or anxiety	18†	9.0†	4.7†	318‡
Relaxed	13	4.3	5.8	271

* Nine subjects.
† $p = <0.01$.
‡ $p = < 0.02$.
Levels of significance are of the same magnitude when the values for anger and/or anxiety are compared with either relaxation or depression during the hypnosis sessions.

OBSERVATIONS

Compared with control measurements, the initiation of the hypnotic state had minimal or no effect on the physiologic variables (Table 1 and Figs. 1 and 2) except for a decrease in oxygen consumption. Respiratory

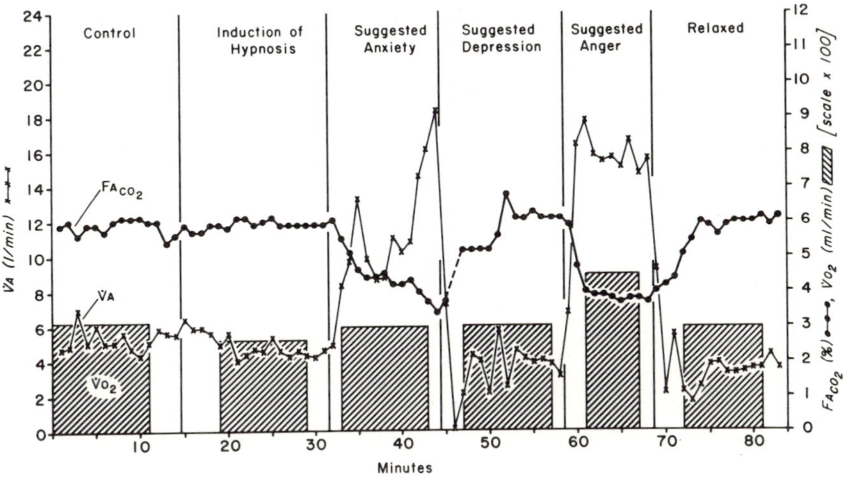

Fig. 1. Similarity between hypnotic suggestion of depression and deep relaxation and physiologic results of mixed emotional responses in Subject 1. Hyperfunction response to relatively pure anger and anxiety is clearly illustrated.

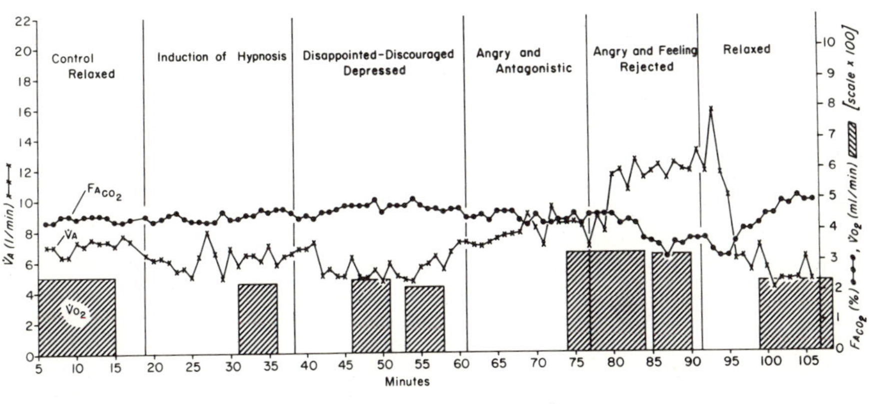

Fig. 2. Hypofunction in response to hypnotic suggestion of depression and hyperfunction with suggestion of anger. In Subject 2, suggested anger regarding his mother's rejection of him was associated with mild attack of asthma.

hyperfunction, characterized by an increase in alveolar ventilation and oxygen uptake and a decrease in carbon dioxide concentration, followed suggestions of anger, anxiety, and exercise. In contrast, respiratory hypofunction, characterized by decreased alveolar ventilation and oxygen uptake and increased carbon dioxide concentration followed suggestions of depression and deep relaxation.

The magnitude of the response appeared to depend upon the depth of hypnosis and the significance of the events used as the stimulus. During the experiments the concentration on suggested topics was in many cases so strong that there was amnesia for the suggestion after the experiment. The trauma of suggested emotional events was severe enough in one subject to warrant termination of the experiment. The emotional responses to hypnotic suggestion varied from minimal to those which were difficult to terminate by suggestion of relaxation. During the experiments the subjects were generally unaware of changes in respiration.

Suggestion of Emotionally Laden Experiences

As illustrated in Table 1 there was a statistically significant difference between respiratory measurements taken during suggestion of deep relaxation and depression and measurements taken during anxiety or anger. The following are detailed descriptions of individual protocols.

SUBJECT 1. Subject 1 was a 25-year-old medical student. As shown in Fig. 1 the sequence of the experiment was changed from that used in other subjects in that suggestion of depression rather than relaxation was used as the stimulus to terminate the anxiety reaction. This was done in order to validate the physiologic similarity between the suggestion of relaxation and depression. Action-oriented states could be terminated by the suggestion either of relaxation or depression.

Anger was aroused by the revival of thoughts of a guard at one of the hospitals who had insulted and berated the subject. He desired to take aggressive action and commented, "I would like to have hit or hurt him. . . . If I hadn't feared getting in trouble I would have smashed him."

Anxiety was evoked by asking the subject to recall a situation in which he was waiting for his professors to ask questions which he feared he could not answer. He felt as if he were being "put on the spot" and did not know how to respond. His subjective reaction was characterized by the following statement: "I wish this were over and I could get out of here." In addition to thinking of the above, he also recalled a meeting with a professor who had always seemed particularly unreceptive to the student's personal ambitions, unmindful of his feelings. His reaction to this man was that of feeling acutely tense and anxious and "wanting to get away." However, he also felt overwhelmed and somewhat discouraged and depressed as the professor had the power of greatly influencing the student's future. The net result was a mixed reaction of depression and anxiety with anxiety predominating.

During suggestion of depression he was asked to revive his thoughts of possibly failing in medical school and the accompanying feelings of being discouraged and overwhelmed. He felt as if he were unable to take action and could do nothing to better himself. Accompanying the feeling of discouragement and self-abasement was a mild feeling of anxiety over what he would do if he actually did fail. Once again there resulted a mixed reaction. This time, however, depression predominated.

COMMENT. In this subject the oxygen uptake did not change between anxiety and depression. The alveolar ventilation fell and the $F_{A_{CO_2}}$ rose as expected. These findings—shown in Figure 1—perhaps can be explained on the basis of the mixed emotional reaction producing a mixed physiologic response. Several other subjects displayed this same type of physiologic pattern with a mixed emotional reaction. In the absence of a mixed emotional reaction, ventilation and oxygen uptake invariably fluctuate in the same direction. The changes in oxygen uptake appear to occur in relation to changes in muscular activity during the measuring period as indicated by observed behavior and muscle potentials on the electrocardiograph. This is illustrated by the physiologic reaction of increased oxygen uptake of this subject to suggested anger, also shown in Figure 1.

SUBJECT 2. Subject 2 was a 25-year-old tuberculous patient with severe emotional problems and known asthma since the age of eight. He had anterior poliomyelitis at the age of 3 months and spent most of his life in hospitals until the age of 16 years. At one time his divorced mother left him in the hospital for nine years (age 7 to 16) without visiting him.

After the induction of hypnosis and deep relaxation he was asked to relive his reaction to being told that he had tuberculosis. His feelings were those of discouragement and depression. He expressed himself as follows: "It's something that can't be helped. . . . I felt resigned because I couldn't do anything about it." As shown in Figure 2, ventilation and gas exchange remained at equal or lower levels than the values found during the induction of hypnosis and deep relaxation.

To elicit anger the subject was first asked to relive a situation in which he felt that one of the staff physicians had falsely accused him of sleeping with one of the female patients. He was not very successful in reviving this situation. He stated: "I flip my lid and it's all over." His general outlook toward the physician who had angered him was as follows: "I tell him what I think of him and that takes a long time. . . . I won't change doctors because I want to make life miserable for that ignorant intellectual."

After the suggestion of the above situation, he was asked to think of how angry and rejected he felt because his mother had left him in a children's hospital for a period of nine years without visiting him. He reacted with clenched fists and was at times openly crying. He had an anguished expression on his face and appeared tense. "It shook me. . . . I looked back and felt like I did when I was there. . . . Nine years is a long time. They might have been busy, but that's no excuse." Recalling this experience provoked mixed emotions of severe anger and mild depression.

During this suggestion period he had shortness of breath and said that he "had a mild attack of asthma." His response to the suggestion of relaxation was not immediate, but after 4 min he relaxed and the attack terminated. No gross wheezing was documented during this experiment. However, this subject had been observed during four previous attacks of typical asthma, and the pattern of high ventilation, high oxygen consumption, and mental anguish was present in each one.

COMMENT. The general pattern of elevated ventilation and oxygen consumption during suggestion of anger and anxiety, as well as decreased or no change from resting values during suggestion of depression and deep relaxation, was duplicated to a greater or lesser degree in the other nine subjects.

Suggestion of Physical Activity

In suggesting exercise the subjects were asked to relive a type of physical exercise in which they had actively participated. This varied from mild calisthenics in the tuberculous subject to running a race, playing tennis, or climbing a mountain in the medical students. As shown in Table 2, there were statistically significant changes in respiratory variables during the period of suggestion as compared with relaxation.

Table 2. Suggested Exercise Compared to Initial Relaxation (11 Subjects)

	RR	$\dot{V}_A$ (L/MIN)	F_{ACO_2} (%)	$\dot{V}_{O_2}$ (ML/MIN)
Relaxed	13	4.3	5.8	271
Exercise	21*	12.7†	4.0‡	377†
Relaxed	12	4.3	5.5	269

* $p = 0.01$.
† $p = <0.01$.
‡ $p = <0.001$.

Figure 3 shows the continuation of the experiment on Subject 1. The stimulus used with this subject was the suggestion of a grueling hike. Throughout the suggestion period the subject was told to exert himself to his utmost. As shown in the illustration, there was an immediate and sustained increase in ventilation and oxygen uptake which was similar to the response to the suggestion of anger or anxiety shown in Figure 1.

Figure 4 shows the response of Subject 2 to the suggestion of exercise.

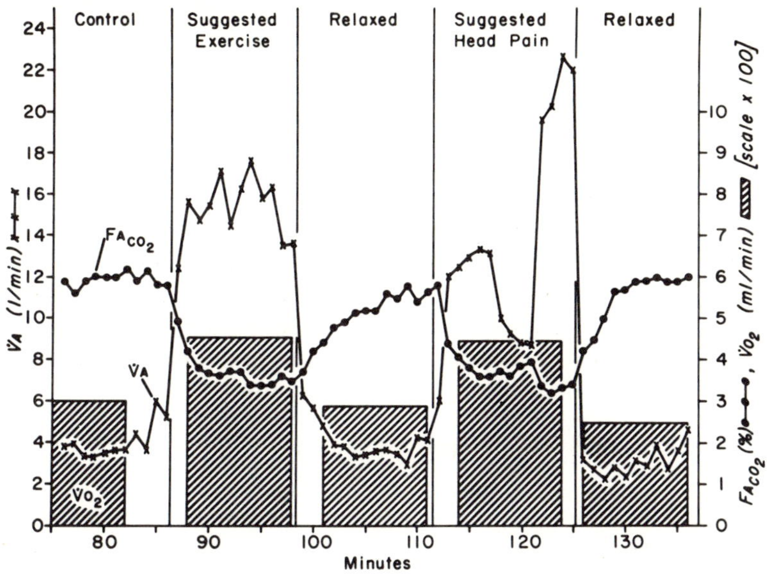

Fig. 3. Continuation of experiment in Subject 1. Hyperfunction response to suggested exercise and head pain. These physiologic changes are identical to response to suggested anxiety and anger.

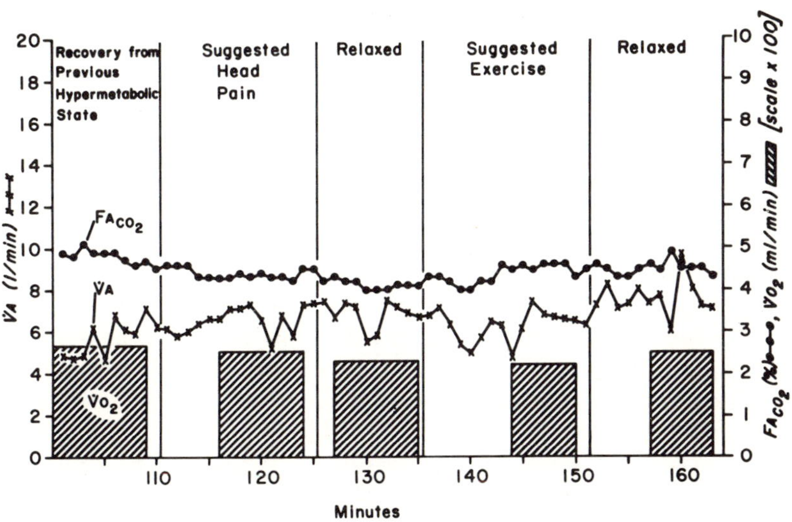

Fig. 4. Continuation of experiment in Subject 2. There is relative lack of change in pulmonary physiology following suggested head pain and exercise. Subject was not traumatized by head pain and had never experienced heavy exercise. This is in contrast to his response to depression and anger (Fig. 2).

This subject had never exercised vigorously and said that he did not know what it was like. He spent a good share of the suggestion period thinking of how he wanted to be like the "rest of the guys." He thought of calisthenics in the hospital and what it was like trying to cut a limb off a tree, but he had difficulty *reliving* these experiences.

COMMENT. In general, the suggestion of exercise evoked responses when the individual had experienced heavy exercise. Although Subject 2 did not respond to the suggestion of exercise (Fig. 4), he showed a strong reaction to the suggestion of a situation which was accompanied by anger (Fig. 2). In contrast, the response of Subject 1 to suggested exercise was duplicated to a greater or lesser degree in the nine other medical students.

DISCUSSION

In all 11 subjects the use of hypnosis produced rapid changes in psychologic orientation and in 10, the reliving of active exercise experiences. The respiratory hyperfunction when anger, anxiety, or exercise was suggested can be seen as an attempt to prepare the individual for action by making more oxygen available for gaseous exchange. Conversely, the lack of change in ventilation found with suggestion of deep relaxation and depression is compatible with the absence of action-oriented behavior.

Although numerous studies have differentiated the physiologic change occurring with various emotions, there is as yet inadequate research focused on determining the similarities and differences of exercise versus anger or anxiety, and depression versus sleep or deep relaxation.

In evaluating the responses occurring with the reliving of an exercise experience, consideration needs to be given to the fact that feeling changes are common accompaniments and that part of the reaction observed may be related to emotion. The combination of reactions is illustrated by Subject 1 (Figs. 1 and 3), who, on the suggestion of reliving an arduous hike, felt that he was aggressively exerting himself and experiencing some anxiety about the dangers and his ability to compete with his fellow mountaineers.

The reliving of the head pain experience was always accompanied by a personality reaction. In 10 of the 11 subjects there were overt emotional expression and an accompanying physiologic response. The emotions were most frequently anxiety and anger. For example, one subject recounted that he was restless and anxious and that he developed a backache when reexperiencing the headache. Another subject felt anger at having to undergo the discomfort. In the eleventh subject there was denial or repression of emotion and no physiologic response.

Such divergent psychologic reactions as anger and depression involve contrasting adaptive physiologic responses. During emotion such as anger the emphasis is on expending energy in performing or preparing to perform some type of task. During an emotion such as depression the emphasis may be on conserving or building up of energy stores. The same type of differentiation applies to deep relaxation or sleep versus exercise.

SUMMARY

In a group of 11 subjects, it has been shown that elevated ventilation and oxygen consumption follow hypnotic suggestion of situations eliciting anxiety or anger, exercise, and head pain. Hyperfunction occurred only on suggestion of a stimulus which was meaningful to the subject. In the absence of a psychologic reaction, no physiologic change was evident. With anger, anxiety, and exercise there was orientation toward action.

In contrast, it was shown that with suggestion of depression there was no change in respiratory variables over that of deep relaxation indicating a reaction of hypofunction. With depression and deep relaxation there was no action orientation. Mixed emotional responses were accompanied by mixed physiological responses.

13

Hypnotically Induced Facsimile of Noxious Stimulation of the Head

Many studies have shown that hypnotic suggestion of emotion is followed by physiologic and psychologic change. However, the effectiveness of hypnosis in faithfully reproducing actual events appears to be a relatively neglected field of study. The work of Stern et al. demonstrated that it was possible to reproduce specific attitudes and the related physiologic change associated with different diseases in normal subjects. The study by Cobb, Ripley, and Jones showed that the physiologic and psychologic response to hypnotic suggestion of exercise is similar to that of actual exercise. In previous studies similar results were obtained during psychophysiologic studies of the respiratory system in which hypnotic suggestion, nonhypnotic suggestion, and naturally occurring events were used. From this work and that mentioned above it was concluded that the suggested experience closely parallels the actual experience. However, no direct evidence was available. The work reported in this chapter was designed as an exploratory attempt to compare directly the reaction to noxious stimulation of the head with its hypnotically induced facsimile.

A total of 21 experiments was carried out on 11 volunteer male subjects aged 21 to 28. Ten were normal male medical students, and one a patient with tuberculosis. Ten subjects were studied before, during, and after hypnotic suggestion of relaxation, depression, anxiety and/or anger, head pain, and exercise—in that order. The respiratory data on emotion

This chapter is adapted from an article originally published in *Arch Gen Psychiat*, 15:198, 1966, by Dudley, D. L., Holmes, T. H., Martin, C. J., and Ripley, H. S.

and exercise have been previously reported, and the data on head pain was reported in part (see Chapter 11). Only one of the subjects had been previously hypnotized.

The noxious stimulus consisted of a metal headband with 14 adjustable rubber-tipped screws around the circumference. When the rubber-tipped screws were fixed tightly against the circumference of the skull, this device produced an intense pressure headache, generalized physical and mental discomfort, and physiologic change. One subject who did not receive the headband stimulus was asked to recall a previously experienced migraine headache during the hypnosis session.

All subjects were interviewed several days prior to the experiments to allay their fears about the procedures. Prior to the suggestion period hypnosis was induced by eye fixation on a light and suggestion of relaxation and drowsiness. During the induction period the subjects were continually told that they were growing more and more relaxed and that their eyelids were growing heavy. When it became difficult for them to keep their eyelids open, the subjects were told that they should close their eyes and they would then become more deeply relaxed. At that point the subject's arm relaxation was evaluated by lifting the arm as a measure of the depth of relaxation.

After induction, life situations and the headband experience were suggested to the subjects. With suggestion of the headband experience the subjects were asked to "relive the headscrew situation and the pain you experienced." At 2- to 4-min intervals they were told that the pain was getting "more and more unbearable" or "worse and worse." After 10 to 15 min the suggested experience was terminated with suggestion of relaxation.

During the experiments the depth of the trance and response to suggestion were indicated by the subjects' pained facial expressions, the clenching of fists, pounding on the arms of their chairs, and verbal expressions of experiencing pain. They experienced vivid imagery and memories during hypnosis and had posthypnotic amnesia for traumatic events. At the termination of the experiments all subjects were told, "When you awaken you will be relaxed and have a sense of well-being." This suggestion was effective in all cases. During and after hypnosis the subjects were questioned about their feelings, and observations were made of their overt behavioral responses.

All subjects were interviewed before and after the experiments. Notes were kept of their descriptions of their sensations, emotions, and attitudes during the experiments. The two experiences were then compared. The psychologic and physiologic data were recorded by two investigators working independently. Data analysis was done by using Student's t test for paired samples.

Table 1. Actual Head Pain
(10 Subjects)

	RR	$\dot{V}_A$ (L/MIN)	F_{ACO_2} (%)	$\dot{V}_{O_2}$ (ML/MIN)*	Blood Pressure Systolic	Blood Pressure Diastolic	Heart Rate	Skin Temperature (°C)
Control period	13	5.8	5.7	315	128	81	81	29.3
	±9.6	±0.8	±0.63	±28.7	±8.8	±10.9	±13.1	±3.8
Pain period	17	12.0†	4.5†	388‡	155†	102†	88	27.9
	±7.8	±4.5	±0.79	±74.1	±24.6	±19.7	±16.2	±2.5
Recovery period	13	5.3	5.3	294	129	85	74	30.2
	±6.6	±1.1	±0.55	±39.1	±9.4	±10.1	±16.6	±1.8

*Seven subjects.
† $p = < 0.01$.
‡ $p = < 0.02$.
± 1 S.D.

Table 2. Suggested Head Pain (10 Subjects)

	RR	$\dot{V}_A$ (L/MIN)	F_{ACO_2} (%)	$\dot{V}_{O_2}$ (ML/MIN)*	Blood Pressure Systolic	Blood Pressure Diastolic	Heart Rate	Skin Temperature (°C)
Control period	12	4.3	5.5	272	128	81	66	30.8
	±2.4	±1.8	±0.6	±35.6	±11.4	±10.9	±13.6	±1.9
Suggested pain period	25†	10.5‡	4.0§	344‡	130	83	73†	30.6
	±4.7	±4.3	±0.9	±79.2	±13.0	±10.4	±11.9	±1.6
Recovery period	13	4.1	5.3	262	126	81	65	30.8
	±2.7	±1.5	±0.7	±35.1	±13.1	±9.8	±12.1	±1.6

* Seven subjects.
† $p = <0.02$.
‡ $p = <0.01$.
§ $p = <0.001$.
± S.D.

OBSERVATIONS

Actual Stimulation

The response of the ten subjects to actual headband stimulation was generally one of intense action orientation. This was characterized by emotions of anger and anxiety and behavioral responses of restlessness and irritability. The essense of the response was that of an intense desire to act. Associated with the behavioral and emotional changes were significant elevations of ventilation, oxygen consumption, and blood pressure, and a significant decrease in the fractional concentration of alveolar carbon dioxide (Table 1).

The one exception of the above pattern was that of the tuberculous subject, who had had considerable experience with pain. He admitted to little preoccupation with the stimulus even though he admitted awareness of it. He denied being disturbed by the discomfort, but he appeared to be restless and irritable and he asked to have the experiment discontinued when reactions were at a peak level. (More complete data on this subject will be presented in the case reports.)

Suggestion

As shown in Table 2, the respiratory response of the 10 subjects to suggestion of the headband experience is similar to the actual experience. However, the changes in blood pressure were not reproduced. Instead, there was a significant elevation of pulse rate that was not shown during stimulation with the headband. The emotional and behavioral responses experienced during the actual experience were generally well reproduced. However, the headache itself was reproduced in varying degrees. Table 3

Table 3. Comparison of the Subjects' Impressions of the Actual and Suggested Headache

Subject	Immediately After Suggested Headache	Immediately After Actual Headache	No. Days Between Experiences
1	"I wanted to terminate it. I'd had enough. The painful sensation was a real threat. I was fighting the head pain and was angry with you."	"I wished it were over. I would have done anything to stop it."	431

2	"I felt uncomfortable. I had a headache but couldn't feel the headscrew."	"I felt like getting out of the situation somehow."	4
3	"I relived the pain, but it didn't bother me a bit. I'm immune to pain. I can grin and bear that headband."	"It didn't bother me a bit."	28
4*	"I actually developed a headache and was very happy to get it over with. It was frontal and more on the left side. Great relief afterwards."	"Oh boy! My migraine headaches are excruciating. I often get them when I'm trying to find out whether I can handle situations."	1,000
5	"I was uncomfortable. I resented it. After it was over, it took me a while to realize it was just an experiment, I didn't deserve it."	"I just wanted to get out. I felt very tense and restless."	151
6	"I was trying to hang on until the end of the pain which was much like the actual headscrew application."	"During the final period I had panic. The foremost thought in my mind was 'God Almighty, I've got to get this over with.'"	13
7	"I could kind of feel it. As you reinforced it, I could feel it more and more."	"It seemed almost unbearable. It was the worst pain I ever had. I just wanted to get out."	34
8	"Some head pain was experienced. My stomach got upset as it did with the actual head screw. I clenched my fist and had nasal hyperfunction and dryness of the mouth."	"I really had a terrible headache. The thought passed across my mind to tear it off."	21
9	"I had an uncomfortable feeling with tension in my neck. I squirmed and felt it might be something outside."	"There was some basic challenge to overcome it (the head pain). I had a choking sensation with panic. I just wanted to get out."	39
10	"The pain was hard to bear. It was difficult to tolerate the discomfort much longer."	"It was unbearable. What the hell am I doing here."	37
11	"It was the most real situation of all. I pictured myself with the headscrew. The pain was almost unbearable. The nose clip was also painful."	"It was extremely painful. I tried to concentrate on something else. I wished it were over."	393

* Migraine headache.

compares statements from these 10 subjects after the actual and suggested pain experiences.

Individual Case Reports

The following case reports provide detailed accounts of response to the headache and to its hypnotically induced facsimile. It is of interest that even though the elapsed time between the actual pain experience and the suggested experience varied from 4 to 1,000 days (Table 3), this did not appear to be a limiting factor in the production of emotional, behavioral, or physiological change, or in the reproduction of the headache. This is illustrated by Subject 1 and Subject 2, who underwent the suggested experience 431 days and 4 days after the actual experience, respectively.

Subject 1. Subject 1 was a 24-year-old white male, married medical student. During the course of the experiments he was working in the laboratory as a research fellow. At the first adjustment and tightening of the headband the subject felt alert and tense but experienced minimal discomfort. After 8 min the headband was tightened a second time, and the subject experienced transitory head pain and an increasing feeling of general physical and mental discomfort.

At 15 min the band was tightened a third time. The subject experienced a diffuse, steady, dull pain over the entire head region. During this period he felt tense and restless and kept thinking, "I wish it were off. What did I do it for?" Over the next 5 min the pain and feelings of restlessness steadily increased, and the subject found it impossible to think of anything but the head pain and the urge to terminate it. From 17 to 20 min, the subject was aware of breathing fast and hard and felt numbness and tingling in his hands and arms. He broke out in a cold sweat and was observed to have twitching of the facial muscles. He experienced feelings of helplessness, resentment, anger, and irritation. At 20 min he felt that he could no longer tolerate the stimulus, and the headband was removed.

After removal of the band the discomfort vanished, and the subject was profoundly relieved. At this point he felt as though he had just finished some difficult, demanding physical task.

During suggestion of the head pain experience the subject was easily able to relive the most traumatic portion of the actual experience. It should be noted that the initial tightenings of the headband, which did not produce severe discomfort, were not reproduced. The subject described the suggested pain experience as follows: "I wanted to terminate it. I had had enough. The painful sensation was a real threat. I was fighting the head pain and was angry with you for not ending the discomfort." The physiologic response to actual and suggested headache is illustrated in Figure 1. This subject displayed the best reproduction of blood pressure and pulse rate changes of the ten subjects studied. Changes in skin temperature were not reproduced.

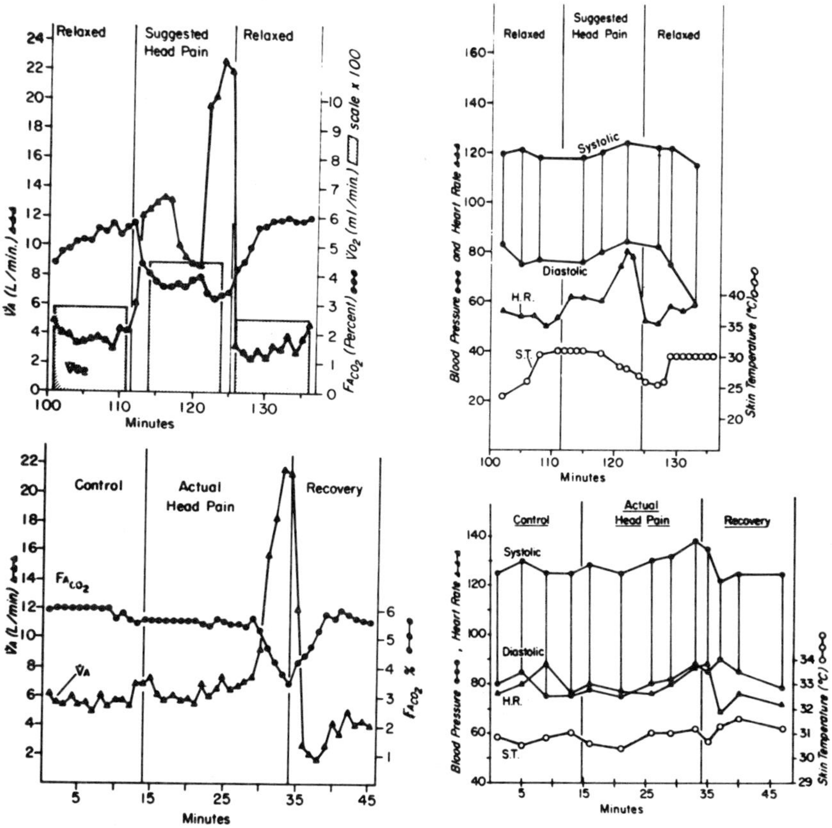

Fig. 1. Physiologic response of Subject 1 to suggested and actual noxious stimulation of the head. Subject displayed good reproduction of respiratory changes and the best reproduction of blood pressure and heart rate changes of any of the subjects. Changes in skin temperature were present during suggested experience but not during actual experience. It should be noted that the last 5 min of headband experience (which is the most traumatic) is portion of experiment which is reproduced.

SUBJECT 2. Subject 2 was a 25-year-old white male, married medical student who reacted to the pain in a manner very similar to that of Subject 1. The pain was constant and dull and extended over the entire upper half of the head. He felt restless and anxious and could not concentrate. He felt that his respiratory rate and blood pressure had increased. He said that he felt "like getting out of the situation somehow."

During the suggested head pain experience the onset of the reaction was prompt and sustained and duplicated the latter part of the actual experience. Subject 2 said that he experienced the headache and felt very uncomfortable but could not feel the headband on his head. He also developed a backache.

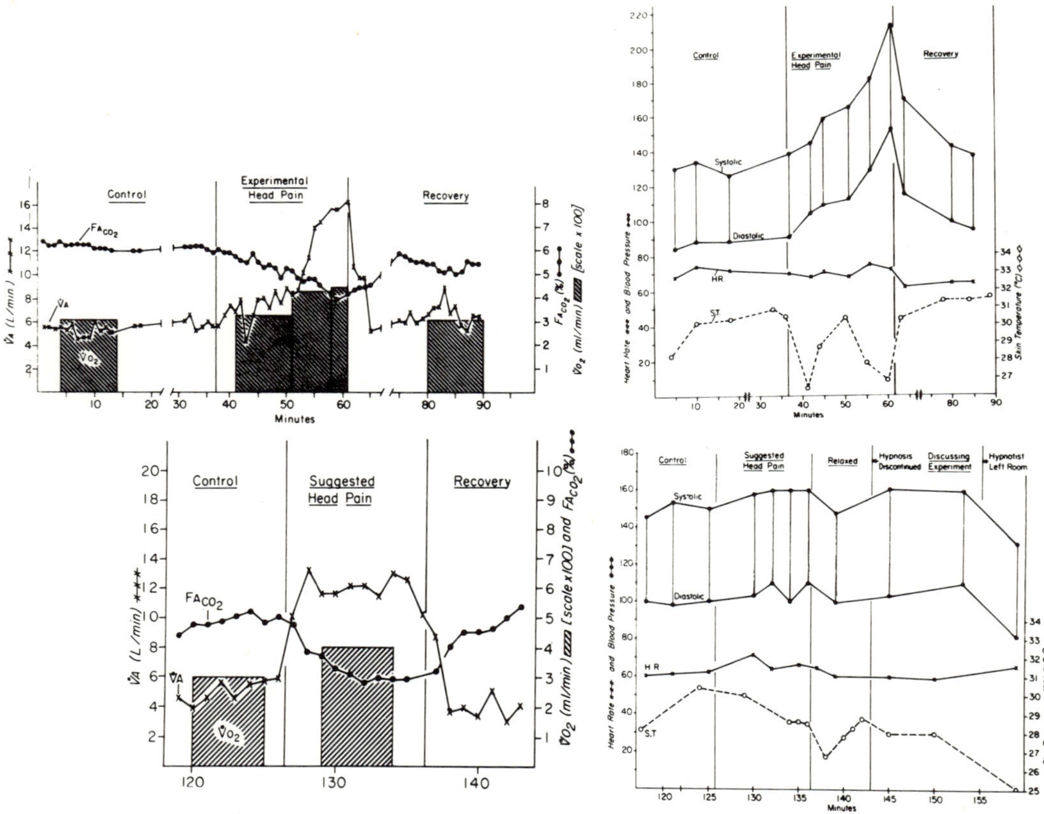

Fig. 2. Physiologic response of Subject 2 to suggested and actual noxious stimulation of the head. Subject had good reproduction of changes in respiration but changes in blood pressure were not reproduced. Pulse rate varied little during either experiment and changes in skin temperature were partially reproduced.

As shown in Figure 2, the respiratory changes were well reproduced, but the changes in blood pressure were not reproduced. Pulse rate varied little during either experiment and changes in skin temperature were partially reproduced.

COMMENT. Even though only four days had elapsed between the actual headband experience and the suggested experience in Subject 2, changes in blood pressure and skin temperature were not reproduced. In contrast, Subject 1—with 431 days between the actual and suggested experience—displayed fair reproduction of almost all physiologic, emotional, and behavioral changes. Thus time did not appear to be a crucial factor in the reproduction of the experience.

SUBJECT 3. Subject 3 was a 25-year-old white, divorced laborer admitted to the hospital with far advanced pulmonary tuberculosis, bronchial asthma, and an irreversible chronic obstructive pulmonary syndrome as well. He had contracted anterior poliomyeletis as an infant and crippling foot deformities had resulted. He was unable to walk until after the first of his surgical operations for correction of the deformities at age seven. After this first of nine operations, he developed a severe attack of asthma which lasted for several days. He has never been free from attacks since. He had experienced much "pain" with the operations and subsequent physical therapy and lived at the hospital until he was 16 years of age. In this setting he dealt with pain by developing drowsiness or emotional detachment.

In contrast to the first two subjects the stimulus made him feel "depressed." He stated, "I just felt something like being down in the dumps." He did not feel like doing anything about the stimulus as he felt that there was nothing that could be done. He admitted getting a little irritated at the height of the experiment but insisted that "it didn't bother me a bit," even though he requested that it be terminated. He withstood the stimulus for 39 min. The longest period any of the other nine were able to tolerate the stimulus was 24 min.

During the experiment he showed minimal to no changes in the fractional concentration of alveolar carbon dioxide, alveolar ventilation, or oxygen consumption. However, marked changes in skin temperature and a moderate elevation of blood pressure were present.

In response to repeated suggestion of the headband experience the subject said, "I relived the pain, but it didn't bother me a bit. I'm immune to pain. I can grin and bear that headband." His response to actual and suggested stimulation is shown in Figure 3. As shown, there was essentially no change in the respiratory variables during actual or suggested headache. The blood pressure and skin temperature changes were not reproduced during the suggested experience.

SUBJECT 4. Subject 4 (not included in the group of ten) was a 25-year-old white, married medical student who did not undergo the headband experiment but was subject to migraine headache. His psychologic and physiologic response to suggestion of a migraine headache was similar to the other subjects' response to the suggested headband experience (Fig. 4). He showed a marked respiratory response but no change in blood pressure, pulse rate, or skin temperature.

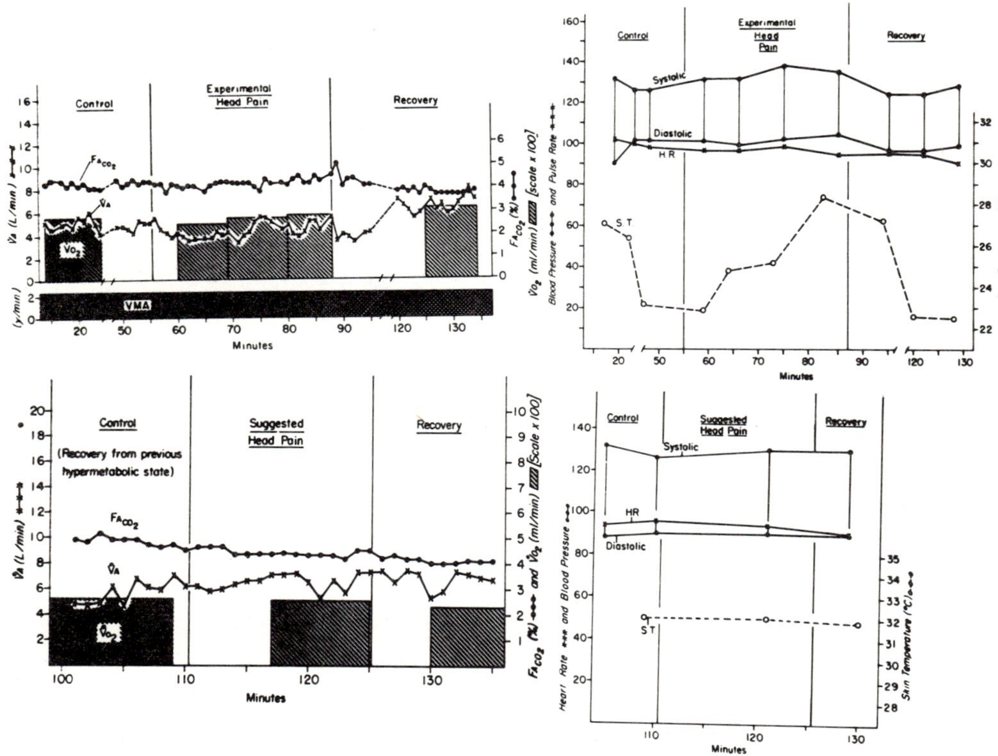

Fig. 3. Physiologic response of Subject 3 to hypnotic reproduction and actual noxious stimulation of the head. As shown, there were essentially no changes in respiratory variables during actual or suggested headache. Blood pressure and skin temperature changes were not reproduced during suggested experience.

During the suggestion he developed a moderately severe frontal headache which was greater on the left. He felt tense and had a pained expression on his face and experienced profound relief when he was told the headache was no longer present.

COMMENT. This last-described subject illustrates that reaction to pain from a bodily response may not differ from that occurring with an external stimulus.

DISCUSSION

In general, respiratory changes in response to headband stimulation were well reproduced during suggestion of the noxious experience, while cardiovascular changes were incompletely reproduced. The emotional and behavioral responses to the actual experience were also well reproduced. However, the headache itself was reported as being reproduced in varying degrees and in one instance in a different location than the actual stimulus. With actual experience of the noxious stimulus the subjects fought to control their reaction. It was only after repeatedly increasing the intensity of

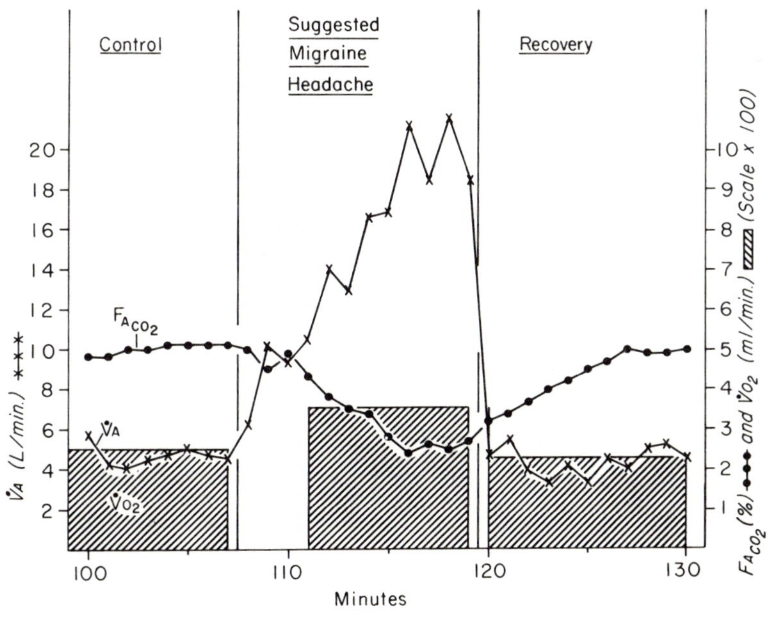

Fig. 4. Physiologic response of Subject 4 to hypnotic reproduction of migraine headache. Psychologic response to migraine experience was similar to other medical students' response to actual and suggested headache.

the stimulus that emotional, behavioral, and physiologic changes became evident. During the suggested experience the subjects concentrated on reliving the most traumatic part of the experience. Consequently the physiologic and emotional changes occurred promptly following the suggestion. Because of the psychologic differences between the actual and suggested experiences, physiologic differences would also be expected. Except for the greater increase in respiratory rate during the suggested experience, the changes in the respiratory system were identical during the two experiences. However, as noted, a considerable difference was found when measurements of blood pressure, pulse rate, and skin temperature during the actual noxious experience were compared with the same measurements during the suggested experience.

Within the small group of subjects studied there was a spectrum of physiologic and psychologic responses to the hypnotic suggestion. Four subjects had good reproduction of head pain, and one had poor reproduction of both emotions and head pain. A very important factor in the production of emotional and physiologic change during hypnosis was the desire of the subject to cooperate. The subjects who appeared to be the most interested and cooperative had the best reproduction of emotional and physiologic change. On the other hand, one subject told the investigator that he was fighting hard to ignore suggested material. This subject had poor reproduction of all parameters of reaction. The length of time between the actual and suggested experience did not appear to be a crucial factor in determining the response to the suggestion. Much more important were the significance that the subject applied to the original experience and his ability and desire to cooperate.

That the psychologic, behavioral, and physiologic responses to suggested headache were not responses limited to the headband experience is shown by Subject 4's response to suggested migraine headache. The response is similar whether it is to an external stimulus or reproduction of an endogenous (naturally occurring) experience (i.e., migraine).

It is recognized that the pain produced by the headband constituted only a part of the stimulus situation. Therefore, as in previous chapters, reference is made to the experiment as a "noxious situation" to include factors in addition to pain which contributed to the total response.

SUMMARY

In a group of 10 male subjects it was found that an actual stimulus with its emotional and physiologic components could, in part, be accurately reproduced during hypnotic suggestion of the experience.

Respiratory and emotional changes were well reproduced, while changes in blood pressure, skin temperature, and pulse rate were poorly reproduced. The headache experienced by all subjects was reproduced in part.

The hypnotic facsimile is seen to resemble the original experience, but is not identical either physiologically or psychologically.

REFERENCES

Cobb, L. A., Ripley, H. S., and Jones, J. W. Role of the nervous system in free fatty acid mobilization as demonstrated by hypnosis, in Physical Activity and the Heart: Proceedings of a Symposium, Helsinki, Finland. Karvonen, M. J., and Barry, A. J., eds. Springfield, Ill., Charles C Thomas, Publisher, 1967, Chapter 16, pp. 192–199.

Dudley, D. L., Holmes, T. H., Martin, C. J., and Ripley, H. S. Changes in respiration associated with hypnotically induced emotion, pain and exercise, Psychosom Med, 26:46, 1964.

——— Martin, C. J., and Holmes, T. H. Psychophysiologic studies of respiration, Psychosom Med, 26:645, 1964.

——— Masuda, M., Martin, C. J., and Holmes, T. H. Psychophysiological studies of experimentally induced action oriented behavior, J Psychosom Res, 9:209, 1965.

Graham, D. T., Stern, J. A., and Winokur, G. Experimental investigation of the specificity of attitude hypothesis in psychosomatic disease, Psychosom Med, 20:446, 1958.

Stern, S. A., Winokur, G., Graham, D. T., and Graham, F. K. Alterations in physiological measures during experimentally induced attitudes, J Psychosom Res, 5:73, 1961.

14

Comparison of Actual Head Pain, Hypnotically Induced Head Pain, and Suggested Head Pain

It has been demonstrated that direct suggestion of a given life event does not produce so great a physiologic response as suggestion with hypnosis. Other authors have shown that hypnotic suggestion is no more effective than direct suggestion without hypnosis. From the preceding chapter it is evident that hypnosis is a relatively good tool for the reproduction of psychophysiologic respiratory changes. In the present chapter, actual noxious stimulation and direct suggestion and hypnotic suggestion of noxious stimulation of the head are compared.

A total of 37 experiments was carried out on 15 volunteer subjects (14 male and 1 female) ages 21 to 28. Fourteen were medical students and one was a patient with tuberculosis. All 15 subjects were stimulated with a metal headband. The stimulus consisted of a band with 14 adjustable rubber-tipped screws around the circumference. When the rubber-tipped screws were fixed tightly against the circumference of the skull, this device produced an intense pressure headache, generalized physical and mental discomfort, and physiologic change. Within 45 min of the actual stimulation the subjects were studied before, during, and after direct suggestion of the headband situation. They were requested to close their eyes and think of how they felt and what they felt like doing during the stimulation. This was repeated several times over a 4- to 8-min period.

At poststimulus periods varying from 4 to 151 days, seven of the subjects were studied before, during, and after hypnotic suggestion of the headband situation. After hypnotic induction, life situations and the headband experience were suggested to the subjects. With suggestion of the headband experiment the subjects were asked to "relive the headscrew situation and the pain you experienced." They were told at 2- to 4-min intervals that

This chapter is adapted from an article originally published in *J Nerv Ment Dis*, 144:258, 1967, by Dudley, D. L., Holmes, T. H., and Ripley, H. S.

the pain was getting "more and more unbearable" or "worse and worse." After 8 to 15 min the suggested experience was terminated with suggestion of relaxation.

The direct suggestion and hypnotic suggestion were done by two investigators working independently. The psychologic and physiologic data were also recorded by two investigators working independently and by the subjects themselves. Statistical analysis was done by utilizing Student's *t* test for paired samples.

OBSERVATIONS

Actual Stimulation

The response of the 15 subjects to actual headband stimulation was generally one of intense action orientation. This was characterized by emotions of anger and anxiety, and behavioral responses of restlessness and irritability. The essence of the response was that of an intense desire to act. Associated with the behavioral and emotional changes were significant elevations of respiratory rate, minute ventilation, alveolar ventilation, oxygen consumption, and a significant decrease in the fractional concentration of alveolar carbon dioxide (Table 1).

Table 1. Comparison of Actual Pain and Nonhypnotic Suggested Pain (15 Subjects)

	RR	$\dot{V}$ (L/min)	$\dot{V}_A$ (L/min)	$F_{A_{CO_2}}$ (%)
Control	10	7.1	5.7	5.8
Pain	13*	14.5†	12.2†	4.3†
Recovery	11	7.3	5.7	4.5
Control	11	6.5	5.0	5.4
Suggestion	14‡	8.3‡	6.3*	5.1*
Recovery	11	6.3	4.9	5.4

* p = <0.05.
† p = <0.001.
‡ p = <0.02.

Direct Suggestion

Also shown in Table 1 is the respiratory response of the 15 subjects to nonhypnotic suggestion of the headband situation. As shown, the response is in the same direction as the actual experience, but is of reduced magnitude.

Table 2. Actual Stimulation and Direct Suggestion (7 Subjects)

		RR					$\dot{V}$ (L/min)					$\dot{V}_A$ (L/min)					F_{ACO_2} (%)				
Rating	Subject No.	Control	Pain	Control	Recall	Recovery	Control	Pain	Control	Recall	Recovery	Control	Pain	Control	Recall	Recovery	Control	Pain	Control	Recall	Recovery
1	4	10	29	12	25	14	6.0	18.8	7.5	10.2	6.7	5.2	15.2	6.1	7.4	5.1	6.2	4.3	5.6	5.0	5.6
2	1	6	16	10	17	8	7.4	20.9	6.0	15.1	4.6	6.6	18.0	4.7	12.0	3.5	5.1	3.6	4.7	3.8	5.6
3	3	9	10	11	12	10	6.1	9.5	6.7	8.1	5.9	4.4	7.6	4.7	5.8	4.3	6.0	5.4	5.8	5.0	5.2
4	2	10	18	12	15	12	7.8	18.0	8.7	9.9	8.4	6.6	14.3	7.0	7.8	6.7	5.7	3.7	5.3	5.2	5.2
5	5	10	11	11	14	12	7.2	17.9	6.3	7.4	6.8	5.9	15.4	4.7	5.2	5.2	5.9	3.6	5.1	5.0	5.3
6	6	9	9	10	13	10	6.5	10.0	6.2	6.3	5.1	5.2	8.5	4.6	4.2	3.6	6.5	5.5	5.9	6.0	6.0
7	7	7	6	8	9	7	6.3	9.2	6.5	6.9	7.2	5.3	8.2	5.1	5.6	6.1	5.7	5.7	5.7	5.6	5.3
Mean		9	14	11	15	10	6.8	14.9*	6.8	9.1	6.4	5.6	12.5*	5.3	6.9	4.9	5.9	4.5*	5.4	5.1	5.5

* $p = <0.01$.

This table shows the physiologic effects of actual pain and suggested pain (without hypnosis) in the 7 subjects who underwent the hypnosis experiment. Levels of significance apply to comparison of the directly preceding control period with the experimental period.

Table 3. Hypnotic Suggestion (7 Subjects)

		RR			$\dot{V}$ (L/min)			$\dot{V}_A$ (L/min)			F_{ACO_2} (%)		
Hypnotist's Rating	Subject No.	Control	Hypnotic Suggestion	Recovery	Control	Hypnotic Suggestion	Recovery	Control	Hypnotic Suggestion	Recovery	Control	Hypnotic Suggestion	Recovery
1	4	16	53	16	7.4	18.9	5.3	5.4	12.3	3.4	5.0	3.0	4.8
2	1	6	31	10	3.7	14.6	3.8	2.7	9.9	2.1	5.9	3.4	6.0
3	3	9	10	9	3.5	14.7	4.2	2.1	13.3	2.6	4.7	3.0	4.6
4	2	11	20	16	5.8	14.4	6.0	4.4	11.8	4.6	6.3	4.4	6.0
5	5	11	42	10	6.3	16.6	6.0	4.9	11.4	4.8	5.4	3.6	6.0
6	6	6	22	6	2.6	6.3	3.6	1.9	3.9	3.0	6.1	5.5	5.6
7	7	6	6	7	5.1	6.5	4.6	4.5	5.3	3.8	6.3	5.4	5.4
Mean		9	26*	10	4.9	13.1†	4.8	3.7	9.7†	3.5	5.7	4.0‡	5.5

* $p = <0.05$.
† $p = <0.01$.
‡ $p = <0.001$.

A rating of 1 signifies that the subject was rated by the hypnotist to have the best reproduction of the pain experience as indicated by vivid recall during the suggestion and posthypnotic amnesia for the event. This judgment was made independently of knowledge of the physiologic data. The subjects were also rated as good, fair, and poor. In this regard Subjects 1 through 4 were rated as good, Subject 5 as fair to good, Subject 6 as fair, and Subject 7 as poor.

Actual Stimulation, Direct Suggestion, and Hypnotic Suggestion

The physiologic data on the seven subjects who were stimulated with direct suggestion, hypnotic suggestion, and the actual headband situation are shown in Tables 2 and 3. As illustrated in these tables, results of hypnotic experience were physiologically similar to those of the actual experience, while the suggested experience was, again, in the same direction but decreased in magnitude. In contrast with the actual and hypnotically suggested experience, the physiologic changes during direct suggestion do not reach statistical significance.

As shown in Table 3, the five subjects rated as good hypnotic subjects —as indicated by vivid recall during the suggestion and posthypnotic amnesia for the event—had good reproduction of the physiologic change. Subject 7, who was a poor hypnotic subject, had a minimal response to the hypnotic suggestion. However, he was also among the poorest responders to the actual pain situation. Subject 3, who was considered a good hypnotic subject, responded to hypnotic suggestion with marked hyperventilation, while his reaction to the actual pain was comparable to that of Subject 7, who had the poorest hypnotic response. Subject 6, who was rated as a fair subject, responded with physiologic changes between those of Subject 7 and the five good subjects.

It should be noted that the hypnotist also rated the subjects from 1 to 7 with 1 being the best subject and 7 the poorest. There was some difficulty in discriminating between the first five subjects, who were considered roughly comparable. However, the difference between the subject rated as 5 and those rated 6 and 7 was obvious—as were their physiologic differences.

With the exception of respiratory rate, physiologic change occurring during the actual stimulation was significantly greater than changes occurring during the suggested experience ($p = <0.05$). Physiologic change occurring during the direct suggestion was significantly less than during the actual or hypnotic experience ($p = <0.05$). The respiratory rate, again, proved an exception. Change in this variable was not significantly different when the actual and suggested experiences were compared. Also, there were no significant differences between change during hypnosis and the actual stimulus—except for the respiratory rate, which was significantly greater during hypnosis ($p = <0.05$; see Table 4).

When the control values prior to the actual experience were compared with control values prior to direct suggestion, the respiratory rate was found to be significantly lower and the fractional concentration of alveolar carbon dioxide significantly higher during the actual control ($p = <0.05$). During the control prior to the hypnotic experience, the minute ventilation and alveolar ventilation were found to be significantly higher than

Table 4. COMPARISON OF CHANGES FROM CONTROL VALUES DURING ACTUAL PAIN, DIRECT SUGGESTION, AND HYPNOTIC SUGGESTION

	ΔRR	$\Delta\dot{V}$ (L/MIN)	$\Delta\dot{V}_A$ (L/MIN)	ΔF_{ACO_2} (%)
Actual	+5	+8.1	+6.9	−1.3
Suggested	+4	+2.3*	+1.7*	−0.4†
Actual	−5	+8.1	+6.9	−1.3
Hypnosis	+17†	+8.2	+6.0	−1.6
Suggested	+4	+2.3	+1.7	−0.4
Hypnosis	+17†	+8.2*	+6.0†	−1.63‡

* $p = <0.01$.
† $p = <0.05$.
‡ $p = <0.001$.

during the control prior to the actual experience ($p = <0.05$). The minute ventilation and alveolar ventilation were also found to be significantly higher during the control prior to the suggested experience as compared with the control prior to the hypnotic experience ($p = <0.05$; see Table 5).

The initial values were also compared with the change in response to

Table 5. COMPARISON OF CONTROL VALUES PRIOR TO ACTUAL PAIN, DIRECT SUGGESTION, AND HYPNOTIC SUGGESTION

	RR	$\dot{V}$ (L/MIN)	$\dot{V}_A$ (L/MIN)	F_{ACO_2} (%)
Actual	9	6.8	5.6	5.9
Suggested	11*	6.8	5.3	5.4*
Actual	9	6.8	5.6	5.9
Hypnosis	9	4.9†	3.7‡	5.7
Suggested	11	6.8	5.3	5.4
Hypnosis	9	4.9‡	3.7‡	5.7

* $p = <0.01$.
† $p = <0.05$.
‡ $p = <0.02$.

the stimulus. There were no correlations between the initial values and the amount of change from this value.

COMMENT

From the data given above, it is evident that physiologic change occurring during direct suggestion is significantly less than that occurring during either the actual stimulus or the hypnotic reproduction. The differences found between control values reflect the subject's varying metabolic state during differing time periods. As there was no correlation between the level of the control values and the response to stimulation, the variation in the control values was not seen as detracting from the results.

Individual Case Reports

The following case reports provide detailed accounts of response to the headache and its suggested and hypnotic reproduction.

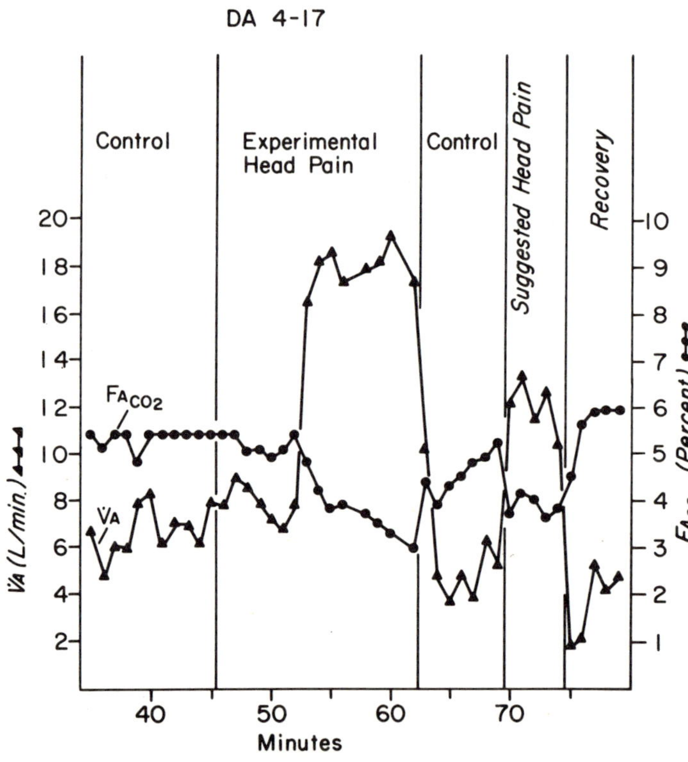

Fig. 1. Actual and nonhypnotic suggestion of head pain in Subject 1. Marked hyperventilation response (greater during actual pain) occurred during both stimuli, which was promptly terminated at end of stimulus period.

SUBJECT 1. Subject 1 was a 21-year-old white male single medical student who was able to withstand the headband stimulation a total of 16 min. After being stimulated 6 min, he began to hyperventilate markedly and later noted, "All I could think about was getting the thing off. I got very restless—a strange tingling or throbbing in my hands—sweaty all over. I wanted to get up and leave." Toward the end he felt afraid and was completely preoccupied with the pain. After removal of the band he reported, "I felt all through." He wanted to be left alone. He gradually relaxed and 7 min after removal he said, "Things are more like before the experiment." He was then asked to close his eyes and think about the pain and his feelings of wanting to do something about it. This stimulus was repeated once and then terminated after 5 min. During this stimulation he said he felt more restless, developed a throbbing sensation in his hands, and hyperventilated. The reaction was terminated promptly when he was asked to relax. Results of this experiment are illustrated in Figure 1.

During the hypnotic suggestion of the headband situation (which occurred five months later) he was asked to "Think about the headband situation and the pain you experienced." This stimulus was repeated in 2-min intervals over a 12-min period. A marked hyperventilation response followed the suggestion which was terminated with suggested relaxation. During the stimulus period he said he felt very uncomfortable and "I didn't like it. I resented it—it was unfair—I didn't deserve it." He pounded the chair and looked very angry. When asked about his feelings after the hypnosis he could not recall them (Fig. 2).

COMMENT. In this very cooperative and suggestible subject the suggested experience is similar to the hypnotic and actual experience.

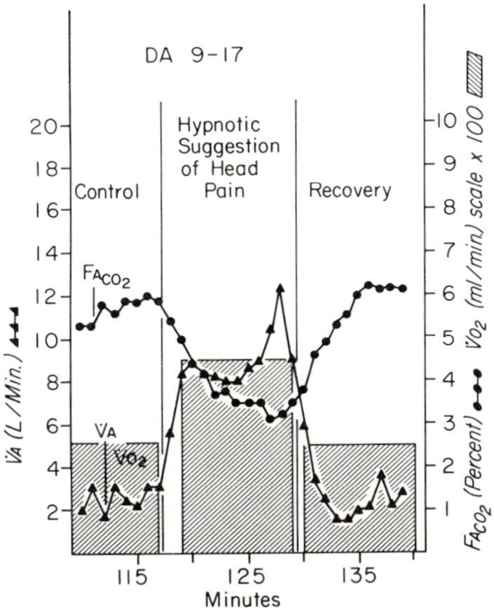

Fig. 2. Response of Subject 1 to hypnotic suggestion of head pain situation five months after actual stimulation. Hypnotic suggestion produced a more intense response than direct suggestion, but otherwise seemed very similar. As shown, a considerable increase in oxygen consumption occurred as well.

SUBJECT 2. Subject 2 was a 23-year-old white male medical student who was able to endure the headband stimulation for 23 min. He began to hyperventilate immediately after the band was placed and hyperventilated more severely as the stimulus was increased in intensity. During the first portion of the experiment he said it "wasn't too bad." Toward the end, as he got progressively more uncomfortable, he noted: "I was getting mad as hell. . . . I felt like grasping the damned thing and throwing it off. . . . I just wanted to get out." After it was removed he felt "great, relaxed." Thirty-nine min after the band was removed he was asked to close his eyes and relax. Three min later he was asked to think of how he felt and what he felt like doing during the height of the headache. This was repeated several times over an 8-min period. A mild increase in ventilation followed the stimulation, which was terminated with suggested relaxation. About this suggestion period he said, "I was mad as hell." He didn't think he could reproduce the headband situation. He said he was uncomfortable and irritable because of the length of the experiment (Fig. 3).

During the hypnotic stimulation he was told every 2 min over a period of 8 min that the "headscrew is being tightened and you are experiencing pain" and "the pain is more and more unbearable." A prompt hyperventilation response occurred which increased in intensity until he was told to relax. Of the hypnotic experience he said, "I felt more pressure than real pain; as you reinforced I could feel it more and more." This experiment is illustrated in Figure 4.

COMMENT. During direct suggestion Subject 2 was unable to relive the headband situation. However, during hypnotic suggestion carried out 34 days later, he had fair reproduction of the headband situation and the physiologic changes.

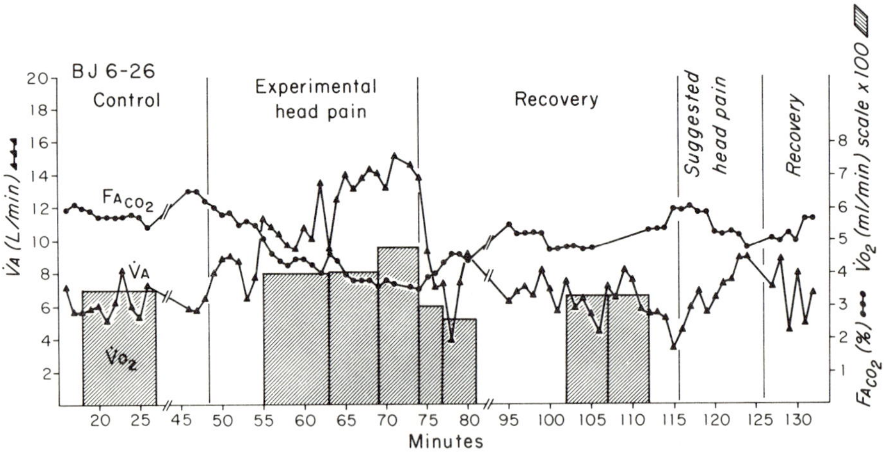

Fig. 3. Hyperventilation and elevated oxygen consumption in response to head pain in Subject 2. Although he responded to suggestion period with hyperventilation, it was secondary to anger and irritability evoked by length of experiment. Headband situation was not relived.

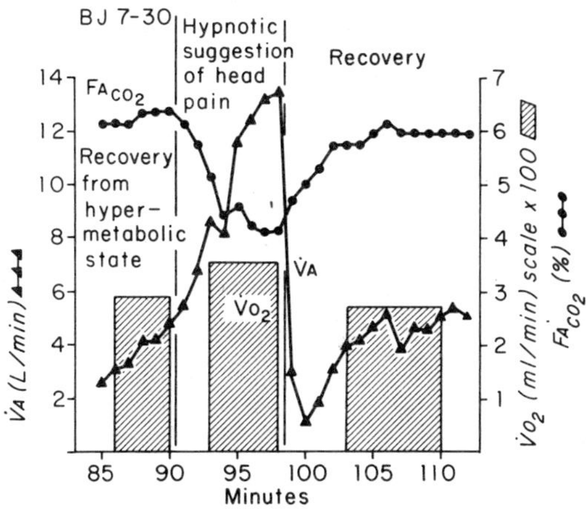

Fig. 4. Hyperventilation and elevated oxygen consumption occurring in Subject 2 one month after actual headband experience.

DISCUSSION

In this study the use of suggestion during hypnosis was compared with direct suggestion without the aid of a hypnotic trance and with reactions to the original stimulus. Although a number of experimental problems were present which make interpretation of the data subject to error, it appears evident that the advantages of hypnosis over direct suggestion were the ease of maintaining relaxation and concentration on the subject matter, and the greater vividness of reproduction of the experimental head pain situation.

Factors which may have influenced the results were the use of two investigators (one for the hypnosis and one for the actual pain and suggestion), the sequence of the experiments, the time lapse between the suggested and hypnotic experiments, and the desire and ability of the subjects to cooperate with the suggestion.

With the use of two investigators—one who was a skilled hypnotist and the other who routinely used direct suggestion but not hypnosis—one might expect a difference in patient response even if the investigators both used the same technique. However, if both suggestion periods were done by the same investigator using different techniques, there is the question concerning whether he could vary his technique enough so that the subjects respond differently to him during suggestion versus hypnosis. If he hypnotized a subject first and did the suggestion several weeks later, there may be rapid induction of a hypnotic trance during the second suggestion period and the direct suggestion would in effect be hypnotic suggestion. If direct suggestion was done first, the following hypnosis experiment may be influenced by prior conditioning and a greater or lesser response result. The sequence of the experiments may thus produce results which indicate that hypnosis is more effective, no different, or perhaps even less effective than direct suggestion.

As the suggested stimulus and actual stimulus were separated by no more than 45 min and the hypnotic stimulus and actual stimulus were separated by 4 to 151 days, it is doubtful that the suggestion period had a significant effect on the hypnosis. Also, the time lapse between the actual stimulus and hypnotic experience does not appear to be an important factor in the production of psychologic and physiologic change during hypnotic suggestion. It can be argued that the direct suggestion was not so effective because it was done directly after the actual stimulation—which, in turn, had a dampening effect on the results. This may be illustrated by Subject 2, who hyperventilated during the suggestion period and was unable to relive the head pain experience because of his anger and restlessness over the length of the experiment. However, the direction of the error in this subject was to produce hyperventilation which was comparable to the response of several subjects to suggestion.

This consideration brings in the factor of desire and ability to cooperate with the suggestion. Regardless of the sequence of the experiments, the different investigators, and the time lag, problems such as those illustrated in Subject 2 were absent during the hypnosis experiments. Therefore, although it may be true that hypnosis is merely an elaborate way of suggesting material and is an entirely voluntary phenomenon, its advantage lies in the ease of maintaining relaxation and concentration on the suggested subject matter. It is possible that the direct suggestion would have yielded similar results if the same element of relaxation and concentration could have been induced without the aid of a hypnotic trance.

From these experiments it would seem that the physiologic response was directly related to the depth of the trance and vividness of reliving of suggested events. This was true to the extent that a vivid hypnotic experience produced a good physiologic response in a subject who had had only a fair response to the actual stimulation (Subject 3). On the other hand, Subject 6—with a poor hypnotic experience and the same physiologic response to the pain as Subject 3—had a poor physiologic response during the hypnosis. The vivid reliving of suggested events is seen as the major differentiating factor between the suggestion with and without hypnosis and is thought to account for the markedly better physiologic response during hypnosis.

The findings in this report are consistent with those of Vanderhoof and Clancy, Kehoe and Ironside, and Graham and Kunish, and in conflict with those of Damaser, Shor, and Orne, Barber and Hahn, and Barber, Chauncey, and Winer. It is important, however, to examine the results of these experimental reports within the light of the considerable differences in methodology. The findings in these experiments are for different physiologic variables, and some variables appear to reflect hypnotically induced emotion better than others. Therefore, the selection of the variable may determine the result and account for the discrepancy. Some variables may be more likely to reflect changes in a given organ system. For example, a subject may increase cardiac output during one experiment by increasing heart rate, and in the next by increasing stroke volume. If the only variable being measured is heart rate, the conclusion will be drawn that cardiac function did not change with the stimulus applied. However, this is obviously untrue as the cardiac output may be the same during both experiments. Therefore, conclusions about the effectiveness of suggestion with and without hypnosis cannot be drawn until multiple variables from several organ systems are involved.

In this regard Vanderhoof and Clancy used peripheral blood flow, Kehoe and Ironside used gastric acid secretion, and Graham and Kunish used skin temperature. These investigators all found hypnosis to be more effective than direct suggestion. Barber and his coworkers used parotid gland excretion in one series of experiments and skin resistance, heart rate, and frontalis muscle activity in another. Damaser et al. also used skin resistance, heart rate, and frontalis muscle activity. Both Barber's and Damaser's groups found no difference between suggestion and hypnosis. It may well be that certain physiologic variables do not differentiate between hypnosis and suggestion, but that other variables do perform this function. The diversity of variables and methodology employed do not permit a definitive statement.

SUMMARY

1. Direct suggestion of a head pain experience was found to be less effective in reproducing the experience than hypnotic suggestion.

2. The above findings are discussed in the light of a number of experimental problems which have direct bearing on the results.

3. It is concluded that hypnotic suggestion and direct suggestion without the aid of a hypnotic trance may give similar results under optimal circumstances. However, circumstances are seldom optimal and the hyp-

notic trance adds to the subject's ability to ignore extraneous material and to concentrate on the suggested material.

4. Certain physiologic variables may differentiate between suggested and hypnotic stimuli while others do not.

REFERENCES

Barber, T. X., Chauncey, H. H., and Winer, R. A. Effect of hypnotic and non-hypnotic suggestions on parotid gland response to gustatory stimuli, Psychosom Med, 26:374, 1964.

——— and Hahn, K. W. Experimental studies in "hypnotic" behavior: Physiologic and subjective effects of imagined pain, J Nerv Ment Dis, 139: 416, 1964.

Damaser, E. C., Shor, R. E., and Orne, M. T. Physiologic effects during hypnotically requested emotions, Psychosom Med, 25:334, 1963.

Dudley, D. L., Holmes, T. H., Martin, C. J., and Ripley, H. S. Hypnotically induced facsimile of pain, Arch Gen Psychiat, 15:198, 1966.

——— Masuda, M., Martin, C. J., and Holmes, T. H. Psychophysiological studies of experimentally induced action oriented behavior, J Psychosom Res, 9:209, 1965.

Graham, F. K., and Kunish, N. O. Physiologic responses of unhypnotized subjects to attitude suggestions, Psychosom Med, 27:317, 1965.

Kehoe, M., and Ironside, W. Studies on the experimental evocation of depressive response using hypnosis: II. The influence of depressive responses upon the secretion of gastric acid, Psychosom Med, 25:403, 1963.

Vanderhoof, E., and Clancy, J. Peripheral blood flow as an indicator of emotional reaction, J Appl Physiol, 17:67, 1962.

15

Comments on the Etiology of Psychophysiologic Changes in Ventilation

There are no studies in the literature which deal with the mechanisms of ventilatory change during varying emotions. There are studies, however, which compare respiratory center sensitivity to inspired carbon dioxide during varying activity levels. Katz found that hypnosis was accompanied by respiratory center depression as measured by the respiratory response to inhaled CO_2 and compared with that in the alert resting state. Reed and Kellogg reported similar findings when they compared the response of sleeping individuals versus awake resting individuals. Identical findings were also reported by Sieker, Heyman, and Birchfield, and by Robin et al. A variety of factors has been proposed to explain the increase in ventilation during exercise. However, the hyperpnea of exercise appears to be best explained by a combination of humoral and neural factors. Bannister, Cunningham, and Douglas provide evidence of an increased sensitivity of the respiratory center to carbon dioxide immediately following exercise which would appear to be mediated through central mechanisms.

It was thought that respiratory center changes during exercise, anger, and anxiety might be similar, and that sensitivity changes during sleep and depression might also be similar, but opposite from the changes found during activation.

It was evident from these studies that minute ventilation and alveolar ventilation could be increased or decreased over long periods of time without any change in the carbon dioxide level. Further, if there are changes in $F_{A_{CO_2}}$, they may be in the opposite direction. Thus a higher or lower level of ventilation is then supported by carbon dioxide levels which are inappropriate if that is the only stimulus involved. In order to explain this situation, it is necessary to think in terms of a primary neurological drive or an increase or decrease in the sensitivity and/or the threshold of the respiratory center to carbon dioxide during the various emotional changes.

OBSERVATIONS

In exploring this problem, two subjects were followed longitudinally during days when they were normal, depressed, or angry. On each day they were studied, subjects were exposed (through a closed system) to concentrations of inhaled carbon dioxide varying from 1.5 to 4.3 percent, while continuous measurements were made of minute ventilation and the fractional concentration of alveolar carbon dioxide. The subjects breathed each concentration a minimum of 10 min to allow for equilibration. Although the data are preliminary, they provide some useful insight into the possible etiology of some of the psychophysiologic changes observed.

SUBJECT 1. Subject 1 was a 60-year-old divorced male with clinical emphysema and tuberculosis. He was exposed to a F_{ICO_2} of 1.64 and 4.30 percent in air. The carbon dioxide was administered from 300-L meteorological balloons. This patient was tested on a "blue" day when he felt tired and "like not doing anything" and was experiencing "low spirits," and on a day when he felt that his spirits were near normal and he was relaxed and comfortable. While breathing air, his minute ventilation was 1 L lower on the "blue" day as compared with the normal day. The 1-L difference was maintained during exposure to the 1.64 and 4.30 percent carbon dioxide. Thus, although ventilation increased during exposure to carbon dioxide, the rise in ventilation with the increasing F_{ICO_2} was parallel. However, when the change in F_{ACO_2} was followed, it was found that at higher levels of ventilation it took very little change in F_{ACO_2} to produce a large change in ventilation on the normal day while large changes in F_{ACO_2} had little effect on ventilation on the "blue" day.

COMMENT. The initial data on this subject indicate that there are probably both a change in sensitivity and a change in the threshold to carbon dioxide with mild depression as compared with a normal or relaxed emotional state.

SUBJECT 2. Subject 2 was a 56-year-old married male with normal pulmonary function and who experienced intermittent anger at his wife. Periods of mild and severe anger were compared with periods of relaxation while he inhaled air and 1.8 percent carbon dioxide. During relaxed periods, the patient's minute ventilation averaged 6 to 7 L/min. During mild anger it averaged 12 L/min and the patient was mildly dyspneic. The F_{ACO_2} was 5 percent during relaxation and mild anger, and 3.5 percent during the severe anger. The minute ventilation increased ½ to 1 L while the subject inhaled carbon dioxide during relaxation. During mild anger, his increase was 2 L/min. However, during severe anger, the patient dropped his ventilation approximately 2 L/min (from 12 to 10) and the $F_{A_{CO_2}}$ increased from 3.5 to 4.5 percent. He also experienced alleviation of his dyspnea and his anger decreased. When inhalation of carbon dioxide was stopped the changes reversed.

COMMENT. It appears that not only is the sensitivity and threshold of the respiratory system changed during emotional states compared with the relaxed, resting state, but also that the changes in sensitivity and threshold may depend both on the amount and kind of emotional change.

DISCUSSION

It is evident from preliminary data that there are fairly wide variations in the threshold and sensitivity of the respiratory system to inspired carbon dioxide during a subject's experiencing various emotions. During a mild depressive reaction, the ventilatory response to inspired carbon dioxide was found to be decreased. During mild anger it was increased. However, during severe anger the sensitivity of the respiratory system to inspired carbon dioxide was found to be greatly decreased—in fact, reversed. During mild depression, it was found that large changes in the $F_{A_{CO_2}}$ produced small changes in ventilation when compared with the resting relaxed state. There was no "severe" depression to compare with the severe anger.

From the above data and from that presented in preceding chapters, it becomes difficult to ascribe to carbon dioxide the primary role of mediating changes in ventilation. The effects of this stimulus appear to be modified considerably by the central nervous system, and a given level of arterial or alveolar CO_2 does not result in a specific amount of ventilation. During hyperventilation reactions (as illustrated in Subject 2), inspired carbon dioxide may reduce ventilation and reduce symptomatology. However, during a similar emotion of smaller degree, inspired carbon dioxide produced an increase in ventilation which was greater than that observed during the resting, relaxed state. A variable which was not investigated in this study was the effect of varying the level of inspired carbon dioxide with different types and intensity of emotional response.

The original speculation concerning the basis of the respiratory hyperfunction and hypofunction seen in the psychophysiologic reactions was that of increases and decreases in respiratory center sensitivity and/or threshold. It was thought that a smaller or larger amount of carbon dioxide in the blood could support a larger or smaller minute ventilation, respectively. During long-term changes in emotion when the metabolism was seen to "catch up" with ventilation, the level of the F_{ACO_2} returned to prestimulus levels. This was thought to result from the adjustment of the respiratory center to a new sensitivity with a return to homeostasis and a Pa_{CO_2} of 40 mm. With the finding that the carbon dioxide drive to ventilation can be decreased or even *reversed* during action oriented conditions, the above does not apply.

Although the picture is very complex it would appear safe to state that cortical drive and respiratory center sensitivity to CO_2 both play important roles in the production of the respiratory changes described in preceding chapters. It is not possible at present to discuss these roles further because of a lack of data; the precise definition of the roles awaits future investigations.

REFERENCES

Bannister, R. G., Cunningham, D. J. C., and Douglas, C. G. The carbon dioxide stimulus to breathing in severe exercise, J Physiol, 125:90, 1954.

Cunnnigham, D. J. C. Some quantitative aspects of the regulation of human respiration in exercise, Brit Med Bull, 19:25, 1963.

Katz, J. Respiratory response to carbon dioxide in the awake and hypnotic state, JAMA, 193:767, 1965.

Reed, D. J., and Kellogg, R. H. Effect of sleep on carbon dioxide stimulation of breathing in acute and chronic hypoxia, J Appl Physiol, 15:1135, 1960.

Robin, E. D., Whaley, R. D., Crump, C. H., and Travis, D. M. Alveolar gas tensions, pulmonary ventilation and blood pH during physiologic sleep in normal subjects, J Clin Invest, 7:981, 1958.

Sieker, H. O., Heyman, A., and Birchfield, R. I. The effects of natural sleep and hypersomnolent states on respiratory function, Ann Intern Med, 52: 500, 1960.

Section IV

Clinical Aspects

The following material consists of a mixture of clinical facts and experimental observations on patients with emphysema and asthma. In general, discussion is limited to the patient with severe debilitating disease. (In Chapter 16, normal patients and those with tuberculosis are included for comparison in a study of dyspnea.) In order better to understand the psychophysiologic and psychosocial variables which are of importance in the maintenance and progression of disability and insufficiency in diffuse obstructive pulmonary syndromes, the experimental observations were conducted during the treatment of the patients. In essence, much of the material represents an attempt to apply the data derived from Sections II and III to clinical evaluation and therapy.

Although there is, of necessity, some separation of medical and psychiatric information in Chapters 20 and 21, every attempt was made at integration.

16

Dyspnea: Psychologic and Physiologic Observations

In previous chapters we have discussed psychologic and physiologic changes in patients with and without respiratory disease. Little was said about the significance of these changes in terms of symptom production.

One of the common symptoms in patients with cardiopulmonary disease is shortness of breath or dyspnea. Dyspnea depends for its identification on the subjective judgment of the patient, and is not definable in terms of blood gas or ventilatory abnormalities. Patients vary in their reports, but the general theme is that of uncomfortable sensations arising in the chest or airway which are interpreted as interfering with the subjects' breathing. The patient feels smothered, breathless, and in need of more air, or that not enough air is available. Some subjects experience dyspnea with minimal or no structural change in their cardiopulmonary system, while others will experience no dyspnea or mild dyspnea with severe structural change. The condition has been reported by normal subjects in association with heavy exercise, increased airway resistance, and periods of undergoing strong emotion. Structural change or damage involving the cardiopulmonary system may well be a sufficient condition for the production of dyspnea, but it does not appear to be necessary for the genesis of the symptom.

The present study was designed to identify some of the respiratory and emotional variables which are associated with the report of dyspnea and which are independent of the degree of cardiopulmonary disease. Student's *t* test for paired samples was utilized for data analysis.

This chapter is adapted from an article originally published in *J Psychosom Res*, 11:325, 1968, by Dudley, D. L., Martin, C. J., and Holmes, T. H.

EXPLORATORY OBSERVATIONS

An exploratory set of observations was made on 16 subjects; they were patients with chronic pulmonary disease who experienced dyspnea frequently. Their ages varied from 29 to 78 with a mean of 53 years. There were three females in the group. Thirteen had DOPS (diffuse obstructive pulmonary syndrome or clinical emphysema) with tuberculosis, one had DOPS without tuberculosis, and two had tuberculosis without DOPS. Those with DOPS were classified according to the criteria listed in Table 1.

Table 1. CLASSIFICATION OF DIFFUSE OBSTRUCTIVE PULMONARY SYNDROME

	DISABILITY*		INSUFFICIENCY†
I	None	A	None
II	Mild dyspnea	B	Arterial hypoxia
III	Moderate dyspnea	C	Arterial hypoxia with hypercapnia
IV	Severe dyspnea	D	Cor pulmonale with any of the above

* Disability is classified on the basis of tolerance levels similar to those used by the New York Heart Association.

† The classification of pulmonary insufficiency has been modified from that suggested by Baldwin, Cournand, and Richards, who used the presence of hypoxia, hypercapnia, and cor pulmonale during exercise to distinguish the different states of pulmonary insufficiency. This laboratory uses any abnormal values found during rest or when the subject is walking at 2 mph. Also, this laboratory no longer uses the above sequence of change—which actually represents the clinical progression of the disease. Instead, "D" has been changed to *acidosis*. The sequence then represents the progression of blood gas changes in the disease. Perhaps more properly, the term "insufficiency" should be replaced by "clinical status" in this table.

Table 2. DYSPNEIC DAYS COMPARED WITH NONDYSPNEIC DAYS (16 SUBJECTS)*

	RR	$\dot{V}$ (L/MIN)	$\dot{V}_A$ (L/MIN)	F_{ACO_2} (%)	$\dot{V}_{CO_2}$ (ML/MIN)
No dyspnea	18	9.5	6.4	5.3	331
Dyspnea	21†	10.1†	6.6†	5.5†	362†

* Data collected in part by Gleeson and Anderson.

† p = not significant.

Mean member of dyspneic days = 3.7; mean number nondyspneic days = 12.3.

Evaluation of pulmonary function was made during days on which the subjects complained of dyspnea and these findings were compared with those on days during which no dyspnea was reported.

Table 2 compares the days on which these subjects experienced dyspnea with days on which they did not. As shown, there was no significant change in the mean levels of any of the five respiratory variables utilized.

Three of these subjects were studied before, during, and after exercise on days on which they reported dyspnea and on days in which no dyspnea was experienced. No difference was found between physiologic response to exercise on dyspneic and nondyspneic days.

Table 3. DOPS CLASSIFICATION AND WALKING VENTILATION INDEX (14 SUBJECTS)

SUBJECTS	DISABILITY	INSUFFICIENCY	WALKING VENTILATION INDEX*
WR	III	A	0.34 to 0.52
C	IV	C	0.54
E	IV	A	0.64
WR	IV	D	1.18
GT	III	B	
R	III	B	
M	II	A	0.60
SE	III	C	0.26
B	II	A	0.50
SH	II	A	
AD	IV	D	0.72
K	IV	B	0.54
GB	III	B	
ET	III	A	

* WVI's were not obtainable on all patients because of technical problems.

Table 3 shows the classification of the subjects with the diffuse obstructive pulmonary syndrome. Patients with a classification of A in the insufficiency scale are seen to experience disability (as measured by their symptoms at rest and exercise) as severe as patients in B, C, or D scale.

FOLLOW-UP OBSERVATIONS

In a follow-up study, observations were made on a group of 20 subjects. Ten were medical students with normal lungs, two were patients with DOPS and tuberculosis, and eight were patients with tuberculosis without DOPS. Their ages ranged from 22 to 49 with a mean of 29 years. There were seven females. These subjects were observed under three separate experimental conditions:

1. The hospitalized subjects were observed daily, and naturally occurring variations in life situations were noted and correlated with dyspnea and measurements of respiratory function.

2. Life experiences which the subjects had previously reported as being associated with the occurrence of dyspnea were suggested. Subjects were first instructed to close their eyes and relax. After relaxation and the recording of control measures these experiences were suggested to the subjects. The suggestion was limited to asking the subject to free his mind of extraneous thoughts and to concentrate on the particular life situation which had been previously associated with dyspnea. The suggestion was restated at 1- to 5-min intervals.

3. A metal headband with 14 adjustable rubber-tipped screws around the edges was used for noxious stimulation of the head. This device produced a pressure headache and physical and mental discomfort when the adjustable screws were fixed tightly against the circumference of the head. As it was the objective of the experiments to utilize the noxious stimulus to produce a significant change in behavior from the control state, time and magnitude of pressure were held as variables rather than constants. The end point of the observation was determined by the subject and was defined as that point at which he felt he could no longer tolerate the experience. Following application of the pressure device to the head, the screws were tightened at intervals of 5 to 8 min until the end point was achieved. Time required to reach the level of intolerance and termination of the noxious stimulus ranged between 18 and 33 min.

In these observations, emotional change was used as an independent variable in an attempt to correlate emotional reactions and dyspnea.

Suggested and Naturally Occurring Events

Table 4 records the response of seven subjects to suggested and naturally occurring events which produced dyspnea and emotion, and the subsequent alleviation of symptoms with relaxation and suggestion of pleasant

Table 4. PSYCHOLOGIC AND PHYSIOLOGIC CHANGES ASSOCIATED WITH DYSPNEA

SUBJECT	EMOTION	RR	$\dot{V}$ (L/MIN)	$\dot{V}_A$ (L/MIN)	V_T (ML)	F_{ACO_2} (%)	$\dot{V}_{O_2}$ (ML/MIN)	BREATHING
WR	Control	14	6.0	4.3	429	5.7		No symptoms
	Anger	26	7.9	5.3	304	5.2		Dyspneic
	Recovery	13	5.2	3.9	400	5.7		No symptoms
	Control	22	6.5	4.4	295	5.5		No symptoms
	Depression	14	4.6	3.1	329	5.9		Dyspneic
	Recovery	14	6.0	4.3	429	5.7		No symptoms
OH	Control	15	5.0	3.8	300	4.6		No symptoms
	Anger	32	7.1	4.6	222	3.9		Dyspneic
	Recovery	13	3.7	2.7	285	5.0		No symptoms
	Depressed	11	3.5	2.9	318	5.5		Dyspneic
	Recovery	13	4.6	3.8	354	5.3		Reduced symptoms
GB	Control	45	10.9	6.4	242	4.6	284	No symptoms
	Agitated (asthma)	52	16.8	11.6	323	6.6	523	Dyspneic
	Recovery	43	12.0	7.7	279	4.4	291	No symptoms
VW	Anger, anxiety	15	9.7	8.5	647	3.5		Dyspneic
	Recovery	13	5.2	4.3	400	5.2		No symptoms
Wal	Irritated, angry	18	11.0	9.0	611			Dyspneic
	Relaxed	13	8.5	7.1	654	4.3		Reduced symptoms
GM	Depressed	15	5.3	3.7	353	4.8		Dyspneic
	Relaxed	13	6.6	5.1	508	5.1		No symptoms
W	Relaxed	13	5.0	3.8	385	5.8		No symptoms
	Depressed	12	4.0	2.9	333	6.1		Dyspneic
Control $\frac{\Sigma}{N}$		18	6.5	4.8	361	5.1		
Dyspnea* $\frac{\Sigma}{N}$		22	7.8	5.7	355	5.0		

* p = not significant.

topics. As shown in this table, dyspnea was associated with hyperventilation, hyperpnea, hypoventilation, decreased ventilation, anger, anxiety, and depression. The physiologic values for control and dyspnea were not sig-

Table 5. SEPARATE ANALYSIS

	RR	$\dot{V}$ (L/MIN)	$\dot{V}_A$ (L/MIN)	F_{ACO_2} (%)
DYSPNEA WITH ANGER AND ANXIETY (5 SUBJECTS)				
Control	20	7.1	5.2	4.9
Dyspnea	29*	10.5†	7.8*	4.6
DYSPNEA WITH DEPRESSION (4 SUBJECTS)				
Control	15	5.7	4.3	5.4
Dyspnea	13	4.4‡	3.2‡	5.6

* $p = <0.05$.
† $p = <0.02$.
‡ $p = <0.01$.

nificantly different for the group as a whole. However, when dyspnea with depression, and dyspnea with anger and anxiety, are analyzed separately significant differences are found (Table 5).

Noxious Head Stimulation

Table 6 shows the respiratory response of seven subjects who experienced dyspnea in response to noxious stimulation of the head. This group consisted of five male medical students, one female patient with pulmonary tuberculosis without DOPS, and one female patient with tuberculosis and DOPS. Their ages varied from 22 to 49 with a mean age of 27 years. As

Table 6. DYSPNEA ASSOCIATED WITH NOXIOUS STIMULATION OF THE HEAD (7 SUBJECTS)*

	RR	$\dot{V}$ (L/MIN)	$\dot{V}_A$ (L/MIN)	F_{ACO_2} (%)	$\dot{V}_{O_2}$ (ML/MIN)†
Prepain	9	6.4	5.2	6.0	344
Pain (dyspneic)	11	10.7‡	9.0‡	4.9§	442
Recovery (no dyspnea)	10	5.9	4.7	5.5	226

* Comparison between prepain and pain periods.
† Three subjects only.
‡ $p = <0.02$.
§ $p = <0.01$.

shown, there are significant changes in ventilation and the fractional concentration of alveolar carbon dioxide. The experimental stimulus was also correlated with anger, anxiety, restlessness, irritability, and an intense desire to terminate the experiment.

Shown in Table 7 is the response of seven similar subjects—matched as to age, sex, and disease—who did not experience dyspnea in response to

Table 7. NOXIOUS STIMULATION OF HEAD WITHOUT DYSPNEA (7 MATCHED SUBJECTS)

	RR	$\dot{V}$ (L/MIN)	$\dot{V}_A$ (L/MIN)	$F_{A_{CO_2}}$ (%)	$\dot{V}_{O_2}$ (ML/MIN)*
Prepain	11	7.1	5.6	5.5	308
Pain	13	14.8†	12.3†	3.9†	404‡
Recovery	10	6.1	4.7	5.3	276

* Five subjects.
† $p = <0.01$.
‡ $p = <0.05$.

noxious stimulation of the head. The physiologic and emotional responses were similar to those of the group that experienced dyspnea, and the respiratory changes were not significantly different.

Table 8. DESCRIPTIONS OF DYSPNEA

SUBJECT		TB. PT.	DOPS	STUDENT OR LAB. TECH.
WR	*Hyperventilation:*			
(No. 1)	Fast and hard breathing. I gasp in the breath and my heart pounds. It is not a choking physical thing.	X	X	
	Just gasping for breath like you're drowning. [Such an effort to get enough air in that she feels pain across the shoulder.] Like swimming as far as you can and then you can't go any further.			
	Hypoventilation:			
	Hard to get the breath in. Like someone were choking me. Heart does not pound. Air is heavy and hard to get in. I forget to breathe.			

HM	*Hyperventilation:*			
(No. 2)	Halfway between the last tightening and the end, it became progressively more as if I were suffocating and could not get enough air in.			X
GB	*Hyperpnea:*			
	Feels as though my airway is being constricted. I feel as though I'm smothering. Feels as though my chest is full and I can't get more air in. Seems like it's hollow inside. Hard for me to inhale. I want to take in a deeper breath, but I can't.	X	X	
Wal	*Hyperventilation:*			
	It makes my chest hurt and I can't hardly breathe. It makes you breathe fast. You have to breathe fast in order to keep from smothering. It smothers me.	X		
VW	*Hyperventilation:*			
	[She felt as though her breathing was labored.] I had a hard time breathing.	X		
GM	*Decreased Ventilation:*			
	I can't get in enough air. I feel somewhat short of breath.	X		
RP	*Hyperventilation:*			
	I felt short of breath—almost like gasping, and began to feel dizzy and slightly nauseated.			X
GN	*Hyperventilation:*			
	I felt short of breath at the very first tightening. I had difficulty inhaling. [Thinks he hypoventilated.]			X
BV	*Hyperventilation:*			
	I felt a little short of breath at times. A little smothered.			X
TS	*Hyperventilation:*			
	Hard to breathe. Very much so. Felt like there was a pressure on my chest. Hard to breathe in. Also hard to breathe out but not as bad. A pain in back of my lungs. Felt a constriction in my chest. Thought that the shortness of breath might be due to the constriction. I couldn't get enough air in.	X		

WH	*Hyperventilation:*		
	I felt as though I was taking in deeper breaths and at the same time felt as though I was hardly breathing. Felt as though I needed more oxygen. Felt short of breath—couldn't get in enough oxygen.		X
OH	*Hyperventilation:*		
	Like smothering. Like something were held over my face. Like there was a weight on my chest which made it difficult to breathe.	X	
	Hypoventilation:		
	Short of breath. Smothering. Like I feel when I want something I cannot have.		
W	*Hypoventilation:*		
	Felt slightly short of breath. Felt like sighing.	X	

Table 8 contains statements made by the subjects to describe their respiratory symptoms. Using their descriptions without physiologic measurements would make it impossible to tell hyperventilation from hypoventilation.

Subject 1. This is the detailed account of intensive observations made on a 49-year-old, three-times-divorced white female commercial artist. The patient was followed over a two-and-a-half year period during which she was studied on 42 separate occasions. She participated in both the initial study group and the follow-up group. Her DOPS was classified as IIIA and her WVI varied from 0.34 to 0.52 on repeated measurements.

The patient's life was characterized by an inability to tolerate close interpersonal contact. She was married three times, the longest of which lasted three years. All marriages were marked by incompatibility in all spheres. She was born on a remote island in Alaska and patterned her life as though she still lived on that island. She continually felt overwhelmed with life and was frantic in her attempts to adjust. Her first episodes of respiratory disease began in childhood with repeated bouts of quinsy and otitis media. In addition, she had typhoid fever and rheumatic fever at ages 7 and 13, respectively. She stated that she was never a well child. Twenty years prior to the study, after attaining some success as a commercial artist, she developed pulmonary tuberculosis. Since that time she was treated intermittently for active tuberculosis and chronic obstructive lung disease. She could not recall when she first began feeling dyspneic, but noted that it became a problem after her first bout with tuberculosis. At the time of this study the patient was unable to climb one flight of stairs and was unable to work because of exertional dyspnea.

On 17 of the 42 days on which she was measured she came to the laboratory feeling dyspneic. When these 17 days were compared with the 25 eupneic

Table 9. 17 Dyspneic Days Compared with 25 Eupneic Days

	RR	$\dot{V}$ (L/min)	$\dot{V}_A$ (L/min)	V_T (ml)	$F_{A_{CO_2}}$ (%)	$\dot{V}_{CO_2}$ (ml/min)
Dyspneic	19	7.5	5.6	444	5.1	280
Eupneic	9*	5.7	4.8	795	5.4	256

* $p < 0.05$.

days, the only significant difference was found to be in the respiratory rate—which was increased during dyspnea (Table 9). No significant changes were noted in $\dot{V}$, $\dot{V}_A$, V_T, $F_{A_{CO_2}}$, or $\dot{V}_{CO_2}$. On 14 of these days she underwent psychologic stimulation with the intent of either producing or relieving dyspnea and she was followed during dyspneic periods. With this approach it was found that

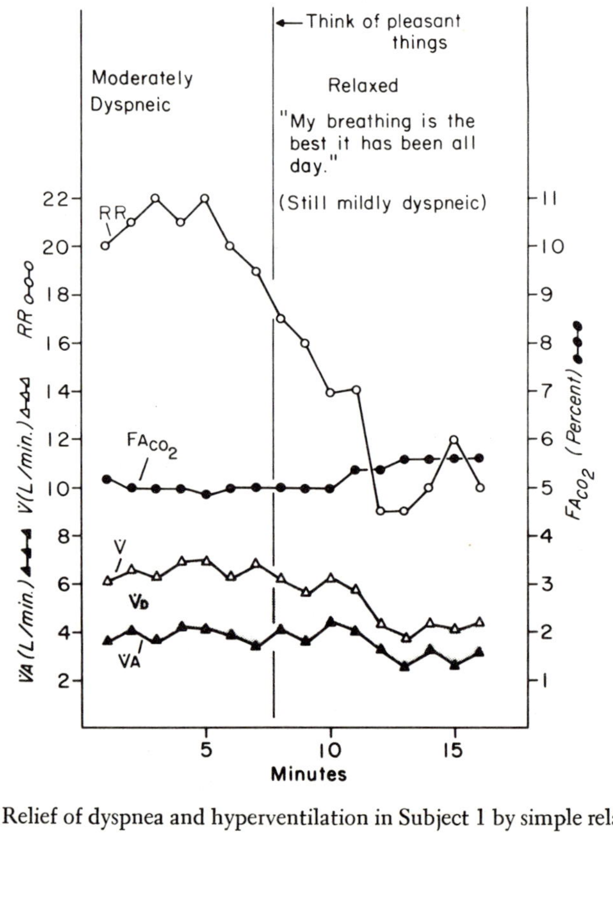

Fig. 1. Relief of dyspnea and hyperventilation in Subject 1 by simple relaxation.

dyspnea which was present at the beginning of an experiment could be relieved by suggestion of relaxation. The relaxation was always followed by change in several respiratory variables (Fig. 1). It was also found that the subject's dyspnea could be relieved by bronchodilators, placebo bronchodilators, 20 percent oxygen in helium, and by 100 percent oxygen. In addition, severe dyspnea was easily produced by the suggestion of life situations that evoked such attacks.

After a careful study of the subject's breathing complaints, it was found that she could describe two distinct "types" of dyspnea. One was described as a panting shortness of breath with fast hard breathing. She gasped for air and her heart pounded. This was described as "not a choking physical thing"—i.e., no impairment of getting the air in and out was perceived. The emotional tone during an attack of this type is illustrated from the following quotes: "Anxious, angry. Terribly angry—but I never do anything. There's nothing I can do. I want to eliminate them [people] from my personal life but I can't do it. Disgusted." An attack of the type described above was precipitated when she was asked to think about people who had provoked her anger and it was associated with hyperventilation (Fig. 2; see also Fig. 7, Chapter 8). Attacks

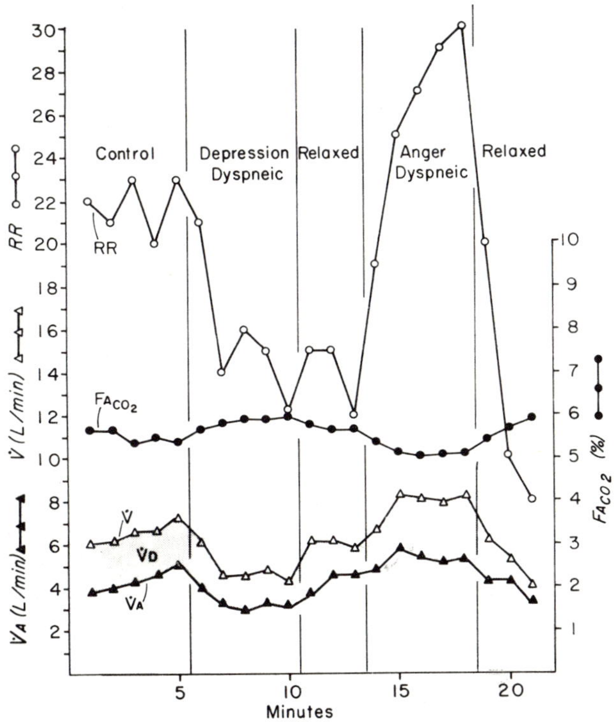

Fig. 2. Dyspnea in association with anger and hyperventilation and depression and hypoventilation. As shown, dyspnea could be readily produced and alleviated with use of simple suggestion. This was true with most of the subjects who experienced dyspnea.

of this type were produced in the laboratory a total of six times, always with the patient at rest (Table 10).

Table 10. Dyspneic Breathing Compared with Eupneic Breathing

	RR	$\dot{V}$ (L/min)	$\dot{V}_A$ (L/min)	V_T (ml)	F_{ACO_2} (%)
	Dyspnea with Anger and Anxiety (6 Experiments)				
Control	15	5.3	3.8	408	5.4
Dyspnea	25*	7.0*	4.5*	287	4.9*
	Dyspnea with Depression (8 Experiments)				
Control	18	6.3	4.9	578	5.4
Dyspnea	20	5.0*	3.6*	349†	5.7*

* $p < 0.01$.
† $p < 0.05$.

Shortness of breath was also described as being choking and smothering. She had "difficulty getting the air in" and the "air felt heavy." Her heart did not pound. She said that she often forgot to breathe when she had this kind of attack. The following quotes from the subject illustrate her emotional tone: "Worried, but not an excited worry. Unhappy. I procrastinate. I feel like doing nothing. What's the use of trying? I feel indecisive. I feel low and depressed and don't give a darn what happens to me. When everything fails and you've exhausted all of your resources." When asked to think of how she felt when she was tired and depressed (hopeless) and at the end of her rope, she exhibited dyspnea and hypoventilated. The respiratory response during this "type" of dyspnea is illustrated in Figure 2 (see also Fig. 8, Chapter 8). Similar attacks were produced in the laboratory a total of eight times, always with the patient at rest (Table 10).

Thinking of her deceased father was consistently associated with dyspnea. She could not remember the time or place of his death and always spoke of him in the present tense. Her father and her relationship to him were described as follows: "There isn't anybody as decent, clean, and perfect as he is. He was the only one who ever understood and accepted me. They [the other children] weren't a pal to him like I was. I was always with him. We would go on hunting and fishing trips together. He was a handsome man, strong, talented. He was a genius and an artist."

Her emotional response to thinking of her father was that of feeling "a terrible loss—a terrible sadness. Nobody in the world can be to me what he was. . . . I have no feelings of committing suicide. . . . I don't feel like doing anything in particular. There's nothing I can do except eliminate it from my mind. Hardly a day passes when I don't think of him. I can't bring him back. I can't bring him back and I can't find anyone to replace him. . . . I know I can't have him so I don't wish for something I can't have. I would give up 90 per-

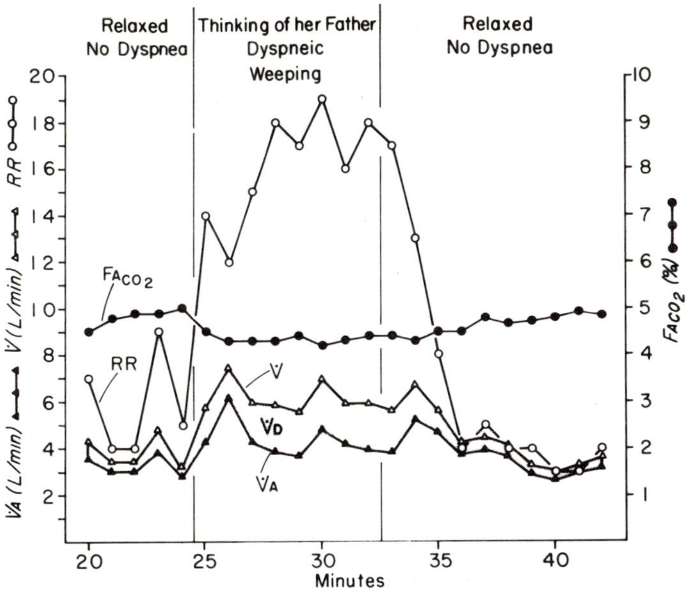

Fig. 3. Dyspnea in association with frustration and hyperventilation in Subject 1.

cent of my remaining life if I could have him back." The loss was felt as acute, sharp, and frustrating and very different from what she described as depression. Her feelings about her father had been getting acute since his death five years previously and she could do nothing to alleviate them. At the time she was studied she experienced visual and auditory hallucinations early in the morning during which her father appeared to be standing at the foot of her bed playing her favorite concerto (which he had written) on his violin. She was preoccupied with death and several months after the completion of these studies she died of an overdose of barbiturates.

In the laboratory, when thinking of her father, she said that she usually breathed more heavily and with more gasping. It was as though she were in an enclosure with no ventilation. Figure 3 shows her respiratory response to feeling frustrated, anxious, blue, and wanting to join him or get him back. The hyperventilation response shown was correlated with severe dyspnea.

In addition to the transient dyspnea experienced with emotion and exertion, this subject had periods of weeks or months when she was dyspneic almost continuously. During her fourth admission the opportunity was present to study her during one of these periods. For eight months prior to admission she had experienced severe abdominal pains which were aggravated by meals and emotional upsets. She also experienced dyspnea which was incapacitating and she was continuously tired, anxious, and frightened. She felt that "everything was over. Nothing picked me up. I was afraid." Self-administered treatment for her pain and nervousness consisted of 100 to 300 aspirin per day and unknown amounts of belladonna, codeine, and phenobarbital. Shortly after admission a large peptic ulcer was diagnosed and self-medication was discontinued. Ulcer therapy and reassurance led to alleviation of her abdominal pain, emotional symptoms, and dyspnea. She also gained 20 lbs over a 7-week period. Figure 6 of Chapter 8 shows the patient's respiratory pattern during and after alleviation of her pain. Drugs, pain, and emotion seem to be the variables present during the above-described episode, which were in turn responsible for the dyspnea. As pain was considered to be the primary stimulus, head pain was used in an attempt to reproduce dyspnea in the laboratory. Prior to the experiment the subject said she felt "very good" and had no dyspnea. As the head pain increased in intensity the patient developed nausea, the urge to vomit, and a severe, sharp, superficial abdominal pain which came in waves and was much more severe than the head pain. She also felt warm, sweat profusely, was dyspneic, "panicky," and developed marked abdominal swelling. For 25 min after termination of the pain, these symptoms gradually decreased in severity. During the poststimulation period she reported that the abdominal pain and nausea were identical to that which occurred when "painful people bother me" (Fig. 4).

COMMENT. This patient was one who had experienced dyspnea for many years in association with emotion, pain, and exercise. She illustrates the wide variety of stimuli which may be used to produce or alleviate dyspnea, and the association of dyspnea with physiologic change from the resting values for any particular day. It is important to note that the disability she experienced was largely secondary to emotional change and the associated physiologic change. When periods of emotional turmoil were not present, she was able to function adequately with minimal disability. To date this has been the experience with patients who have mild insufficiency and severe disability.

SUBJECT 2. This subject was a 28-year-old white male married medical student with normal pulmonary function and no history of pulmonary disease, who volunteered for the noxious stimulation experiment. At the first adjustment

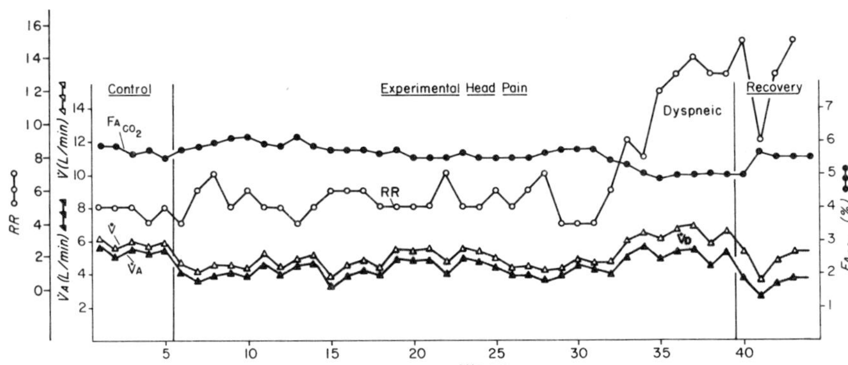

Fig. 4. Production of dyspnea in Subject 1 during noxious stimulation of the head.

and tightening of the headband the subject said that he experienced an unanticipated feeling of terror and being trapped. The pain was diffuse at first. There was an increased wetness of the eyes and a feeling that the eyes were protruding. The pain soon became focal and could be denied, leaving only a feeling of pressure.

As the experimenter approached the subject to tighten the band a second time, the subject wondered "what advantage there was to making the pain excruciating." This was 6 min after the band had been first tightened. At 11 min the band was tightened a third time. After this last tightening the subject experienced increased salivation, a tight feeling in the throat, tearing of the eyes, a feeling that the eyes were protruding, hypermotility, a feeling of suffocation, and moderate hostility toward the experimenter. As the experiment neared the tolerance point at 16 min, the subject became increasingly short of breath ("I felt as if I were suffocating and could not get enough air in"), increasingly hostile, began to hyperventilate, showed increased blood pressure and pulse rate, and could no longer tolerate the pain. At this time his thoughts were as follows: "To hell with this. Let me out of here. Enough! Enough! Enough!" At this point the subject felt that he had lost awareness of his surroundings. Eighteen minutes after the band had been placed on his head it had to be removed.

After the removal of the band the subject felt a "profound feeling of relief" and the discomfort vanished. At this point he felt as though he had just finished some difficult, demanding labor. This experiment is illustrated in Figure 5.

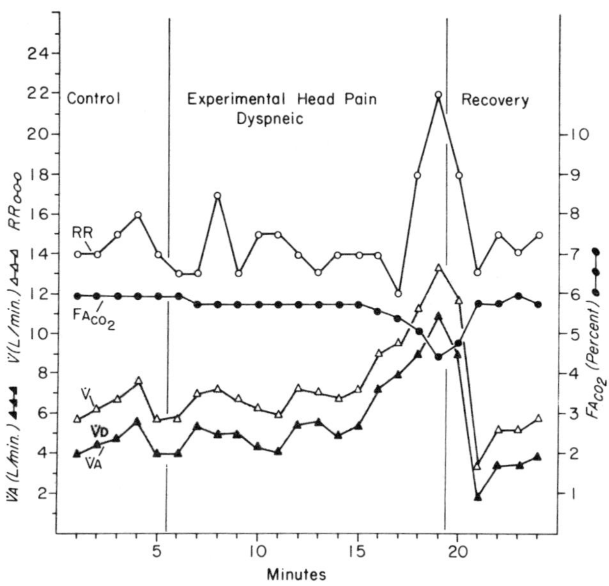

Fig. 5. Production of dyspnea in Subject 2 during noxious stimulation of the head. In contrast to Subject 1, he had no respiratory disease and normal pulmonary function. Subjects who experienced head stimulation without dyspnea had identical physiologic changes to those shown in this figure.

COMMENT. In this subject, dyspnea was correlated with hyperventilation, irritability, restlessness, anger, and anxiety. In contrast to the previous subject he had no pulmonary disability and no pulmonary disease.

DISCUSSION

In this investigation an exploratory group of subjects with pulmonary disease showed no significant relationship between respiratory variables on dyspneic and nondyspneic days. However, in a follow-up study when a subject's emotional state was manipulated and observed it was found that dyspnea was associated with both emotional and physiologic change and was not limited to patients with pulmonary disease. With depressive emotion the subjects experienced dyspnea in association with decreased ventilation or hypoventilation. With strong action-oriented behavior—such as anger and anxiety—the subjects experienced dyspnea in association with hyperpnea or hyperventilation. The relative ease with which dyspnea could be produced in some subjects was illustrated by Subject 1. In this subject any change in resting ventilation was associated with the complaint of shortness of breath. The mechanism by which the change was produced could vary (i.e., exercise or emotion) but the end result was always the same (i.e., disability). The lack of correlation between dyspnea and respiratory variables in the exploratory group is seen to be secondary to variability in levels of function. As dyspnea is associated with either an increase or decrease in respiratory function, mean changes would not be significant. This is complicated by the observation that dyspnea is associated with a change in respiratory function from the mean for a given day. Thus the resting level of ventilation may be higher or lower than that found on a previous or subsequent day when dyspnea was experienced. However, dyspnea is not experienced without a change in the level of resting respiratory function for that day. A further problem is the association of dyspnea with minimal respiratory changes in some subjects, while the same level of dyspnea will not be produced until large respiratory changes have resulted in another subject. This appears to be related to the degree of pulmonary insufficiency. However, all patients with pulmonary insufficiency do not experience dyspnea.

The phenomenon of dyspnea is usually explained by a decrease in the functional capacity of the respiratory system, by an increase in the demand upon the system, or both. According to this concept, dyspnea seems to be experienced when there is some inappropriateness in the ability to supply oxygen versus the metabolic need. However, many biochemical, physiologic, neurologic, and anatomic explanations have been proposed, but none is all inclusive. Dyspnea in our subjects was found to be present with physiologic and psychologic change without regard to pulmonary insufficiency, blood gas changes, or to the work of breathing. Thus certain measurements correlate well with dyspnea in certain patients, but no test or group of tests accounts for this symptom in all people. Indeed, the same changes were noted to be present in subjects who did not experience dyspnea.

The respiratory changes themselves are seen as adaptive biologic responses. Hyperventilation, associated with anger and anxiety (action-oriented responses), is seen as preparation for an increase in metabolism and physical activity. Hypoventilation, associated with depression and similar emotions (nonaction-oriented responses), is seen as preparation for a decrease in metabolism and physical activity. The above responses occur in all subjects—regardless of the functional or structural state of their lungs—but are not necessarily associated with dyspnea. On superficial examination there appears to be little difference between subjects with and without dyspnea. As numerous studies have shown a lack of consistent relationship between physiologic variables and the experience of dyspnea it is suggested that dyspnea may depend upon past conditioning experiences which influence perception of signals arising from the cardiopulmonary system. Events such as breath holding, excessive crying, congestive heart failure, and allergic and infectious events, etc., may lead to the association of physiologic change with threatening experiences in which dyspnea is produced. These people are then hypersensitive to changes in the cardiopulmonary system which other people are unaware of or which do not produce unpleasant symptoms. Although certain individuals experience dyspnea with minimal physiologic change without insufficiency, and others with severe insufficiency do not experience dyspnea, it is assumed that most people with severe life-threatening limitations in cardiac or pulmonary function will be dyspneic. This communication illustrates the association of dyspnea with minimal non-life-threatening changes in pulmonary function which lead to incapacitation. In at least some of these patients dyspnea is related to physiologic change induced by commonly experienced emotions. The steps in control of this symptom would appear to be reassurance that the symptoms are not an indication of impending doom and the reduction of anxiety, anger, or depression-producing situations.

SUMMARY

1. In an initial study group of 16 subjects no correlation was found to exist between dyspnea and the absolute levels of several respiratory measurements.

2. In a follow-up study of 20 subjects dyspnea was found to be associated with change in both the psychologic and physiologic spheres. More meaningful data were found because both physiologic and psychologic measurements were made in addition to registering the subject's breathing complaints. Dyspnea was found to be associated with both the hyperventilation and hyperpnea associated with anger and anxiety, and with both the hypoventilation and decreased ventilation associated with depression. The direction of change seemed unimportant, but a change in both areas occurred at both the onset and relief of dyspnea.

3. The two factors which always seemed associated with dyspnea in this study are psychologic and physiologic change. However, no explanation can as yet be offered as to why subjects with seemingly identical emotional and physiologic change do not experience dyspnea, or why its description differs with the same subject at different times and between subjects.

REFERENCES

Anderson, R. W. Psychic Influences in Pulmonary Ventilation. Medical Thesis, University of Washington School of Medicine, Seattle, 1960.

Baldwin, E. deF., Cournand, A., and Richards, D. W., Jr. Pulmonary insufficiency. III. A Study of 122 Cases of Chronic Pulmonary emphysema, Medicine, 27:243, 1948.

Banyai, A. L., and Levine, R., eds. Dyspnea—Diagnosis and Treatment. Philadelphia, F. A. Davis Co., 1963.

Campbell, E. J. M., and Howell, J. B. L. The sensation of breathlessness, Brit Med Bull, 19:36, 1963.

Comroe, J. H., Forster, R. E., Dubois, A. B., Briscoe, W. A., and Carlson, E. The Lung, 2nd ed. Chicago, Year Book Medical Publishers, 1962.

Dudley, D. L., Holmes, T. H., Martin, C. J., and Ripley, H. S. Changes in respiration associated with hypnotically induced emotion, pain, and exercise, Psychosom Med, 24:46, 1964.

——— Martin, C. J., and Holmes, T. H. Psychophysiologic studies of pulmonary ventilation, Psychosom Med, 26:645, 1964.

Fletcher, C. Dyspnea: The physiological mechanism of dyspnea, Trans Med Soc London, 74:55, 1958.

Gleeson, F. G. The Relationship of Mood, Dyspnea and Pulmonary Function Studies in Respiratory Cripples. Medical Thesis, University of Washington School of Medicine, Seattle, 1958.

Grace, W. J., and Graham, D. T. Relationship of specific attitudes and emotions to certain bodily diseases, Psychosom Med, 14:243, 1951.

Martin, C. J., and Hallett, W. Y. The diffuse obstructive syndrome in a tuberculosis sanatorium: I. Etiologic factors; II. Incidence and symptoms. Ann Intern Med, 54:1146, 1961.

Pace, W. R., and Martin, C. J. Pulmonary physiology in clinical practice: IV. Interpretation from office testing, Northwest Med, 62:266, 1963.

Wasserman, A. J., and Patterson, J. L. Physiologic observations during induced dyspnea, Circ Res, 9:1059, 1961.

17

Dyspnea: Psychophysiologic Treatment and Evaluation

In previous chapters it was shown that dyspnea is associated with both emotional and physiologic change in patients with and without lung disease. With depressive emotion, dyspnea was associated with hypoventilation or decreased ventilation. With anger and anxiety the subjects experienced dyspnea in association with hyperventilation or hyperpnea. The respiratory changes were seen as adaptive biologic responses. The hyperventilation and hyperpnea associated with anger and anxiety were seen as preparation for an increase in metabolism and physical activity. The hypoventilation and decreased ventilation associated with depression were seen as preparation for a decrease in metabolism and physical activity. In subjects with chronic lung disease and pulmonary insufficiency, these reactions were noted to contribute to hypoxia, hypercarbia, and acidosis.

The above-noted psychophysiologic responses may also occur in the absence of dyspnea. Because dyspnea occurs in the absence of cardiopulmonary disease—but appears to be consistently related to measures of respiration—it was postulated that structural damage may be a *sufficient* condition for the production of dyspnea, but is not *necessary* for the genesis of the symptom. It was further postulated that dyspnea is dependent on reactions to ongoing experiences and past conditioning experiences. Subjects who experienced dyspnea were seen as being hypersensitive to changes in the cardiopulmonary system which other people were unaware of or which did not produce unpleasant symptoms. Once dyspnea is present, the resultant emotional changes produce positive feedback which increases and perpetuates the dyspnea. This is seen as being responsible for a large part of the disability experienced by patients with chronic obstructive lung disease.

It was thought that with the use of a "desensitization" or "deconditioning" technique or traditional psychotherapy the emotions experienced in response to the dyspnea could be diminished or abolished, and thus one could interrupt the feedback. Subsequently a pilot investigation was carried out on three patients.

The treatment of the three patients varied but the goal was the same in all cases: the reduction or abolishment of dyspnea and observation of the resulting change in adjustment. All treatment was done while the subjects were hospitalized. Changes were documented by direct observation in all cases, by the Minnesota Multiphasic Personality Inventory (MMPI) in two cases, and by blood-gas and gross ventilatory measurements in two cases.

The gross ventilatory measurements consisted of the vital capacity, the maximal breathing capacity, and the maximal expiratory flow rate. The blood gas measurements consisted of the partial pressure of oxygen (Pa_{O_2}), the partial pressure of carbon dioxide (Pa_{CO_2}), and pH. These measurements were resting values obtained while the subjects were breathing air.

Subjects 1 and 2 received intensive expressive psychotherapy and Subject 3 received hypnosis. Psychotherapy was aimed at expression of feelings and conflicts, reassurance, support, problem-solving, and (to a limited degree) "desensitization." Hypnosis was directed strictly at symptom reduction with no attempt at exploratory psychotherapy. Variations in methods used with the different patients will be outlined in the case reports.

OBSERVATIONS

Case Reports

SUBJECT 1. Subject 1 was a 68-year-old single Irish Catholic male who was admitted to the hospital for treatment of his chronic lung disease. Pulmonary function studies revealed a maximal expiratory flow rate of 60 L/min, a maximal breathing capacity of 28 L/min (35 percent of predicted), a vital capacity of 2.6 L (78 percent of predicted), a minute ventilation of 14.1 L/min, a Pa_{O_2} of 58 mm Hg, and a Pa_{CO_2} of 50 mm Hg. The arterial pH was normal.

The patient had retired at age 62 from his job as a stock clerk, with a pension of $141 per month. Over the next four years his friends and family died or left the state, leaving him completely alone except for a niece in a distant city. During this time, he began to feel lonely and experienced a few episodes of dyspnea but was able to engage in his usual sources of satisfaction—such as long walks, betting on the horses, ball games, and movies. He led his usual, relatively isolated, independent life of his own choosing. At 66 he was run down in the street by an automobile driven by a striptease dancer from a local burlesque theatre. Both legs were broken and he was taken to a county hospital. The dancer had no insurance and quickly left the state. He was hospitalized for six months, after which he had complete recovery of function. While in the hospital he paid his total savings of $500 for his care. On discharge he was presented with an additional bill of $3,500. He attempted to pay this bill at the rate of $15 per month out of his pension, but found that this necessitated his skipping several meals each week and curtailing his activities. In addition, the money owed was increasing each month because of interest of approximately $20 per month. He was threatened by bill collectors and legal action. He received a bill at the first of each month for the total amount.

For approximately one year in the above setting he felt comfortable from the middle to the latter part of the month. However, when he received the bill at the first of the month he said, "I lost my breath. I got nervous and excited. All upset all around, I felt like I was all alone. Like the whole world was on my neck. I couldn't do anything. I couldn't go no place. I didn't know what to do. I just didn't care for anything." His dyspnea was severe during these periods and he was convinced he was dying. At first these symptoms were limited to the first of the month, but after one year they were almost continuous. In addition he developed nausea, vomiting, chest pain, headache, vertigo, and abdominal pain when confronted with the bill. In trying to control the dyspnea he would become completely immobile for hours at a time. The slightest motion would produce a great increase in his dyspnea and fear.

By the time he was admitted to the hospital for treatment he was completely incapacitated and walking was limited to approximately five steps. He was convinced that his pension would be taken away to pay for the hospital bill and he would be left destitute.

He was hospitalized for a total of three-and-a-half months, during which time he was first treated with bronchodilators, intermittent positive-pressure breathing, and mild sedation—with no improvement. When it became obvious that maximal medical therapy left him completely incapacitated, the last three months were directed toward intensive psychotherapy aimed at desensitizing him to the county hospital bill and the feelings it generated. He rapidly developed a close working relationship with a therapist, and when separated from the therapist for one week during the middle of his hospitalization he developed pneumonia and a feeling of hopelessness. With the return of the therapist the feeling of hopelessness left and the pneumonia which had previously not responded to antibiotics cleared up in several days.

While the subject was in therapy, receiving the monthly statement from the county hospital was associated with a marked increase of his dyspnea, severe anxiety, headache, nausea, vomiting, chest pain, abdominal pain, and abdominal distention. In the midst of his misery he was encouraged to bring the statement to his therapist's office. He would tearfully place it on the desk and receive reassurance that he did not have to pay it. An attorney who was then called agreed that he did not have to pay. This information was transmitted to the patient. The bill was then torn up in front of the patient and thrown in the waste basket with the comment that it was worthless. A similar procedure was carried out on the first of each month for the three-and-a-half months of hospitalization. In the periods between receipt of the bills he received individual and group therapy. On discharge he was able to discuss the bill freely with only mild symptoms. In addition he could slowly walk approximately one half to one mile on level ground. He experienced mild dyspnea during the walking but continued anyway. The receipt of the bill no longer elicited incapacitating symptoms.

In spite of his obvious symptomatic improvement he had become increasingly suspicious and withdrew from interpersonal contacts. Prior to psychiatric intervention he was very dependent and incapacitated. At that time significant scores on the MMPI were limited to the Hs and D scales. After psychiatric intervention he scored outside two standard deviations in the L, F, Hs, D, Hy, Pd, Pt, and Sc scales (Fig. 1). For the year following discharge he became increasingly isolated and suspicious, but was relatively comfortable physically. He returned to his old habit patterns and appeared to be doing well. He would not visit the therapist although he maintained communication through another patient whom he trusted. He had no recurrence of his severe dyspnea which originally caused his hospitalization.

At discharge, his maximum expiratory flow rate was 80 L/min, maximum breathing capacity 29 L/min, vital capacity 3.2 L, minute ventilation 12.2 L/min, Pa_{O_2} 60 mm Hg, and Pa_{CO_2} 40 mm Hg. The pH remained normal. These data indicate mild improvement from admission with a small increase in the maximum expiratory flow rate and vital capacity. However, most significant is the Pa_{CO_2} of 40 in the face of a smaller minute ventilation than was present on admission. Previously, with mild exercise (2 miles per hour on level ground for 45 sec), his Pa_{O_2} dropped from 58 to 50 with no change in the Pa_{CO_2}. On discharge, with identical exercise, his Pa_{O_2} remained unchanged and the Pa_{CO_2} dropped from 40 to 37. The drop in minute ventilation and response to exercise indicate an increased efficiency of gas exchange with very little if any change in the disease status.

COMMENT. This patient had always led an independent, isolated life with minimal interaction. He had a severe diffuse obstructive pulmonary syndrome and in addition was exposed to a situation in which he was forced to interact in more and more depth and with more and more emotional in-

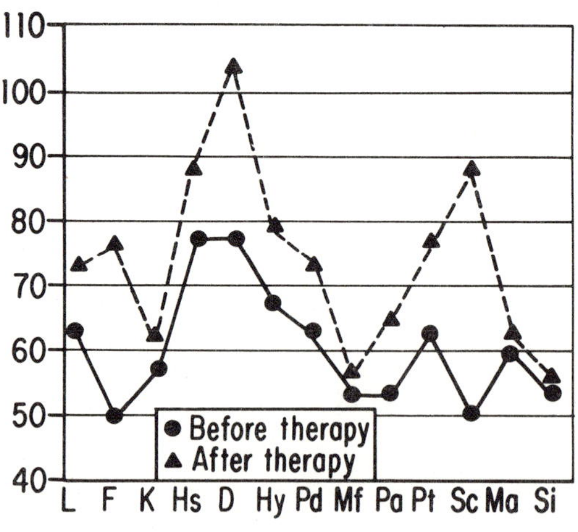

Fig. 1. MMPI profile on Subject 1 before and after treatment. Despite deterioration in MMPI, he was more comfortable and able to maintain himself outside hospital setting with minimal dyspnea in face of severe chronic lung disease.

volvement. In this setting he developed a variety of psychophysiologic symptoms including severe dyspnea. Once started, the symptoms perpetuated themselves and led to increasing discomfort as the patient tried unsuccessfully to solve his financial problems. During the period of maximum symptomatology he was trying hard to engage in the necessary kinds of communication which would remove the financial burden. This involved assuming a pattern of behavior which was very uncomfortable, and his symptoms became incapacitating. The symptoms, in turn, produced anxiety and depression which provided feedback that increased and perpetuated the symptoms. With solution of the financial problem his symptoms reverted to controllable levels; he reverted to his previous more comfortable life style and the MMPI profile changed to a markedly abnormal picture.

Subject 2. Subject 2 was a 40-year-old twice-divorced male piano player and card dealer who entered the hospital with severe dyspnea and fear of dying. He was convinced that "My life was in danger—physiologically speaking something was wrong." He had no pulmonary or cardiac disease.

The patient was a college graduate and former real estate broker, with a lifelong feeling of suspiciousness of others, who had given up his occupation after his second divorce 12 years earlier. Since that time he had lived the life of a gigolo. He always chose a woman with an advanced college degree (master's degree or better), lived with her for two to three years, and then left her for another. His usual way of operating was for the woman to bring in the money and for him to take care of the apartment or house and supply a good share of the social life. The association was open and he had always felt free to break it off at any time.

Prior to the episode which brought him to the hospital he had spent three years living with an attractive woman administrative chief who held a master's degree. They had recently bought a house together and she was pressuring him to marry her, which he had no intention of doing. However, she had him tied up financially as the house was in her name and all of his money was invested in the house. This produced a great deal of anxiety and an urge to terminate the affair. As the above situation was progressing he obtained a sacred mushroom.* After he took it he slowly developed a fear that his mistress would "do something to me while I was out." He then induced vomiting and discharged the mushroom. The fear persisted and he went to a hospital emergency room "so that I would be safe." The above incident was quickly forgotten. One month later he was working on a refrigerator and punctured a metal tube. Freon spurted from the hole and struck him in the face. He continued to work on the refrigerator for several more minutes and then went to dinner which his mistress had prepared. At that time he wondered if she would try to poison him. As he was waiting for dinner he felt a numbness and tingling in his arms and became frightened. He "commanded" his mistress to take him to a hospital emergency room where he presented with severe dyspnea and weakness. He was told he was in good health and that the freon was harmless. However, he was convinced that "I was either wounded or dying." "The doctor said, 'There's

* Found to be most likely a cactus bud containing mescaline.

nothing wrong with you,' and I thought, 'The hell there isn't. I'll take care of me if you don't. I could have heart trouble.' "

At that point he decided abruptly to change his life style to avoid death from heart trouble. He stopped his heavy smoking, drinking, gambling, and playing the piano in bars and wondered about leading a "normal married life." However, the dyspnea and weakness persisted and were accentuated when after several visits to several hospital emergency rooms he manipulated a physician into saying that his symptoms could kill him. He withdrew even further from his usual ways of operating and his fear of dying and dyspnea increased. Two months after being struck with the freon gas he was admitted to a hospital with increasingly severe episodic attacks of dyspnea and fear and was essentially incapacitated.

He was treated with psychotherapy which consisted of verbalization of his feelings, reassurance, support, and much explanation. Initially he was convinced that the hyperventilation and dyspnea were going to kill him and that it was related to "too much sugar." The self-prescribed cure consisted of taking vitamins and a variety of health foods. He early recognized that his fear of being harmed was in some way associated with ventilation and the accompanying symptoms. However, he was unable to use this information in any constructive fashion. Because of his increasing fear and dyspnea he was started on low doses of Mellaril which he accepted very reluctantly and discontinued as soon as he felt better. After he felt secure with his therapist it became evident that he was struggling very hard to "play it straight." He had isolated himself from his usual sources of satisfaction (i.e., gambling, women, drinking, and piano playing) in order to try becoming a model citizen. After being in therapy for six months, he felt secure enough to manipulate his mistress out of her share of the house. He terminated his relationship with her and felt a great sense of relief. He then slowly began to re-establish his former life. At the same time he refused to see his therapist except at his own bidding and refused all medications. He started

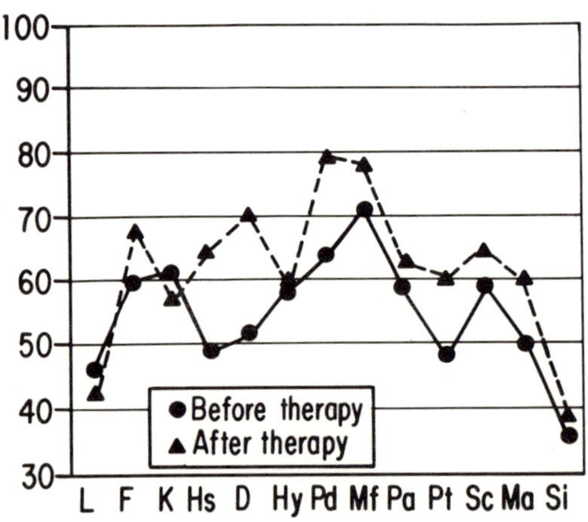

Fig. 2. MMPI profile on Subject 2 before and after treatment. As with Subject 1, MMPI deterioration was followed by improved ability to function and in this case an absence of dyspnea. In contrast to Subject 1, Subject 2 had no lung disease.

drinking heavily again, gambling, dealing cards in a casino, and manipulating women. Over the year since terminating therapy he has become involved with a woman with a master's degree who is married to a man with a Ph.D. degree. His interest was in taking her away from her husband because "she's perfect for me." At the same time he was involved in a scheme of buying a girl from the Far East as a "bride," thinking that he would be able to train her to satisfy his needs.

At a year posthospitalization he was almost back to his old ways of operating and he completed an MMPI and sent in a requested letter to his therapist telling him how he felt, and then left for Europe and parts unknown. He ended his note by saying, "My current fear is that brain damage or mental breakdowns could be progressive—based on fear. I hope it's not too tough a nut to crack by learning how to live."

The first MMPI done on this patient in the midst of his complaints showed a significant Mf scale only. One year later after resuming his former way of life and attaining comfort, the D, Pd, and Mf scales were significantly elevated (Fig. 2).

COMMENT. This subject illustrates the identical kind of problem presented in Subject 1, but without the complicating lung disease. The subject was forced into a new life pattern characterized by "going straight" by external circumstances. He responded to this by becoming very anxious and angry. These emotions led to the development of dyspnea which in turn produced more anxiety and thus increased and perpetuated the dyspnea. With a return to his old life style the dyspnea disappeared. The change in life style in both Subjects 1 and 2 was associated with a "sicker" MMPI. However, it was also associated with physical and apparent psychologic comfort.

SUBJECT 3. Subject 3 was a 60-year-old former car salesman with a long history of chronic obstructive lung disease and passive aggressive behavior. The patient was admitted to the hospital because of increasing dependency and incapacitation. His laboratory studies at that time revealed a maximum expiratory flow rate of 60 L/min, maximum breathing capacity of 21 L/min (24 percent of normal), a vital capacity of 1.4 L (41 percent of normal), a Pa_{O_2} of 47 mm Hg, a Pa_{CO_2} of 56 mm Hg, and a pH of 7.36. The patient's chief complaints were those of increasing weakness and severe incapacitating dyspnea at rest.

The subject's behavior on the ward was characterized by negative responses to all attempts to help him, as well as by increasing dependency. Despite his apparent ability to move about in relative comfort in his own room, he demanded that he be taken care of as if he were a small child. Any attempts to increase his independence were met by anger and increasing dyspnea and cyanosis. (Anger is associated with an increase in oxygen consumption which, in severe chronic lung disease, is not compensated for by increased ventilation. Over a period of five weeks he was treated with a series of eight hypnotic trances during which it was suggested that the dyspnea was associated with relaxation, comfort, and pleasant experiences. The patient was easily hypnotized and responded readily.

After the suggestion treatments the patient appeared happier, more comfortable, and less anxious. He became more cooperative, but in a very passive manner and with little initiation of activity. His dyspnea decreased but he appeared to have stopped struggling to stay alive. Despite what appeared to be an improving emotional climate his blood-gas picture deteriorated and he died of apparent respiratory acidosis six weeks later. The blood-gas profile just prior to being placed on an automatic breathing device revealed a pH of 7.30, Pa_{CO_2} of 60 mm Hg, and a Pa_{O_2} of 31 mm Hg.

COMMENT. On reviewing the patient's social situation the following sequence of events came to light. As the patient's chronic lung disease progressed he began having marital difficulties which resulted in divorce. After the divorce he found himself unable to work and soon spent all of his funds for living expenses and medical bills. His ex-wife took him back when he was in a dependent position. However, she did not want to marry him and both experienced a great deal of guilt over the relationship. After the reconciliation he used his respiratory symptoms to insure that she would not leave him. Threatened loss of her care led to feelings of anxiety, anger, and depression—which increased and perpetuated his dyspnea. She responded to this by spending more time caring for him because of a realistic fear of his dying during an attack of dyspnea. Finally she could tolerate the situation no longer and he was admitted to the hospital. During the hospitalization he used the same techniques to control the nursing staff that he had used with his ex-wife. It was evident that he did not expect her to take him back and that she did not want him back. However, she continued to come to the hospital to take care of a number of his personal needs. While visiting him she was uncomfortable and apparently experienced a good deal of guilt over what she was doing. This was accentuated because she had formerly worked on the ward as a nurse's aide and felt her responsibilities strongly.

When this patient was treated with hypnosis he responded with a decrease in his dyspnea, anxiety, and anger, and became a more pleasant patient. However, he seemed to have given up struggling to live and passively accepted death. It was as though he had traded his passive-aggressive life style for one of giving up. It is postulated that a socially oriented treatment course which had enabled him to solve the problems surrounding his relationship to his ex-wife would have led to a continuation of his life. This case would be seen as one in which symptomatic treatment alone was destructive.

DISCUSSION

From the data collected on these patients it is evident that symptom removal or reduction is a complex operation which may involve major changes in life adjustment. The dynamically oriented therapist would state that these data support the concept that the treatment objective is to clarify underlying problems. This clarification is in turn used to change ongoing adjustment with its associated symptoms. Treatment aimed at symptom removal alone would be seen as frequently leading to the development of new symptoms as a manifestation of the unclarified underlying problem. This concept is challenged by some behavioral therapists who tend to aim their therapy at symptom relief alone and claim symptom abolishment without symptom substitution. The symptom is seen as a conditioned response which is relieved by "deconditioning" or "desensitization" techniques.

Both viewpoints are seen as being too constrictive, and are not in keeping with developments in the behavioral sciences. From Groen's studies it is seen that the "niche" that an individual chooses to fit into in life necessarily produces and solves problems and represents only one of several alternatives. In general it represents the best compromise between the individual's needs and wants and his adjustmental abilities. He may pay a price for adjusting the way he does. This price is illustrated by Graham's work on attitudes. As Graham has shown, specific attitudes toward life are associated with physiologic change in a particular organ system. It is postulated that the physiologic change in turn produces disease. The disease is manifest by symptoms appropriate to the organ and represents the price. Successful "desensitization" would be seen as occurring only in the face of a change or adjustment in life style. Abolishing symptoms, therefore, would not necessarily produce new symptoms. It would depend upon the attitude that the patient developed after readjusting. Treatment failures by "desensitization" or traditional psychotherapy would be seen as having been directed at people with a limited number of alternative behaviors or life styles.

Graham's attitude-specificity formulation of disease development provides the structure for understanding the association of certain psychologic attributes and a given disease, but it leaves open the question of how to determine who will and who will not develop a given disease with a given attitude. Part of the answer would appear to be given by the concept of life change units as developed by Holmes. In the use of his quantitative method a powerful association between the onset of a variety of diseases and preceding life change has been demonstrated. By combining the work of Holmes, Graham, and Groen an opportunity is provided to view disease as the result of a genetic predisposition, a life adjustment pattern characterized by specific attitudes, and the clustering of life change. With this in mind symptoms become secondary phenomenon. The argument as to whether they can be removed with or without solving underlying problems becomes meaningless. Symptom removal in the face of high life change would likely result in new symptoms. However, symptom removal in the face of low life change would probably not lead to new symptoms. Attention is diverted from the "underlying problem" to the ongoing total life adjustment. The underlying problem is a part of the ongoing adjustment. Solving this would be seen as identical to "desensitization" or "deconditioning" of a symptom and would lead to new symptom formation if done during periods of high life change.

In the three dyspneic patients presented it would appear impossible to separate alleviation of the symptom from the total life adjustment. Treatment was aimed at the specific problem in Subject 1, at the new adjustment pattern in Subject 2, and at the symptom in Subject 3. Regardless of the approach a new or altered life style resulted from treatment which was directly associated with symptom relief.

Symptoms are thereby not seen as simple conditioned responses or as expressions of underlying problems. They are a by-product of adjustment in which conditioning or some psychologic problem may play a part.

SUMMARY

Case histories of three patients are presented which illustrate the changing behavioral patterns which accompany symptomatic change. Disease and the accompanying symptoms are presented as being a by-product of a way of life and as not being amenable to change without some change in that way of life.

REFERENCES

Baldwin, E. DeF., Cournand, A., and Richards, D. W., Jr. Pulmonary insufficiency: I. Physiologic classification, clinical methods of analysis, standard values in normal subjects, Medicine, 27:243, 1948.

Dudley, D. L., Martin, C. J., and Holmes, T. H. Dyspnea: psychologic and physiologic observations. Presented at the 123rd Annual Meeting, American Psychiatric Association, May 1967 (Abstract p. 205 of Proceedings).

——— Martin, C. J., and Holmes, T. H. Psychophysiologic studies of pulmonary ventilation, Psychosom Med, 26:645, 1964.

Goldsmith, J. R. A simple test of maximal expiratory flow for detecting ventilatory obstruction, Amer Rev Tuberc, 27:180, 1958.

Grace, W. J., and Graham, D. T. Relationship of specific attitudes and emotions to certain bodily diseases, Psychosom Med, 14:243, 1952.

Graham, D. T. Health, disease and the mind-body problem: Linguistic parallelism, Psychosom Med, 29:52, 1967.

——— Lundy, R. M., Benjamin, L. S., Kabler, J. D., Lewis, W. C., Kunish, N. O., and Graham, F. K. Specific attitudes in initial interviews with patients having different psychosomatic diseases, Psychosom Med, 24:257, 1962.

——— Stern, J. A., and Winokur, G. The concept of a differing set of physiological changes in each emotion, in Explorations in the Physiology of Emotions, Psychiatric Research Reports #12. Washington, D.C.; American Psychiatric Association, 1960, pp. 8–15.

Groen, J., Bastiaans, J., and Van Der Valk, J. M. Psychosomatic aspects of syndrome shift and syndrome suppression, in Psychosomatics. Booij, F., ed. New York, Elsevier Publishing Co., 1957, pp. 33–59.

Holmes, T. H., and Rahe, R. H. The social readjustment rating scale. J Psychosom Res, 11:213, 1967.

Martin, C. J., and Hallett, W. Y. The diffuse obstructive pulmonary syndrome in a tuberculosis sanatorium: II. Incidence and symptoms, Ann Intern Med, 54:1136, 1961.

Pace, W. R. Pulmonary physiology in clinical practice: V. Arterial blood gas analysis, Northwest Med, 62:350, 1963.

Rahe, R. H., and Holmes, T. H. Life crisis and disease onset: I. Qualitative and quantitative definition of the life crisis and its association with health change. In preparation.

Yates, J. A. Symptoms and symptom substitution, in Behavior Therapy and the Neuroses. Eysenck, N. J., ed. New York, Pergamon Press, 1960, pp. 22–27.

18

Death and Long-Term Adjustment in Irreversible DOPS

With increased knowledge in the classification and treatment of clinical emphysema, it might be assumed that we could predict the outcome and reverse the progression of this lung failure. To some measure this is true. For a population of known severity of DOPS, the risk of death is known (Chapter 4). The expiratory flow rate, the blood gases, and the membrane permeability have all been shown to have predictive potential. That the progression of the DOPS can be halted is unknown at this time. That the airway obstructive mechanism can be repaired is doubtful, and within the classification categories there is little or no ability to predict the clinical outcome from physiological variables.

To date, reported studies have ignored psychologic and social data that might be of benefit in predicting the outcome within categories as well as providing a significant treatment modality. Psychosocial variables have been shown to be important to onset, prognosis, and treatment of other chronic diseases and it seemed logical to add these variables to the evaluation and prognosis of emphysema. It was assumed that the ability to respond to treatment and maintain oneself outside a hospital setting was determined by psychosocial assets as well as by the severity of the obstructive syndrome. Further, it was assumed that treatment failures and patients with a poor prognosis have few psychosocial assets and few physiologic assets and thereby inadequate defenses against environmental inputs. Everyone dies; hence it was postulated that the patients with low psychosocial assets would die sooner than those with high psychosocial assets.

Forty subjects between the ages of 25 and 81 years of age (mean age 58) with moderate to severe clinical emphysema were studied. The group

This chapter is adapted from an article in press in *Psychosomatic Medicine*, 1969, by Dudley, D. L., Verhey, J. W., Masuda, M., Martin, C. J., and Holmes, T. H.

was composed of 5 females and 35 males. All subjects were followed with psychiatric observation while conducting their daily routine and more intensively during the process of dying. The procedure followed was that of daily or weekly interviews with discussion of symptom levels and feeling states. Out of the 40 selected subjects only one refused to participate fully.

All patients were clinically stable at the beginning of the study. In the month prior to the study, baseline blood-gas and gross ventilatory measurements were collected on all subjects. Psychosocial variables were estimated with the Berle Index. Data on which to score the test were derived from the initial evaluation by the ward physician and the patient's subsequent performance.

The Berle Index is a test which furnishes a general quantitative assessment of total psychosocial assets. The test is divided into three parts. The first is composed of objective data (worth 20 points), the second is concerned with facts about the patient's family and interpersonal relationships (worth 30 points for females and 28 for males), and the third is an evaluation of past performance, personality structure, and attitude toward his illness (worth 40 points). In general, patients scoring below 60 percent have not shown symptomatic improvement. The final ratings of the Berle's were made by an investigator who had no knowledge of the clinical course or the physiologic data.

LONG-TERM ADJUSTMENT

The Defense

As a group, these subjects were observed to use denial, repression, and isolation as defense mechanisms. The stated reason for the resulting behavior was that they could not afford to allow incoming stimuli to produce emotional change because of the subsequent subjective distress. The patient's attempts to insulate himself from his surroundings led to numerous misunderstandings with the staff which in turn led to greater use of the defenses. Failure to adequately utilize these defenses was associated with increasing symptoms and physiologic deterioration in many subjects.

TESTING THE DEFENSE

To demonstrate the effectiveness of the psychologic defense mechanisms in reducing the impact of environmental stimuli, six DOPS subjects and six medical students were stimulated with a headband which was known to produce a severe headache and respiratory hyperfunction in normals. As illustrated in Table 1, the DOPS subjects and normals had significantly different responses. Respiratory hyperfunction was seen in the normals and a mild respiratory hypofunction in the DOPS subjects (Table 2).

Table 1. HEAD PAIN: MEAN CHANGE FROM CONTROL VALUES*

	ΔRR	$\Delta\dot{V}$ (L/MIN)	$\Delta\dot{V}_A$ (L/MIN)	ΔF_{ACO_2} (%)	$\Delta\dot{V}_{O_2}$ (ML/MIN)
DOPS	−1.5	−0.8	−0.8	−0.1	−14
Normal	+4.3†	+4.9‡	+3.9‡	−0.8†	+95†

* 6 DOPS subjects compared with 6 normal subjects.
† $p = <0.05$.
‡ $p = <0.025$.

Table 2. RESPONSE TO HEAD PAIN

	RR	$\dot{V}$ (L/MIN)	$\dot{V}_A$ (L/MIN)	F_{ACO_2} (%)	$\dot{V}_{O_2}$ (ML/MIN)
		MEDICAL STUDENTS (6 SUBJECTS)			
Control	9	6.8	5.7	5.9	319
Pain	13	11.7*	9.6*	5.1*	414†
		DOPS PATIENTS (6 SUBJECTS)			
Control	20	8.2	5.9	5.0	303
Pain	19	7.4†	5.1†	4.9	289

* $p = <0.02$.
† $p = <0.01$.

The lack of activation in the DOPS subjects was seen as being secondary to the successful use of denial and repression. An additional physiologic load was thereby shunted from a failing organ system. The verbal productions of the emphysema and normal subjects regarding the experience are compared in Table 3.

As a further step in testing the defense system, 12 subjects were subjected to an intensive group therapy experience in which emotional changes were unavoidable. Seven subjects were unable to tolerate the therapy. The emotional changes produced physiologic decompensation and increased symptom levels which they could not adjust to. These patients refused to

Table 3. VERBAL PRODUCTIONS INDICATIVE OF DIFFERENT PSYCHOLOGIC RESPONSES FOUND IN THE TWO GROUPS

Normal Subjects

1 "I just wanted to get out."
2 "I felt like grasping the damned clamp and throwing it off."
3 "I felt like getting the damned thing off, throwing the mouthpiece off and getting up."
4 "I felt like getting out of the situation somehow."
5 "I just wanted to get the whole thing over with."
6 "The thought flashed through my mind to tear the thing off."

DOPS Subjects

7 "It did not seem to bother me a bit."
8 She felt an intense pressure which she felt she could tolerate.
9 It felt "heavy and tight" but was not painful.
10 "It felt like a tight hat in the wind. It was not unpleasant."
11 "It was like a tight hat." He denied any discomfort.
12 "It was like a tight hat." "I wanted to do nothing—just what the doctor suggests." "There was nothing unpleasant so it must have been pleasant."

As illustrated, the normal subjects saw themselves as being in a threatening situation in which action was an appropriate response. The DOPS subjects denied being threatened or that action was appropriate.

attend the therapy meetings in defiance of their physicians' orders. When they were not allowed to use denial or repression in the therapy situation the only recourse was isolation. If this defense had also been overcome it

Table 4. COMPARISON OF PATIENTS WHO HAD A POSITIVE GROUP PARTICIPATION (5) AND PATIENTS WHO HAD A NEGATIVE GROUP PARTICIPATION (7)

	BERLE INDEX	%VC	%MBC	MEF	pH	Pa_{CO_2}	Pa_{O_2}
Positive	68	92	62	128	7.44	41	64
Negative	44*	61	36†	73‡	7.43	44	59

* $p = <0.005$.
† $p = <0.05$.
‡ $p = <0.025$.

is postulated that complete physiologic decompensation and death would have rapidly occurred. As shown in Table 4, the subjects who could not tolerate the therapy had significantly fewer physiologic and psychosocial assets.

The Symptoms

The symptom of concern in this presentation is dyspnea. In Chapters 16 and 17 we have delineated some of the emotional variables which influence the subjective complaint, shortness of breath. As noted, any change from a relaxed and relatively neutral emotional state was associated with increased dyspnea. There did not appear to be a difference between depression, anger, anxiety, resentment, etc. The major factor appeared to be rapid environmental change. Once dyspnea was present a feedback mechanism appeared to operate which intensified and extended the incapacity produced by the original stimulus. The dyspnea led to anxiety or depression, which produced more dyspnea and presumably more physiologic change, which in turn produced more dyspnea. The mechanism was self-perpetuating and was seen as being responsible for a large part of the disability seen in many of the patients.

Most patients recognized the role of emotional change in producing symptoms and would go to great lengths to avoid experiencing emotional change of any kind. When emotional change was experienced, the subjects' attempts to readapt depended on whether activation or inactivation had been induced. If activation had occurred they tried to "slow down everything—thoughts and action." If inactivation (withdrawal) had occurred, they tried to speed things up and become more activated. Only by successfully counteracting the induced changes in activation were they able to remain comfortable. Most patients viewed changes in energy levels as "wasted energy," which they needed to avoid.

DYING

Group Observations

At the termination of an 18-month observation period, 24 subjects were alive and 16 were deceased. Of the 24 living subjects, 14 had been discharged and 10 remained hospitalized. When the values of the mean of the deceased group were compared with the entire living group and the hospitalized group, significant differences were limited to the Pa_{CO_2}. When the deceased group was compared with the discharged group, significant differences were limited to the Berle Index Part 3 and the total Berle. At termination of 48 months, 29 subjects were deceased and 11 were still alive. Only one of the 11 living subjects remained in the hospital from the original hospitalization. When the deceased subjects were compared with the living subjects significant differences were limited to the %VC,* the Berle Index Parts 2 and 3, and the total Berle (Tables 5 and 6).

* %VC or %MBC indicates percent of normal corrected for age and body size.

Table 5. Deceased Subjects Compared with Living, Hospitalized, and Discharged Subjects: 18 Month Follow-up (40 Subjects)

	Deceased (16)	Living (24)	Hospitalized (10)	Discharged (14)
%VC	63	66	69	65
%MBC	36	44	45	43
pH	7.42	7.42	7.43	7.41
Pa_{CO_2}	48	42*	40*	43
Pa_{O_2}	58	63	62	64
Berle Index:				
Part 1	12	12	13	12
Part 2	20	20	19	20
Part 3	18	22	17	25*
Total	50	54	49	57†
Berle Index Total plus %MBC	86	98†	94	101†

* p = <0.01.
† p = <0.05.

Table 6. Deceased Subjects Compared with Living Subjects: 4 Year Follow-up (40 Subjects)

	Deceased	Living
%VC	62	72*
%MBC	39	45
pH	7.41	7.43
Pa_{CO_2}	45	43
Pa_{O_2}	61	59
Berle Index:		
Part 1	13	11
Part 2	18	23*
Part 3	18	26†
Total	49	60*
Berle Index Total plus %MBC	88	105†

* p = <0.05.
† p = <0.01.

In a further analysis in which chi square was utilized, the %MBC was chosen as the one physiologic variable which best reflected total pulmonary performance. The total Berle was used as the best reflection of psychosocial assets. With the use of this type of analysis the only significant difference between the deceased and living group was limited to the %MBC at the 18-month follow-up period. There were no significant differences between the deceased and discharged groups. Both the Berle and %MBC, however, gave trends in the direction of a low Berle and %MBC being associated with death, and a high Berle and %MBC being associated with life. The Berle and %MBC values were therefore added. With use of this value, significant differences were found between deceased and living subjects at 18 months and 48 months and between the deceased and discharged at 18 months (Table 7).

Table 7. χ^2 Distribution (40 Subjects)

Subjects	MBC $<>$ 41%	Berle $<>$ 60%	MBC + Berle $<>$ 101%
Deceased compared with living (18 months)	$p = <0.05$	$p = <0.70$	$p = <0.02$
Deceased compared with living (48 months)	$p = <0.50$	$p = <0.10$	$p = <0.01$
Deceased compared with discharged (18 months)	$p = <0.20$	$p = <0.20$	$p = <0.02$

COMMENT. Although of little predictive significance, when used independently %MBC and the Berle Index were found to be additive factors. This is seen as best representing reality. It is doubtful if any physiologic or psychosocial factor provides good predictive data by itself except in extreme cases. It is the interaction of the psychosocial and psychophysiologic factors with the physiologic factors which provides for a good or a poor prognosis.

Acceptance of the Study

All subjects who were asked to enter a study of dying while in the process of dying were very accepting. One of the patients summed up the prevalent attitude: "I think it is high time we throw some light on the subject and study it together. I can face anything I understand much easier than something I do not."

SUBJECT 1. Subject 1 was a congenial 81-year-old widowed, white male, who had lived a comfortable, relatively solitary life and entered the hospital because of gradually failing health. He considered this hospitalization to be the end of the line as he could not care for himself or tolerate nursing-home care. He was ready to die and spent the last few months occupied with sedentary recreational activities. Death to him was consistent with the natural evolution of his life, and he seemed to look forward to it. He was seldom in any kind of physiological or emotional distress, but he was very tired.

SUBJECT 2. Subject 2 was a 44-year-old white, divorced male, who had no community ties. He was a sensitive, lonely man who was unable to form meaningful personal relationships. He had never been able to stay in one spot and face responsibilities and had therefore been continually on the move. He initially presented to the hospital with severe DOPS which made it impossible for him to continue his peripatetic ways. He was frightened, hopeless, and had little confidence in the hospital or its doctors. His primary goal appeared to be to die, as he could not see readjusting to a new life style. His increasing respiratory difficulty generated severe fear and he referred to this as "fear of death itself." The fear appeared more related to what would be done to him in the process of dying, and the possible pain involved, than to the actual fact of dying, which did not appear so threatening as living.

SUBJECT 3. Subject 3 was a 62-year-old white married male, who entered the hospital with severe DOPS (after being treated for a depressive illness at another hospital). At the time he entered the hospital he had no other place to go, and was unable to work. He was a deeply sensitive, rigid, bitter man. His wife could no longer care for him or tolerate him and he was determined to die regardless of what the doctors did. During the course of his hospital stay he became more and more overwhelmed and hopeless as he realized that the medical staff would not permit him to die in peace. He stated that he had "given up" and that he was fighting the doctors and consciously not cooperating. He stated that he was a "burden to himself and his family" and could not see that living was a reasonable course of action.

Despite his feelings about the staff he remained polite until his life was almost ended, when he became abusive. His clinical course appeared stable until he developed increasingly severe feelings of hopelessness during the last several months of his life. With the onset of these feelings his clinical course deteriorated and he soon died. The process of dying did not appear to be uncomfortable; however, the power struggle with the staff and relatives was very distressing.

SUBJECT 4. Subject 4 was a 60-year-old widowed Catholic female who had been almost continually hospitalized for 16 years with drug-resistant tuberculosis and severe DOPS. For the preceding several years she had been largely confined to her room and to bed because of her DOPS. Approximately one month prior to the start of the study she had decided to die. This decision had followed the mass resignation of part of the staff because of the threatened closing of the institution. New personnel were hired and she said, "They don't know the procedures and are not awfully efficient. This is nerve-wracking."

Although she recognized that she could stay alive if she chose, she said that she was "ready to die" and had "given up." She was comfortable with this decision but was worried that it might be interpreted as suicide. She felt that although her mind was ready she did not know how to stop her body. In the process of dying, which she maintained was very comfortable, she feared that someone would reverse the process or that she would lose her mind. Although she feared death, the struggle to live was so difficult under the present circumstances that she feared it more. The fear of having the dying process reversed was very practical, as she said that having this done was one of the most uncomfortable things that had ever happened to her. In her words, "I felt like screaming." This was in a woman who had an enormous tolerance to pain and discomfort. During the process of dying she was concerned that she continue to contribute to the research project she had joined, and that those around her understand what was happening to her. Above all she wanted to "die with dignity."

She was followed with daily psychiatric interviews during the last two weeks of her life. The sequence of events was as follows:

10–5

"I have given up. I am ready to die." She was willing her body to die, but said she had not found the right combination yet. She felt that she was withdrawing from the world and refused to take sustenance from it. She became nauseated easily and her food did not digest well. She noted that people seemed to avoid her since she had made it plain that she was going to die.

10–6

She was being taught relaxation techniques because she refused to have medications to decrease anxiety or pain as she feared it would interfere with her intellectual functioning. She refused hypnosis for the same reason.

10–7

No change.

10–8

She stopped breathing and was started on an automatic breathing machine through a tracheotomy. The patient said that she "felt like screaming" during the revival procedure. Being unconscious was comfortable and it was the change to consciousness which was perceived as uncomfortable. Received the last rites.

10–9

She still could not breathe unassisted but did not want the automatic breathing machine discontinued. It was kept going for the remainder of her life. She would have preferred that it had not been started. She said she had been able to utilize relaxation techniques to keep discomfort at a minimum. She wanted to stay alert and refused medications which might impair her reasoning ability. She was very much in the driver's seat and wanted to stay there.

10–10

She remained alert and stated that this was the way she wanted to die. Appetite was almost gone.

10–11

Thirst and appetite were almost completely gone. She was still alert and no intravenous fluids were given. Some of the nursing staff thought we were willing the patient to die, which we had no right to do. They stayed with the patient continuously to make sure she did not die. Explanation and reassurance did nothing to decrease this reaction.

Comatose in the afternoon but awakened with mild external stimuli. She felt she would have died if left alone. The comatose period was peaceful and relaxing. Again, awakening was very painful.

10–12

She wanted to be sure we had all the data we needed. Wanted to know if her impending death depressed me. When I said yes, she gave me "psychotherapy" and said she was glad she did not have my job. She now felt she had been successful in completely shutting off her body and death was just a matter of time. She did not want the automatic breathing device shut off, but on the other hand, she did not want any other "devices" used to keep her going. Except for suctioning and some pain on swallowing, she was comfortable and relaxed. She stated that death was a natural biological event and she was ready for it. "Somewhat of an adventure." She feared last minute resuscitation attempts on the part of the medical staff.

10–13

Weakness was increasing and she now had short comatose periods when she could not move or talk, but could hear. She felt like sleeping continuously. She was pleasant and had a keen mind, although she felt it was deteriorating. When not sleeping she was constantly uncomfortable because of the suctioning and the tracheotomy tube. She denied fear at this point. She stated that the process she was experiencing was very much like "getting prepared for something." The closest she could come was that it was a natural biological process which prepared you for something—"like getting ready for a long winter nap." Again stated that being revived made her feel like screaming and she preferred not going through it.

10–14

Consciousness was fading. Almost no intake or output for the past 24 hrs. BP 30/0 and pulse 130. She stated that she was ambivalent about dying now, but that there was no fear and she was comfortable. She was very cold to the touch and felt cold.

10–15

A mild increase in thirst and appetite. Numerous moist rales in the left chest and occasional pain in that area. She was much more alert than at any time over the past several days. She was very upset to learn that it was Sunday as she thought it was still Wednesday. At this point the "giving up" process appeared comfortable. Again stated that attempts to revive her made her feel like "screaming" and she feared this more than anything.

10–16

Appetite and thirst were gone again. Still in control, but appeared to be losing her will to do so.

10–17

She was confused and disoriented and knew it. Her time sense and ability to recognize common objects were gone. She was frightened that she might be losing her mind and needed much reassurance and support.

She wanted to give up control and wanted the doctors to use their own judgment with medications and treatment because she felt she was too confused to make adequate decisions. She was very relieved when this was done.

She said she did not fear dying, but that the confusion was frightening and she felt she needed help in facing it. I informed her that I would have to leave the state for several days and she was very upset.

10–18

I said good-by to her. She was very weak and could barely summon enough energy to smile. She slept most of the time and said that everything was all right and that she was comfortable.

10–19

She slept deeply all night. She awoke at 8 A.M. alert and not confused. She had a comfortable day and required no medication. At 8 P.M. she coughed several times and died.

COMMENT. Death in these subjects was not in itself uncomfortable or even particularly threatening. The subjects seemed to regard death as part of the natural evolution of life and the dying behavior itself was regarded as a comfortable and even pleasant experience. However, the interaction of the patient with the environment in which dying occurred produced extreme feelings of discomfort. These reactions were not related to the dying, although that was the interpretation of those observing the patient. They were related to the inability of those surrounding the patient to come to terms with his death. One patient summed up the negative feelings of those around her as follows: "They are resentful. They do not want to face facts. They prefer to hang onto hope. I do not really blame the poor dears. They have all worked very hard—above and beyond what they needed to do."

Mention should also be made of the fact that very few patients wanted to die alone. They needed the same or more human contact during the process of dying as they did while functioning in society. A few patients prefer to die alone and their feelings should be respected as well.

DISCUSSION

The chronic lung disease patient is seen as overutilizing repression, denial, and isolation in order to insulate himself from disturbing inputs which increase his disability and discomfort. These defense mechanisms are seen as necessary to his survival, and failure of them leads to physiologic and psychologic decompensation.

Psychosocial and psychophysiologic variables are seen as being of the utmost relevance and pertinence in the prognosis and treatment of emphysema. Patients with many psychosocial assets are seen as more effective in protecting themselves from dangerous symptoms or behaviors and are more likely to proceed with a realistic appropriate treatment program. They are, therefore, better able to cope with an unprotected (nonhospital) environment. From the data presented, psychological assets are seen to be as important as the physiologic assets in treatment and prognosis.

In these people, the importance of being able to deal effectively with the environment is difficult to overemphasize. From a psychologic point of view, the respiratory system is very reactive. People who have a great number of affective changes also have great variation in the dynamics of respiration. This variability is almost always associated with increased disability and insufficiency. People with few psychosocial assets—or, in other words, a limited number of coping behaviors—experience more affective changes than subjects with many psychosocial assets. This is another way of saying that people who do not know how to adapt are more likely to get angry, anxious, or depressed in their attempts to adapt.

Patients with few psychosocial assets also have difficulty understanding what is expected of them or complying when they do understand. This is particularly so when some change in behavior or occupation is required during rehabilitative procedures. Social changes of any kind are tremendous threats as these patients have few or no alternative behaviors. Lack of compliance to a therapeutic program seems to be directly proportional to the amount of behavioral and vocational change required. Learning to deal with the patient with few psychosocial assets is important because they seem to constitute the great majority of problem patients or those needing rehabilitation. In general, patients with high psychosocial assets do not need rehabilitation or can rehabilitate themselves with little or no assistance. The utilization of psychologic defenses is seen as varying from patient to patient in the degree and effectiveness of their use, depending on the psychosocial assets available to the patient. Attacking the patient's defenses is seen as highly destructive and can result in cardiopulmonary decompensation and death.

Dying behavior is seen as a realistic response on the part of the patient to his total life situation. It is usually triggered by specific social events which are difficult or impossible for the patient to accept. Dying is seen to be a type of goal-directed behavior which is accompanied by a variety of emotions and their physiologic counterparts. These emotions are usually related to environmental situations and not to the dying behavior itself. Dying is described by the articulate patients as comfortable and relaxing and is exceedingly difficult to give up once it is started. As described by one patient, "It's like getting ready for something. Like curling up for a long winter's nap." This patient also described her feelings when this behavior was halted by the doctors as among the most uncomfortable she had ever had: "I felt like screaming."

Although the actual process of dying is relatively comfortable, the emotions generated by interaction with those around such patients can be very distressing. Interestingly, these emotions are sometimes related to fear of what would happen to them in terms of resuscitative procedures and to power struggles between the patient who insists on dying and the hospital staff and relatives who refuse to grant the patient the right to die or even talk about death.

It is recognized that death from an acute disease presents as more of a crisis situation. However, it is thought that the giving up of life is no more uncomfortable in those situations than it is to the patient with chronic lung disease. The trauma of death is in the eyes of the beholder and not in the actual experience of the dying person.

REFERENCES

Berle, B. B., Pinsky, R. H., Wolf, S., and Wolff, H. G. A clinical guide to prognosis in stress diseases, JAMA, 149:1624, 1952.

Dudley, D. L., Holmes, T. H., and Martin, C. J. Dyspnea: Psychologic and physiologic observations, J Psychosom Res, 11:325, 1968.

——— Verhey, J. W., Masuda, M., Martin, C. J., and Holmes, T. H. Long-term adjustment, prognosis, and death in irreversible diffuse obstructive pulmonary syndromes. Psychosom Med, (in press).

Hawkins, N. G., Davies, R., and Holmes, T. H. Evidence of psychosocial factors in the development of pulmonary tuberculosis, Amer Rev Tuber Pulmon Dis, 75:768, 1957.

Holmes, T. H., Hawkins, N. G., Bowerman, C. E., Clark, E. R., and Joffe, J. R. Psychosocial and psychophysiologic studies of tuberculosis, Psychosom Med, 14:134, 1957.

——— Joffee, J. R., Ketcham, J. W., and Sheehy, T. F. Experimental study of prognosis, J Psychosom Res, 5:235, 1961.

Pattison, E. M., Rhodes, R. J., and Dudley, D. L. Psychosocial and psychophysiologic aspects of group psychotherapy in the diffuse obstructive pulmonary syndrome. In preparation.

19

Life Situations, Emotions, and Reversible DOPS

Much has been written about the disease bronchial asthma, which, because of its multiple etiology, can be considered from a variety of points of view. With the development of the theories of allergy, the study of asthma received new impetus, and much has been added to our information about the condition as a result of this work. However, the knowledge obtained from the study of specific sensitization has failed to illuminate the basic pathophysiology in many cases. At present it may add to an understanding of the condition to consider it as a syndrome which may be caused by a multiplicity of factors, rather than as one resulting from only specific allergens. Furthermore, there are individuals with asthma in whom no specific sensitivity to such extrinsic factors as inhalants can be demonstrated. Others, in whom skin sensitivity exists, do not always have symptoms when the test substances are inhaled. On the other hand, symptoms may be present under circumstances in which there is no exposure to such substances. Considerable evidence has accumulated which indicates that psychobiologic factors are of great importance in the production and propagation of symptoms of asthma.

In 1926 Ziegler and Elliott concluded from a study of a small series of patients that in a limited number of people without a history of protein sensitivity attacks of bronchial asthma seemed to be induced by "psychic stimuli." Halliday reported the result of the examination of 30 consecutive patients whom he saw because of their asthma-induced disability as showing evidence of some psychoneurotic difficulties during the period preceding the first attack of asthma. McDermott and Cobb, in a survey of 50 unselected cases, found that a 2-hr interview with the patient revealed "emo-

This chapter is adapted from an article originally published in *J Nerv Ment Dis*, 108:380, 1948, by Treuting, T. F., and Ripley, H. S.

tional factors" in 37 instances. In the present study, attention has been directed toward situations which might be threatening to the patient, his emotional response to them, and the relationship between his personality reaction and the precipitation of his symptoms.

MATERIAL AND METHOD

A total of 51 subjects were studied, of whom 28 were females and 23 males. Skin tests were performed on them with extracts of six substances which are common causes of allergic reactions in this vicinity: ragweed, kapok, dust, cottonseed, timothy, and feathers. In this group, 28 subjects had positive reactions to one or more of these substances, while 23 had negative reactions. Detailed histories were obtained from these individuals, with emphasis on personal and family history and the past and present psychophysiologic aspects of the subject, so that a more complete understanding of the psychodynamic factors could be gained. There was a history of disease commonly ascribed to allergy—asthma, hay fever, urticaria, eczema—in other members of the family in 31 subjects. Significant situational conflicts were elicited in all 27 subjects in which opportunity to explore this aspect of the problem was available. There appeared to be a greater incidence of upper respiratory disease among the asthmatics than would be found in an average sample of the population.

The physical findings consisted primarily of the characteristic rales, rhonchi, and wheezes of asthma at some time during the period of observation. Laboratory studies in general revealed an eosinophilia above 3 percent in 34 subjects. Thirty of the subjects had chest x-ray films which revealed pulmonary abnormality, emphysema being most frequently reported. Although 33 had sinusitis by radiological evidence, only 3 presented a complaint of nasal congestion.

The age of onset of asthma was distributed as follows: age 1 to 10 years, 11 cases; age 11 to 20 years, 7 cases; age 21 to 30 years, 13 cases; age 31 to 40 years, 15 cases; age 41 to 50 years, 3 cases; age 51 to 60 years, 1 case; age 61 to 70 years, 1 case. There were 17 unmarried subjects and 34 who were or had been married. Seven of the group had been married twice.

Observations were made on the relationship between the skin reactions and the occurrence of symptoms. In 19 subjects there was no information available on this point. In 30 subjects, the data did not seem to establish any connection between the skin tests and the symptoms of asthma. In the remaining two subjects, the symptoms occurred at times when the subject was exposed to the substance to which his skin had reacted positively. Seasonal variation was definitely observed in five subjects, seemed probable in seven, and was unknown in two subjects; the other 37 subjects had asthma without relation to the season of the year.

With emotional reactions the opposite was true. In 36 subjects, symptoms occurred in certain situations and following certain emotional reactions on the part of the subject. The situations usually involved other members of the family or some aspect of the subject's work. In 12 subjects, there was evidence that emotional factors played a role. In two subjects, there was no apparent correlation between the symptoms and emotional factors; and in one subject, there was no available information, as the subject flatly refused to discuss her problems.

Five subjects who were skin-sensitive to pollen extracts were exposed to the pollen by inhalation during interviews in order to determine whether this noxious stimulant so applied had the ability to produce symptoms. Thirteen of the subjects in this series received sodium amytal (sodium isoamylethyl barbiturate) in amounts ranging from 0.1 to 0.5 g, administered intravenously. The technique of the amytal interview was used in an attempt to obtain a better understanding of the personality reaction. It was also given during an attack of asthma, with reassurance, in an attempt to abolish the attack.

RESULTS

Personality Features

As a group, these subjects were immature in their behavior. They were egocentric, seclusive, and moody, with depression as the predominant mood, particularly during periods of asthma. The emotion associated with the asthmatic attack was frequently not clear. This was especially true at the beginning of treatment; later, in many of the subjects under psychotherapy, as there was less repression, the associated emotional state became more evident.

These subjects frequently displayed great conscientiousness, as a means of obtaining the praise and prestige for which they felt so much need. It was necessary for them to do things better than the others in their group in order to decrease their tension and anxiety and increase their feelings of security. There was a need also to hold on to what they had, even if such a policy should appear shortsighted on the face of it, and an inability to share with others. This characteristic was perhaps most notable in the relationship of these subjects to their siblings.

The subjects showed an overdependence on others and had great difficulty in achieving the needed independence and in assuming responsibility. One subject, for example, expressed great resentment toward a superior who told him exactly what to do, and with whom he frequently argued over points of procedure. However, when he was placed in a different situation with a supervisor who gave him complete freedom of decision and no argument, he was much more unhappy and uncomfortable. This possibility illustrates another point about these people—their need to assert themselves and to stick by their opinions without regard to the rightness or wrongness of their positions. This reaction was even more noticeable in the younger subjects; as the symptoms of asthma diminished, their behavior became more overtly maladjusted. One subject, aged 14, became extremely unreasonable, taking the opposite position to that assumed by any other member of the family in any discussion and arguing until made to leave the room. His relations with his older brother had been none too good originally, but they now became severely strained, so that the two boys were forbidden to play ping-pong together because of their constant quarreling. Another young subject of eight expressed his rebellion against authority by doing the opposite of whatever his mother told him. His table manners also showed some deterioration, so that he was very restless at the table and had to be scolded frequently.

Asthma also developed in situations where the subject felt that his security was threatened. Thus one subject developed asthma while in the Army at a time when he was about to be sent overseas. Another subject did fairly well in the Army so far as his asthma was concerned until after his marriage. Then, when it seemed likely that he was to be sent to a school for special training in Military Government, which would mean going overseas after the end of the war, he developed such severe asthma that he had to be hospitalized, so that his new orders were canceled. There were many examples to indicate that in situations in which the subject felt more secure, the asthma became less troublesome. Thus one young man, a graduate student, had many and frequent asthmatic attacks during a period of difficulty with his studies. When this was resolved and he felt more secure, his asthma became better, and his marital adjustment also improved.

The following examples may stress some of these personality features and give a clearer idea of the way these people behave.

SUBJECT 1. Subject 1 was a 24-year-old housewife who complained of attacks of wheezing with dyspnea, which began when she was a child of two, but had only become troublesome in the previous two and a half years. She was the youngest of five children, of parents of Italian descent and Roman Catholic religion. She had always been extremely close to her mother, who was oversolicitous.

As a girl, she had always "loved night clubs and excitement." She began to go out often with young men when she was 17, and fell in love regularly. As soon as the courtship grew serious, however, she would find herself unable to decide to marry her suitor.

Two and a half years before she sought treatment, she became pregnant, while still unmarried, and had an abortion performed at two months. The incapacitating attacks of asthma began at that time. She benefited by the opportunity to talk these things over with a sympathetic listener, and her symptoms improved.

Two years later she was admitted to the hospital with asthma, a few weeks after her marriage. She had entered into matrimony after the usual amount of indecision, spent the weekend with her husband, and developed severe asthma. She returned to her mother and he, to his. When seen, she was depressed and anxious. She had found it especially hard to leave her mother, on whom she had been very dependent, and had difficulty getting accustomed to marriage and making plans for her own establishment. While in the hospital, she decided to return to her husband, and did so, feeling happy and content and without symptoms (Fig. 1).

COMMENT. This woman illustrates the overdependence which was seen almost invariably, and the inability to establish independence and

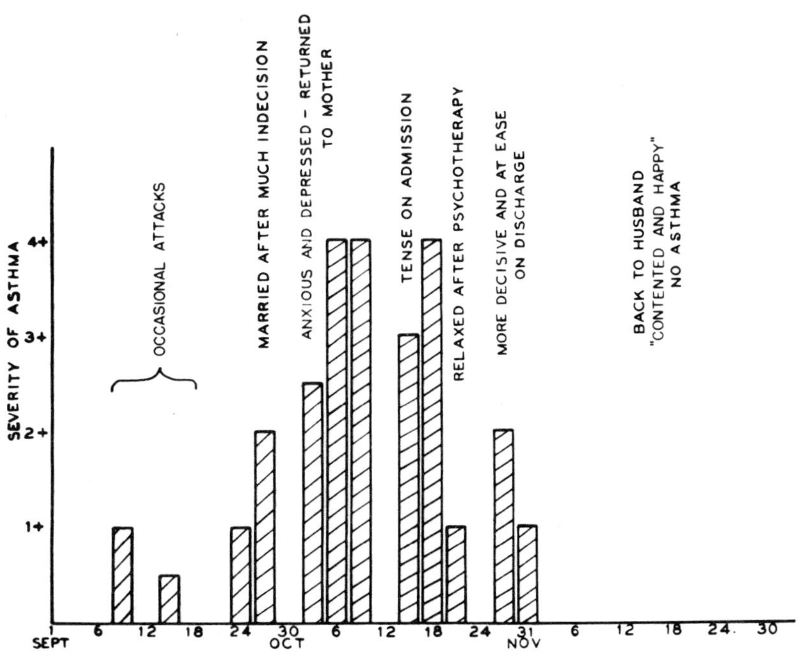

Fig. 1. Occurrence of asthma during period of conflict and indecision, associated with mounting tension and anxiety. With resolution of problem and attendant feelings of contentment, symptoms subsided.

adult self-sufficiency. She further illustrates the characteristic indecisiveness and the difficulty of making a satisfactory sexual adjustment.

SUBJECT 2. Subject 2 was a 21-year-old hospital employee who had had asthma since the age of two years. He was the only child of American-born parents of German-Czechoslovakian extraction. His father, now dead, had been an alcoholic, violent while drunk, who paid little attention to his son at other times. His mother was a suspicious, complaining woman, who reminded her son constantly of his obligation to look after her, and also blamed him and his illness for the death of her husband.

The subject had had one six-month period, three years earlier, during which he was entirely free from symptoms. He had been ill in bed with asthma, and had risen to investigate the sounds of commotion in the kitchen. There he discovered that his father had died very suddenly.He was shocked by this event, and his wheezing disappeared entirely. Because his asthma had left him, he enlisted in the Navy, but after being away from home for a few months, he began to worry about his mother, and about being away from her. His symptoms returned, and he was discharged.

About two years later, he made another abortive attempt to establish his independence. After much indecision, he decided to become engaged to the young woman with whom he had been going out, and also decided to travel to Colorado, perhaps to live. After a week, the girl broke the engagement, but he was still resolved to take the trip in any event. On the eve of his departure, he had a violent quarrel with his mother, in which she charged him with deserting her, among other things. At this time his symptoms of asthma were of 4-plus intensity, and he left for Colorado in this setting. Once on the train, his asthma disappeared, but shortly after his arrival, he began to worry about his mother, developed more symptoms, and decided to return home. His asthma subsided as soon as he arrived there (Fig. 2).

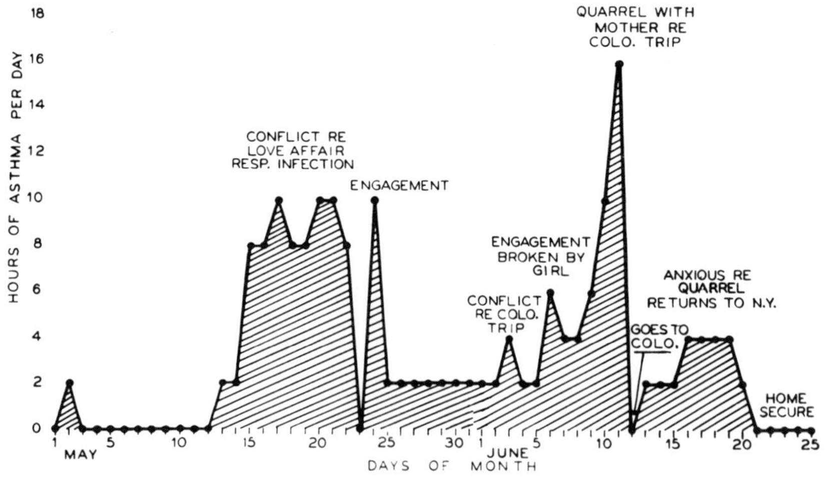

Fig. 2. Asthma associated with attempt to leave home and establish independence. Symptoms improved upon return to home and mother.

Later, after much conflict, he decided to continue his education at an out-of-town college. This time he seemed to have established more independence, and was away for one year with little difficulty.

COMMENT. Again, the great dependency of these individuals is illustrated. Making a decision seemed to help. The subject's immaturity and tendency to make decisions and plans which were not well thought out are also evident. Symptoms developed at an early age, and undoubtedly served to bring him some attention which he would not otherwise have received from his rejecting parents.

SUBJECT 3. Subject 3 was a 23-year-old Jewish fur dealer who gave a history of asthma as a child, and then no further difficulty until three months before admission. He was the oldest of three children, born to immigrants from Austria. His father had died the preceding autumn, while the subject was in the Navy and away from home. His relationship with his father had been punctuated by violent quarrels, but he felt that he loved him all the more for it.

The subject did not learn of his father's death immediately, and felt guilty because he had enjoyed himself at the time. When he returned home he assumed his father's place in the family, and found that he got along well with everyone as long as they did what he told them. It was necessary for him to give up his plans to study law and to take over the management of the fur business. He felt resentful that his younger brother should be able to continue his education, but at the same time he was proud of the position of authority in which he found himself.

When he was given sodium amytal intravenously, he was well relaxed, and breathing quietly and easily through unclogged nasal passages. However, he spoke of his sorrow and guilt at his father's death, and while so speaking he began to wheeze and develop symptoms of nasal congestion. Diversion by neutral and more pleasant topics resulted in prompt clearing of the asthmatic symptoms but the nasal obstruction, although it diminished, remained somewhat longer (Fig. 3).

COMMENT. The role played by feelings of guilt and sorrow in the development of symptoms is well brought out here. Outstanding is the ambivalent attitude displayed toward a situation in which the subject finds himself forced to assume a position of responsibility.

SUBJECT 4. Subject 4 was a 57-year-old office worker who had complained of asthma for the past seven years. She had been born in this country of Russian-Jewish parents, and was the sixth of nine children. Both parents were now dead. Her father had worked as a tailor, and was described by the subject as intelligent, philosophical and kindly, and presumably a rather distant individual. Her mother, on the other hand, was irritable, self-pitying, illiterate, and kinder to strangers than to her own family. There had been little outward show of affection in the family, and the subject felt that she had been ignored by the others.

She had been a timid, withdrawn child, who was overshadowed by her sisters, who were physically and socially more attractive. At the age of 26 years,

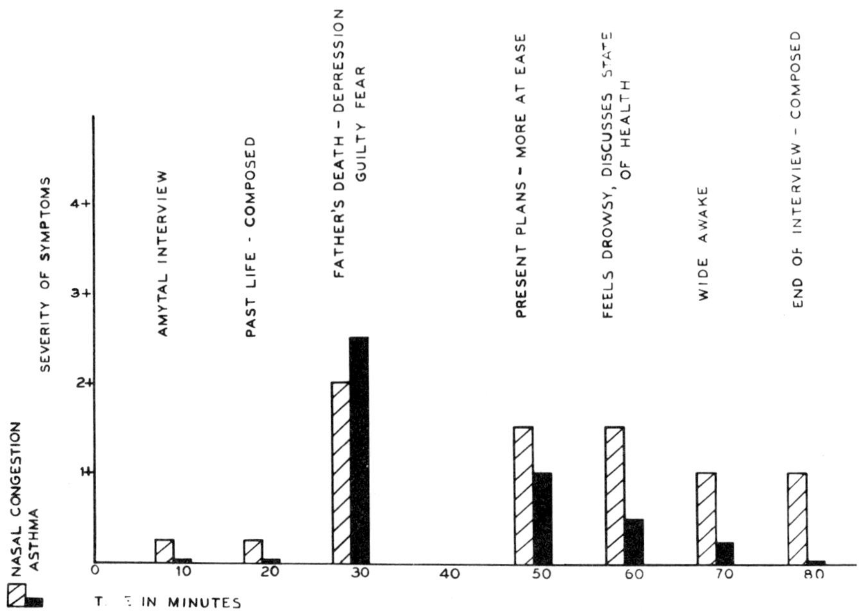

Fig. 3. Precipitation of asthmatic attack and occurrence of swelling and hypersecretion with nasal obstruction during interview (under intravenously administered sodium amytal) dealing with troublesome conflict.

she married an ineffectual, incapable but stubborn man, the first who had asked her. There were two children from this union, a girl, who seemed to have inherited her father's stubbornness, and a boy, who was the subject's favorite. The son had died eight years previously, and this marked the final break in the marriage which had been deteriorating through the years. Separation followed shortly thereafter, and divorce two years after that.

When first seen, the subject's principal problem seemed to be her daughter, who lived in the same building, but had little to do with her mother. When the subject came for an amytal interview, she seemed at ease and was breathing quietly. However, after she had received the injection, she developed noisy, loud wheezing when she began to speak about her daughter in injured and resentful terms. After being diverted by other topics a return to this subject produced wheezing again, but less than before (Fig. 4).

COMMENT. This subject illustrates the role played by resentment, and the need to be the center of attraction. She emphasized her dislike at being ignored. She also provides an example of the perpetuation of a pattern. She had been rejected by her mother, and had in turn rejected and been rejected by her daughter. Once more there is an example of marital maladjustment.

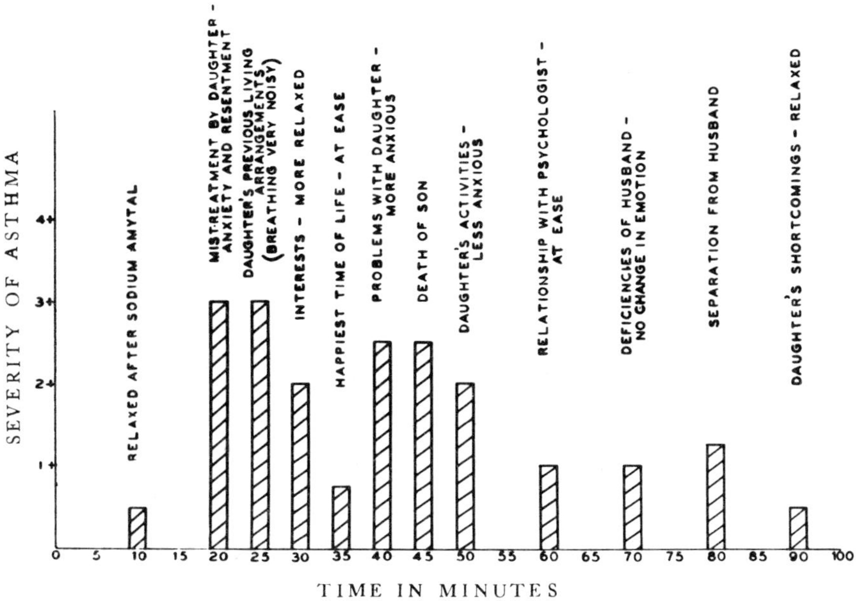

Fig. 4. Development of asthmatic breathing correlated with changes in topic during interview under intravenously administered sodium amytal.

Sexual Adjustment

Sexual activity in these subjects revealed many features in relation to the occurrence of asthmatic attacks. In one male subject of 21 years, the act of masturbation, which was accompanied by a great sense of guilt, was followed by an asthmatic attack on many occasions. In another subject, a boy of 16, the act of masturbation was the occasion for severe scolding and threats from his parents, particularly his father. When he began to have nocturnal emissions following the cessation of masturbation, asthma developed in a setting of fear that his parents would not believe that these were spontaneous and would scold him for disobedience. Several subjects had had overt homosexual relations and others had unusually strong attachments to members of the same sex. No direct relationship between homosexual experiences and asthmatic attacks was noted; however, in one young male subject masturbation accompanied by homosexual fantasy was repeatedly followed by wheezing.

Heterosexual maladjustment was present in most subjects who discussed sex freely. One subject who had not reached a climax for many years had a disappearance of asthmatic attacks after she began to have satisfactory orgasms. Another subject dated the onset of her asthma to an abortion performed before marriage. When she was married, there was such an exacerbation of symptoms that on her wedding day she went to live with her mother and her husband returned to his family. A third subject, married at 31 for the first time, developed such severe asthmatic attacks three days after her marriage that her husband took her home and remained separated from her thereafter. Some of the subjects carried over into their marriages the sibling rivalries and insecurities of their childhood, and these were applied in their relationship with their own children. A male subject, aged 41 years, who had previously had asthma only during the ragweed season, began having asthma of a perennial type following the birth of his son, of whom he was extremely jealous. He complained that since the advent of the baby, his wife had less time to devote to him and they were no longer as close as they had been.

Relations to Parents

The relationship of these subjects with the mother or mother-figure seemed to follow a consistent pattern. About half of the subjects admitted feeling "closer" to the mother than to any other member of the family; some of the others described their feelings toward their mothers in terms of resentment and hate. The "close" relationship was not a warm one, but rather a dependent one with feelings of hostility in the subject toward the mother who kept him tied to her without giving him sufficient affection and understanding in return. The dependency was frequently instilled in the subject by stirring up feelings of obligation and guilt. Thus the mother of one subject, herself an emotionally sick woman, reminded her son continually of his duty toward her and blamed him and his illness as the cause of his father's death. Another mother, whose eight-year-old son had asthma, managed to dominate her family by means of her headaches and seemed to derive considerable satisfaction from the fact that whenever she became ill her son developed symptoms of asthma. A third mother, who had gone out to business when her children were quite small and was a brisk, efficient woman, was quite surprised when her asthmatic son stated that the kind of mother he would have liked to have had was a woman like that painted by Whistler. This relationship was one from which the subject usually tried to break away without complete success. One married young woman, aged 33, lived with her two children in her mother's home while her husband lived with his parents. They were able to spend only week-ends together. This condition was ascribed to the housing situation. When a separate living establishment was found to which the subject was able to move with her husband, she developed asthmatic attacks. The first young man referred to in this paragraph had severe asthma while in the Navy when he began to think about being away from his widowed mother and home, and was discharged for this reason. Four years later, a trip to Colorado for a vacation—and also as an occasion to assess the locale's virtues as a possible future residence—was made without the maternal blessing. After he had been gone only two or three days, he began to worry about his mother and the circumstances under which he had left her, and his asthma became troublesome again, clearing up only after he reached home.

The fostering of independence at an early age in the child by the mother revealed another facet of the mother-child relationship. One subject, a young man of 26 years, now married and with a son of his own, sought help for his asthma somewhat reluctantly, because his mother had recommended it. She was apparently a forceful, capable person, who had raised her children without much help from their father, following a separation and divorce. She had early taught her children to be independent so that they were able to dress and otherwise care for themselves at a very early age. The subject expressed considerable resentment that he had been forced into such an independent position while still an infant—and, interestingly enough, his mother, who was being psychoanalyzed, likewise expressed regret that she had made her children self-sufficient while they were still so young.

One subject awakened with an asthmatic attack on several occasions while having a dream which she interpreted as meaning that she feared she was being abandoned by her mother. She had to have someone to lean on and became quite depressed after this dream. This is one of the few examples in this series in which a subject awakened with an asthmatic attack after an alarming dream, although this phenomenon has been reported by many investigators.

Relations to Siblings

There was an equal distribution of the subjects between oldest, middle, and youngest sibling positions. In only three instances was the subject an only child. Where there were siblings there were usually instances of rivalry and competition with one or more of the group. In one boy of eight, the symptoms of asthma began at the age of two years, following very closely upon the birth of his younger brother. As the children had grown up, it had been a complaint of the family that the subject did not play with the younger sibling and refused to share with him. Another young subject, aged 14, had exacerbations of his asthmatic attacks on such occasions as his older brother's birthday and during a period in which the whole family was busily engaged in helping the brother with his college application blanks.

Attitude Toward Body

The physical activity of the subjects with asthma also was studied. Although in a few subjects there seemed to be diminished activity as a result of the asthma, in the great majority of the subjects there was no indication that the disease hampered their physical outlets. In fact, the evidence suggested overactivity and restlessness. Particularly among the younger subjects there was an interest in tennis, skiing, bowling, and dancing, and the youngest enjoyed running and rolling in the snow. Narcissism was evident in the great preoccupation with physical appearance and the need to look well. The young subjects expressed repugnance at the application of the term "skinny" to their bodies, and made every effort to avoid this unpleasant stigmatization by such devices as weight-lifting and body-building exercises. It was believed that the asthmatic subjects had a great need to excel and to be looked up to, and to be considered "normal" in every respect by their contemporaries and colleagues. Probably because of such needs, they tended to play and work harder than other people.

Attitude Toward Odors

Dunbar, in discussing the analysis of three patients with asthma and hay fever, mentioned as one feature a great interest in the sense of smell. In two of the subjects in the present study, the sense of smell seemed to play an unusually important part in the development of their illness. One mentioned the odors of perspiration and of urine, at a time when he was staying in a dormitory with several other men whose personal hygiene was none too efficient, as causing his chest to feel tight and his breathing to become difficult. The other placed considerable emphasis on gasoline fumes, upon which he blamed the attacks which he had while in the city. This same individual also made much of the stuffiness of a steam-heated room in which the windows could not be opened because of his young son. He frequently timed his attacks with the approach of dusk.

Alternation of Reaction Patterns

A relationship between asthma and crying has been observed many times. It has been reported that many patients with asthma were formerly weepers, and that with the suppression of crying, the typical attack of wheezing and dyspnea occurred. A woman in her mid-thirties reported a very severe siege of asthma which she felt was caused by her becoming upset over an unexpected dispossession notice which she received from her landlord. She felt so "nervous" that she cried, and after she stopped crying she began to wheeze. Another female subject reported an alternation of symptoms of a different sort. During the period of observation she developed urticaria, and with the appearance of the hives, her asthma disappeared. Then, as the urticaria subsided, the dyspnea and wheezing recurred. A third subject became psychotic, and with the development of hallucinations and delusions, the asthma symptoms tended to disappear.

Specific Emotional Reactions

Intense emotion—usually fear and rage—was frequently accompanied or followed by asthma. This has been observed also in situations in which feelings of guilt have been prominent. One subject reported the onset of her illness after her house burned down. A male subject of 23 years first developed asthma when his father died and it became necessary for him to give up his plans to study law and take over his family's fur business. Under intravenous sodium amytal, the subject developed wheezing when the topic of his father's death was introduced. Another subject, a doctor, developed asthma when a patient whom he had been treating for asthma died. At this time he had intense feelings of guilt over his fancied improper treatment of his patient and fears concerning his own health. Also reported has been the seemingly contradictory situation in which a severe emotional shock resulted in the disappearance of an asthmatic attack. One young male subject was ill in bed with asthmatic bronchitis and asthma at the time of his father's sudden death from a coronary occlusion. The subject arose from bed to investigate the disturbance which this event created downstairs, and his asthma ceased at once and did not recur for three months. In this case, shock seems to have been the first response; grief appeared somewhat later. As the subject himself said, "I didn't believe it when he died. I bawled for a long time after I went to the funeral parlor." In numerous instances, subjects reported attacks of asthma following quarrels with various members of the family group. The situation here involved anger, which was suppressed, resulting in feelings of frustration.

Depression was almost universal in all subjects during attacks of asthma. A smaller group of subjects was in a state of depression most of the time, and considered their disease with a great deal of concern. In fact, anxiety was a prominent part of the symptom picture in 31 cases. Most of these people felt that asthma hampered their activities in general, and kept them from working; one of these, a man aged 34, married and soon to become a father, still felt that he was unable to work even though he had not had an attack in some time. On the other hand, several of the subjects displayed a lack of concern which very closely resembled the indifferent attitude of the hysteric. These individuals were deeply repressed, and in some cases this suggested that the asthma might be a conversion manifestation. A few derived evident satisfaction from the attacks and the attention they brought them. Sometimes asthma seemed to provide an escape from unpleasant situations. Thus, one female subject to whom sexual relations with her husband were most distasteful, found that her attacks made her too sick to have intercourse. In one of the young adolescent subjects it was clear—regardless of whether he was conscious of it—that because of his asthma he was not punished for his various misdeeds. His mother revealed very clearly that she was afraid that if she scolded or otherwise punished him he might develop an attack of asthma. Another subject was able to soothe her injured pride at not being invited to a party by having an attack which would have prevented her from attending in the first place. One man used the asthma as an excuse for taking morphine; one, who later developed a psychosis, felt that it was "not natural" and suspected a woman of his acquaintance of having put a hex upon him.

The Rorschach test was given to five subjects. While this group was scarcely large enough to permit a generalization, and such varied reactions were obtained that no clear-cut pattern of behavior emerged, features of both anxiety and hysteria appeared prominently in the individuals tested.

Experimental Procedures

Five subjects who displayed a 2- to 4-plus sensitivity to various pollen extracts were exposed to the appropriate pollen in a concentration of 50 to 100 gr/cm^2 by inhalation during interviews. This was a quantity sufficient to produce symptoms. The pollen was circulated in the room by a fan and without the knowledge of the subject. Although with each subject there had been a history, in the beginning, either of purely seasonal asthma or of exacerbation of attacks during the pollen seasons, in no instance did asthma develop under these conditions. There were numerous instances, however, in which, during a routine interview—sometimes for so ordinary a purpose as taking a history—subjects who entered the room breathing quietly began to wheeze when their life problems were first touched upon.

This same procedure has been carried out with nose reactors (subjects with vasomotor rhinitis). In one subject who displayed a 3-plus skin sensitivity to ragweed pollen extract, exposure to the pollen resulted promptly in both objective and subjective evidence of increased nasal congestion and secretion. At the time of this experiment, the subject was depressed and worried, and felt hopeless about her situation, as all of her problems seemed to have assumed overwhelming proportions. When the experiment with the pollen was repeated subsequently, there was no response from her nasal mucous membranes. This time, some of her problems had been resolved and she felt more secure and hopeful about the future.

Sodium amytal was given, or offered, to only 14 of the 51 subjects. Of these, one refused the injection. In six of the subjects, no symptoms of asthma were present either before or during the interview. One of these individuals continued to be as evasive under sodium amytal as he had been without it; one talked freely and his muscle tension was relaxed; one became extremely restless and writhed on the couch while the interview was being conducted; and one showed no effect following the first injection and seemed suspicious and never fully relaxed during the second injection. In five subjects with no symptoms before injection, wheezing developed when topics to which the subject was known to be emotionally sensitive were introduced into the discussion, as has been described by Ripley and Wolf. A woman, aged 57 years, divorced from her husband and living in the same apartment building with her only living child, a daughter whom she had rejected and who had withdrawn from her, developed severe wheezing when the discussion was brought around to this daughter and the ways in which she had failed to live up to earlier promise in the subject's eyes. When diverted by more neutral topics, the wheezing subsided only to recur to a lesser extent when she again spoke of her daughter. A male subject, aged 23 years, was interviewed while under the influence of sodium amytal. At the beginning of the interview there were no signs or symptoms of asthma, and the onset of his illness and his plans for the future were discussed without any change; however, when the interviewer spoke of the death of the subject's father and the guilt and sorrow he felt because this event had taken place while he was away in the Navy, a marked change occurred and the man's previously quiet breathing became extremely noisy. Coincidentally, his nose became obstructed. When he was diverted by other topics, both of these symptoms tended to disappear, although the nasal obstruction persisted somewhat longer.

In one subject who seemed to be suitable, hypnosis was used during a period of repeated asthmatic attacks. He became relaxed and breathed more easily, and felt subsequently that he had learned by this experiment that a large part of the discomfort of his attacks resulted from his tension. He was able, thereafter, to abort or ameliorate attacks by the process of relaxation.

Modifiability of Symptoms

Of these 51 subjects, the majority had had at least one hospital admission while in status asthmaticus. Practically all had received adrenalin, aminophyllin, and the new antihistaminic preparations, with symptomatic relief only. More than half received desensitizing injection therapy, and one-third of the subjects had had various operative procedures performed on the nose or throat. The group of 24 who received psychotherapy over periods of time ranging from several months to two years responded most satisfactorily of all. The criteria for improvement included diminution in the frequency and severity of the attacks, and a change in the subject's attitude toward his illness and his interpersonal relationships.

Of greatest benefit among the psychotherapeutic procedures have been allowing the subject to ventilate his feelings to a physician with a sympathetic, supportive attitude, and analysis of past and present patterns of reaction. The objective has been to understand the motivations and mechanisms of disturbed pathophysiologic function and to institute therapy aimed at altering the disordered pattern in order that the subject may achieve greater utilization of his capacities and find greater satisfaction in a more normal integration. The understanding of the total response can be useful in giving the subject a comprehension of what has been happening to him, so that perplexity may be replaced by a grasp of the dynamic forces at work. When they were first seen the subjects showed a tendency to deny and not understand possible relationships between their symptoms and their emotional reactions and life situations; however, through psychotherapy many were able to see relationships which they were able to use profitably in accepting or changing troublesome life situations. In general, those who developed self-confidence and emancipation from excessive childlike dependency and acquired a capacity to tolerate or deal with unchanged life situations showed the greatest improvement.

DISCUSSION

The tendency in recent years has been to search for the cause of asthmatic attacks among those factors which can produce a reaction in the form of a wheal and a flare when introduced into or otherwise placed in contact with the skin. However, it is not always possible to produce this effect in the skin of the patient with asthma. In addition, even those individuals who demonstrate such skin sensitivity do not always have symptoms when in contact with these substances, and may have quite severe symptoms on other occasions when the allegedly responsible allergens are not present. In the present study, exposure of five subjects with positive skin reactions to pollen extracts in an amount of the pollen sufficient to produce symptoms resulted in no change in physiologic state.

In many instances, asthmatic attacks have developed in a setting of emotional conflict, or have been attendant upon some strong emotional experience. During the course of a history-taking interview, patients have developed asthmatic wheezing and dyspnea while discussing their difficulties. Allergic sensitivity may be altered by the emotional state of the individual. At the time of their exposure to the pollen, the five subjects were all in a state of relative security after receiving reassurance and an opportunity to ventilate their feelings. The nose reactor likewise developed no evidence of increased nasal congestion and secretion when her outlook was more hopeful, although previously marked changes had occurred when she was overwhelmed by her conflicts and problems. Faulkner had observed through the bronchoscope actual widening of the bronchial lumen when pleasurable topics were discussed and a constriction when unpleasant matters were introduced.

In the view of Wolff, the bodily changes which take place with various difficult life situations and their accompanying emotions are part of an integrated protective pattern. The symptoms of bronchial asthma may thus be considered as constituting an effective means of "shutting out" and "shutting in," which limits the individual's participation in the situation about him; " 'Shutting out' then becomes part of an overall reaction of nonparticipation and its 'shutting in' aspect may include the repression of resentments and conflicts." When this reaction pattern has been maintained for long periods, the personality and behavior exhibit certain features. Essentially, these individuals are repressed and defensive, and have great difficulty in discussing personal matters. A great need for love and affection is prominent. Their behavior may vary from a show of bravery in the face of overwhelming troubles to self-pity and childlike whining and whimpering.

Crying seems to have especial significance in the development of the symptoms of bronchial asthma. An interesting alternation of weeping with asthma—or a history of copious weeping superseded by asthmatic attacks when crying was no longer acceptable to the patient—has been frequently reported. Greenacre suggests that the extravasation of water from the body may represent, basically, an expression of aggressive defense. Saul has observed that at the basis of the production of symptoms in an allergic individual is an intense, unsatisfied longing for love, which is like the infantile-dependent kind of reaction a child has for its mother. When this relationship is threatened—either by actual separation or by danger of estrangement because of some temptation to which the patient is exposed—there is a tendency to cry out, which is suppressed. It has been pointed out by French and Alexander that because the asthmatic patient has not acquired a considerable degree of independence and emotional self-sufficiency, there is a constant conflict between the urge for aggressive independence and the overwhelming need for parental approval and affection. The asthmatic attack seems to have the significance of a cry for help.

SUMMARY AND CONCLUSIONS

In the present series of unselected subjects, it has been evident that the development of asthmatic attacks has been related to the subject's life situations and that such attacks accompany emotional reactions. Some of the subjects have had positive skin reactions, some have not. In general, it has been concluded that there was little, if any, correlation between the specific attacks of asthma (during the period of observation of these subjects) and the reaction of the skin. Five subjects who were skin-sensitive to pollen extracts were exposed to the pollen by inhalation during interviews. Although in each case there was either a history, originally, of purely seasonal asthma, or of exacerbation of attacks during the pollen seasons, in no instance did asthma develop under these conditions; however, on numerous occasions during the course of an ordinary interview for the purpose of obtaining a history, subjects who came in breathing quietly began to wheeze and develop the physical findings of the typical asthmatic attack.

The disturbance of the subject's dependent relationship upon the mother or some mother-figure was the commonest conflict situation associated with the development of episodes of bronchial asthma. All of the members of this group of subjects revealed marked insecurity and a great need for protection and affection from some parent or parent-figure. Generally, they were of good intelligence, but emotionally were quite immature. The subjects were egocentric, seclusive, and moody. They were seemingly incapable of expressing their feelings freely in their general interpersonal associations and their sexual relationships. Conscientiousness was frequently employed as a means of satisfying the need for praise and prestige and thus decreasing anxiety and tension. Conspicuous in the precipitation of attacks was anger which was not openly expressed and was followed by feelings of frustration and inadequacy. When emotions were ventilated, symptoms were less severe. The symptoms of asthma and the personality and behavior of the subjects seemed to constitute an effective means of "shutting out" and "shutting in," and were employed by them as an integrated pattern of defense.

In one instance, hypnosis was used as a means both of obtaining relaxation and of implanting the suggestion that the subject would feel better thereafter. In this particularly suitable subject these results were obtained, and the effect persisted and was discernible in the change in the subject's attitude toward his illness. Thirteen of the subjects received sodium amytal in amounts ranging from 0.1 to 0.5 g, administered intravenously. This technique was used with subjects in whom it seemed desirable to obtain further information about the dynamics of the personality reactions. When it was given to subjects during an attack of asthma, it was found that by inducing feelings of security signs and symptoms could be ameliorated or dispelled. When it was given to those who were asymptomatic at the time, wheezing and difficult breathing appeared when topics to which the subjects were emotionally sensitive were introduced into the interview.

Therapy was directed toward allowing the subject to ventilate freely with full support and reassurance from the physician, with the aid of the usual medications which are used for the symptomatic relief of asthmatic attacks generally. The subject who acquired a capacity to tolerate or deal with difficult life situations showed the greatest improvement. In those who developed self-confidence and emancipation from excessive childlike dependency there was a coincident amelioration of attacks.

REFERENCES

Dunbar, H. F. Psychoanalytic notes relating to syndromes of asthma and hay fever, Psychoanalyt Quart, 7:25, 1938.

Faulkner, W. B. Influence of suggestion on size of the bronchial lumen; bronchoscopic study and report of one case, Northwest Med, 40:367, 1941.

French, T. M., and Alexander, F. Psychogenic factors in bronchial asthma, Psychosom Med Monogr, 4, 1941.

Greenacre, P. Pathological weeping, Psychoanalytic Quart, 14:62, 1945.

Halliday, J. L. Approach to asthma, Brit. J Med Psychol, 17:1, 1937.

McDermott, T., and Cobb, S. A psychiatric survey of 50 cases of bronchial asthma, Psychosom Med, 1:203, 1939.

Ripley, H. S., and Wolf, S. The intravenous use of sodium amytal in psychosomatic disorders, Psychosom Med, 9:260, 1947.

Saul, J. Some observations on the relations of emotions and allergy, Psychosom Med, 3:66, 1941.

Treuting, T. F., and Wolf, S. Unpublished data.

Wolf, S., and Ripley, H. S. Studies on the action of intravenously administered sodium amytal, Amer J Med Sci, 215:56, 1948.

Wolff, H. G. Protective reaction patterns and disease, Ann Intern Med, 27:944, 1947.

Ziegler, L. H., and Elliott, D. C. The effect of emotion on certain cases of asthma, Amer J Med Sci, 172:860, 1926.

20

Medical Management of Diffuse Obstructive Pulmonary Syndromes

GENERAL PRINCIPLES

Similar principles apply to the treatment of both reversible and irreversible DOPS. They consist of the promotion of tracheobronchial hygiene and rehabilitation of the chronically ill (see Chapter 22). Tracheobronchial hygiene depends primarily upon supporting the protective mechanisms of the respiratory tract and requires attention in all patients with respiratory disease. Those chronically afflicted require specific instructions to help in preserving these mechanisms. Equally important to the respiratory cripple is a rehabilitation program to reclaim physical conditioning and some self-sufficiency. Motivation in these programs requires enthusiasm on the part of therapists, education of the patient in the course of the disease, and teaching him to handle the symptoms without panic.

Tracheobronchial Hygiene

THE MUCOCILIARY ESCALATOR. Resting man inhales approximately 12,000 L of air daily that is humidified at 37°C. Within the air are variable amounts of dust, fumes, smoke, and bacteria. The larger particles are strained out of the air by the hair within the nasal vestibule. Foreign material is also removed by gravity, diffusion, and impact in the nasal cavity. Bypassing the nasal airways by mouth breathing permits foreign material to reach the lower respiratory tract. Particles inhaled that are 2 to 10 μ in diameter are deposited principally in the trachea and bronchi and must be cleared by the mucociliary stream. Fumes, vapors, and other particles less than 2 μ in diameter may reach the alveoli. Some of these substances remain in the air and are exhaled; others are cleared by the macrophages or lymphatic drainage.

Drying of the respiratory epithelium inhibits ciliary action. These small whips located on the cell surface beat in a fluid medium beneath the blanket of mucus that lines the airways (Chapter 3). This mucous escalator moves toward the glottis at 1 cm/min, powered by the cilia. Dehydration of this layer following excessive fluid loss or inadequate fluid intake is common in respiratory cripples. Cold, dry air aggravates the dehydration of the tracheobronchial tree. The respiratory epithelium may lose 3 to 4 k cal and a pint of water daily, depending upon the temperature of ambient air and its water content. Thick, stringy mucus is difficult to raise, increases the airway resistance, aggravates cough, and promotes the maldistribution of inspired air. These patients are advised to keep their homes warm (greater than 65°F) day and night. They must not sleep with open windows at night. The humidity of the house should be kept close to 60 percent by using open pans of water, well watered plants, or furnace humidifiers in winter months. Such patients should drink 2½ L of fluid a day.

Certain pharmacological agents diminish cilial action. By a mechanism as yet unknown, tobacco smoke decreases cilial action and lung clearance. Excessive use of alcohol depresses cilial action. The acute alcoholic with stupor doubly endangers his respiratory tract. Foreign material is more likely to be aspirated and poor mucociliary clearance will promote a high incidence of pneumonia, lung abscess, and bronchitis in these patients. Barbiturates and atropine-like drugs slow cilial action. Patients with significant respiratory disease should avoid tobacco, alcohol, barbiturates, and atropine.

Chilling of the skin also stops mucociliary flow. The housewife who runs out to hang clothes on the line in a cold wind subsequently has diminished lung clearance for a considerable length of time. Agricultural workers, lumbermen, transportation workers, and those employed in refrigeration plants, machine shops, construction work, and the fishing industry, for instance, are subject to whole body chilling. The occupation may aggravate the respiratory disease and call for a change which is difficult or impossible for many patients in the older age groups to accept.

Overloading the protective mechanism will aggravate respiratory disease. Particulate matter in cigarettes and other forms of tobacco can be completely avoided on the decision of the patient (stop smoking).

Community air pollutants from which urban dwellers suffer can be removed from most homes through the use of filters. Occupational pollutants in the form of smokes, fumes, and dusts can be avoided by a change in occupation. This may require retraining, a decrease in salary, a change in habits, and a loss of retirement benefits. The elderly man with irreversible DOPS finds it hard to make such an adjustment and motivation toward this end requires both the skill of the physician and cooperation of the family. Bacterial pollutants in the inspired air are best handled by avoidance. The patient should not attend conferences, meetings, theatres, and other crowded gatherings, particularly in the winter months.

Aerosol Therapy

Patients with reversible and irreversible DOPS will benefit from the use of medicated aerosols. In bronchial asthma, use of such medication may be limited to the period of bronchospasm. In the reversible DOPS of middle age and in irreversible DOPS aerosols should be used several times every day.

Aerosols may have a pharmacological action that can be obtained by other methods of administration, as well as by agents that are locally useful. The method of administration determines the effectiveness of the aerosol. Aerosols are commonly given in: a single breath device that uses some propellant (e.g. freon) or a nebulizer with a hand bulb; a multiple breath program that uses a nebulizer with a source of compressed air or oxygen; or an intermittent positive-pressure breathing valve with pressure applied during inspiration ($IPPB_I$). Single-breath devices administer a dose of a drug to the respiratory epithelium. This agent acts pharmacologically as it would by any other route of administration. If the pharmacological action is effective the patient gets relief from symptoms. Aerosols administered in a single-breath device should not be expected to have appreciable local action in the airways. Tracheobronchial hygiene is better served by the use of larger volumes of inspired mist over a longer period of time. Nebulizers with a source of compressed air or IPPB valves deliver aerosol over a period of 15 to 20 min; this adds 2 to 4 cc of water to the respiratory tract, which aids in liquefying mucus. The patient is encouraged to raise sputum during the treatment, and aerosol will thereafter enter parts of the lung that would otherwise not be treated. Agents that act locally upon sputum and bronchial mucosa are thereby more effectively distributed.

$IPPB_I$ serves to hyperventilate the patient and is used in treating the respiratory cripple with carbon dioxide retention. To be effective the work of breathing must be relieved; $IPPB_I$ increases the ventilation to the well ventilated areas of the lung. It is doubtful that the distribution of inspired gas is altered with IPPB unless the inspiratory flow rates are materially slowed. Slower, deeper breaths improve oxygenation and carbon dioxide elimination. If IPPB is used for 15 to 20 min in an effective manner, CO_2 increases and arterial Pa_{CO_2} falls. Within 5 min of discontinuing the treatment, however, the carbon dioxide will be at the pretreatment level. Unless a reversible component of the airway obstruction is present, intermittent use of $IPPB_I$ does not alter the chronic state. The use of these valves once or twice daily is of little value in the treatment of carbon dioxide retention.

Some severely crippled patients develop a marked dependency upon the $IPPB_I$ apparatus. They are anxious and fear the onset of shortness of breath. The $IPPB_I$ valve must be available for any breath that they may feel is difficult or panic develops. The patient relates his symptoms and past history around the mouthpiece of the valve, pausing every few words to take a short rapid inspiration. The avidity with which they seek the mouthpiece and the facial expression while on the valve reminds one of the nursing infant. These patients must be weaned from this crutch and motivated to develop a more effective program in tracheobronchial hygiene. The success obtained in motivating these patients depends upon the basic personality of the patient and his dependency.

MEDICAMENTS. Aerosols commonly contain adrenergic drugs as bronchodilators. The drugs that act upon the beta receptors most effectively relieve bronchoconstriction. Isoproterenol, a beta actor, is commonly employed. Epinephrine and vaponephrine which act at both the alpha and beta sites are also used, with more side effects. As a decongestant of the bronchial mucosa, phenylephrine may be added to the aerosol (0.25 percent).

Other medicaments that have been used in aerosols to improve the tracheobronchial hygiene include wetting agents, detergents, and mucolytic agents; they are of little value when intermittently administered for 20-min periods. The best wetting agent is continuous steam, as provided by a hot pot. The same treatment given by cold or ultrasonic nebulizers will often aggravate the patient's symptoms. Acetylcysteine has been used as a mucolytic agent, but it is probably more effective if administered directly into the tracheobronchial tree. Antibiotics, enzymes, expectorants, and corticosteroids have been administered by aerosol, but they are not recommended in this form.

WITH OTHER ROUTES OF ADMINISTRATION. Certain medicaments are given by tablet, injection, or enema to relieve bronchospasm, treat infection, and diminish allergic manifestations. These agents include bronchodilators, antibiotics, corticosteroids, and antigenic materials.

Bronchodilators are of particular use in reversible DOPS, whether it be bronchial asthma or the reversible DOPS of middle age. A very effective agent is Theophylline (aminophylline) if suitable dosage can be achieved. It acts as a respiratory stimulant and diuretic as well. Approximately 2 g of aminophylline daily are necessary for adequate therapy. Gastric intolerance prevents reaching these levels when the drug is given by mouth. Lufyllin can be given by mouth in doses as high as 1 g daily without causing distress. One gram more can be given intramuscularly or rectally. Lufyllin is less painful than aminophylline when given intramuscularly. Rectal suppositories (0.5 g) may cause proctitis, which can be avoided by using 0.5 g of soluble aminophylline in 25 cc of water as a retention enema twice or three times daily.

Ephedrine compounds are often used as bronchodilating agents. Ephedrine acts on the alpha sympathetic receptors through the release of phenylephrine from storage. Its action is slow as a consequence, and it is ineffectual when phenylephrine storage is depleted. As phenylephrine acts principally on the alpha receptors it is not so effective in relieving bronchoconstriction as Isoproterenol is.

Acute infections aggravate reversible and irreversible DOPS, and antibiotics play an important role in the control of these syndromes. Ogilvy has shown that respiratory infections frequently accompany the deterioration of the patient with bronchial asthma. It seems wise, therefore, to treat the bronchial asthmatic who has repeated attacks of mucopurulent bronchitis. Repeated respiratory infections or mucopurulent bronchitis are part of the reversible DOPS of middle age. Although some authors doubt that the deterioration occurring in reversible DOPS can be prevented by the continuous use of antibiotics, the symptoms of the patient can be relieved. These patients and those with irreversible DOPS who are incapacitated have an increase in dyspnea and may go into respiratory acidosis, becoming acutely and seriously ill, with respiratory infections. It is useful, therefore, to give the patient antibiotics to keep at home, which he can take at the onset of upper respiratory infections. Given for seven days these agents will usually control the infection. Oral penicillin and erythromycin are useful in many patients, although the tetracyclines and ampicillin have had greater popularity (at considerably greater expense).

In severe DOPS, particularly that associated with purulent bronchitis, the respiratory tract may become infected with gram-negative organisms (pseudomonas, proteus, and aerobactor). This is an ominous finding because it is almost impossible to clear these organisms from the respiratory tract. Quite often the infection is suppressed for a short period of time only to have the organism reappear.

Expectorants are time-honored therapy in chronic respiratory disease. Potassium iodide, syrup of Ipecac, and many others are given routinely by many physicians. These agents are probably of little value in the therapy of DOPS if adequate attention is given to the principles of tracheobronchial hygiene as outlined above.

The place of corticoids in reversible DOPS is a matter of argument. There is little doubt that the corticosteroids relieve bronchoconstriction and support the patient in his stressful disease. Allergic manifestations, e.g., the eosinophil count in the sputum, are reduced. However, antigen-antibody formation is not affected by the ordinary doses of corticosteroids. Therefore, the mechanism of the disease, particularly in reversible DOPS (bronchial asthma), is doubtfully affected. More important, however, is the sense of well-being experienced by patients taking corticosteroids. This euphoria is useful in chronic respiratory crippling in which the patient is often depressed, hopeless, and anxious. In reversible DOPS of both types, corticosteroids will usually prevent episodic bronchoconstriction for many years.

While large initial doses of corticosteroids are often used, as little as 15 to 20 mg of prednisone daily may allow the patient with severe asthma to become asymptomatic. In some subjects this will result in hypercorticism (Cushing syndrome, peptic ulceration, and osteoporosis). Hypercorticism can be prevented if no more than 10 mg of prednisone or its equivalent are used daily. An equivalent dose (such as dexamethasone used in an aerosol) may provide some patients with relief of their symptoms.

The incidence of hypercorticism varies from study to study. Peptic ulceration approaches 15 percent in some series. This can usually be prevented by the administration of antacids. As many as 30 percent of patients on long-term corticosteroids develop osteoporosis. This is particularly a problem in elderly women and cannot be prevented by the use of sex hormones.

Intensive Care

If the hallmark of obstructive pulmonary syndromes is retardation of expiratory flow, finis is written in pulmonary insufficiency. Progressive maldistribution of ventilation in relationship to perfusion dictates the natural history of the syndrome. Hypoxemia and later hypercarbia develop, and when the compensatory mechanisms of the blood-buffer-base system are exceeded, respiratory acidosis supervenes. The patient when admitted at this point often has asterixis, is confused, stuporous, and critically ill. Administration of high oxygen concentrations to relieve the obvious difficulty may result in carbon dioxide retention and coma from carbon dioxide narcosis. However, hypoxia can be relieved with complete safety by the administration of small amounts of oxygen. Oxygen given by nasal catheter at a flow rate of 1 to 1½ L/min will improve oxygenation and is quite safe. Inspired oxygen concentrations up to 28 percent may be used with relative safety.

The care of these individuals is beyond the scope of this chapter and has been adequately discussed elsewhere. Suffice it to say a suitable airway for ventilation and suctioning of the tracheobronchial tree must be established. An endotracheal tube or tracheotomy with cuffed tube is best suited to this purpose. Controlled ventilation through this tube is provided by pressure or volume cycled valves. At first automatically set to control respiration, the valves are changed to an assisted ventilation with patient cycling as improvement takes place. Close monitoring of the patient's condition with blood-gas measurements is necessary throughout this period. Attention to sputum removal with tracheal suctioning and frequent repositioning of the patient with percussion of the lung bases is necessary. Nutrients and medicaments necessary for the care of the patient are introduced parenterally through an indwelling venous catheter. This is an extremely stressful period for the patient and his family.

During the period of controlled and assisted ventilation it is important that the attendants at the bedside give assurance and support to the patient and his family. As he improves and his sensorium clears, the therapeutic procedures may be a frightening and anxiety-producing situation. Panic may occur which so affects the respiration as to make it impossible for the IPPB valve to follow the erratic rhythm and widely divergent inspiratory flows. The inhalation therapist may be uncertain about the settings of the valves, therefore, and unwarranted changes may be made in the valve parameters. If an inadequate expiratory flow ensues, the patient becomes more frightened. Consequently it is advisable to use intravenous morphine as soon as the endotracheal tube is in place and IPPB is started. This serves to calm the patient, depress his respiratory drive, and smooth the course of controlled ventilation. During ventilatory assistance, when the patient is cycling the valve, this drug cannot be used. At this point the patient must have considerable reassurance and must be given a means of communicating with his attendants.

Specific Measures Used in Extrinsic Bronchial Asthma

In some patients with reversible DOPS or extrinsic bronchial asthma, hypersensitivity can be demonstrated on skin testing. In these patients desensitization will often prevent further attacks of bronchospasm. They do not receive a permanent benefit, as relapse often occurs when desensitization is discontinued. The majority of patients with reversible DOPS do not show that a specific antigen is responsible for their symptoms.

REFERENCES

Arnoldsson, H. Long-term ACTH in cortico-steroid therapy in bronchial asthma, Acta Alergica, Suppl 6, 1958.

De Vries, K., Witkop, J., Hansen, J. F., and Sluiter, H. J. Hormonal treatment in chronic bronchitis, in Bronchitis: An International Symposium, April 1960, Orie, N. G. M., and Sluiter, H. J., eds. Assen, Netherlands, Royal Vangorcum, Springfield, Ill., Charles C Thomas, Publisher, 1961.

Motley, H. L. The effects of slow deep breathing on the blood gas exchange in emphysema, Amer Rev Resp Dis, 88:484, 1963.

Ogilvey, A. G. Asthma: A study and prognosis of 1,000 patients, Thorax, 17: 183, 1962.

Statement by the Committee on Therapy: Physical adjuncts in the treatment of pulmonary diseases, Amer Rev Resp Dis, 97:725, 1968.

Young, A. C., Martin, C. J., and Hashimoto, T. Can the distribution of inspired gas be altered?, J Appl Physiol, 24:129, 1968.

21

Psychiatric Management of the Diffuse Obstructive Pulmonary Syndromes

The following general impressions apply to both irreversible and reversible DOPS (and, for that matter, to most respiratory diseases). As illustrated in Figure 1, a naturally occurring life change leads to an increase or decrease in activation. The change in activities is associated with increased symptoms and physiologic insufficiency. Disability and insufficiency provide the input for further changes, which in turn will produce more physiologic change and more symptoms. This "vicious cycle" of events is exceedingly difficult to terminate and seems to be responsible for much of the disability and some of the insufficiency seen in these patients. The production of physiologic decompensation by this cycle of events is seen to result from the demands on the pulmonary system being out of proportion to the ability of the system to respond.

Patients with moderate to severe DOPS utilize three main psychologic defense methods. The first defense is to isolate themselves from environmental change. This is readily observable and is particularly evident on wards devoted to the care of the DOPS patient. The second and third methods are through denial and repression. Psychiatric treatment methods must recognize these defenses as necessary to the patient's survival. Without them the patient may experience rapid psychologic and physiologic decompensation and death because his failing or impaired pulmonary system cannot tolerate wide changes in activation levels.

Usually by the time a physician is called in on one of these cases, the patient has moderate to severe disability and insufficiency. At this point several patterns of behavior are manifested which can be very destructive in the patient's struggle to adjust to his disease. Some patients can deal with the increasing weakness, dyspnea, cough, and sputum production in a reasonable and logical manner, with little medical support. They will keep

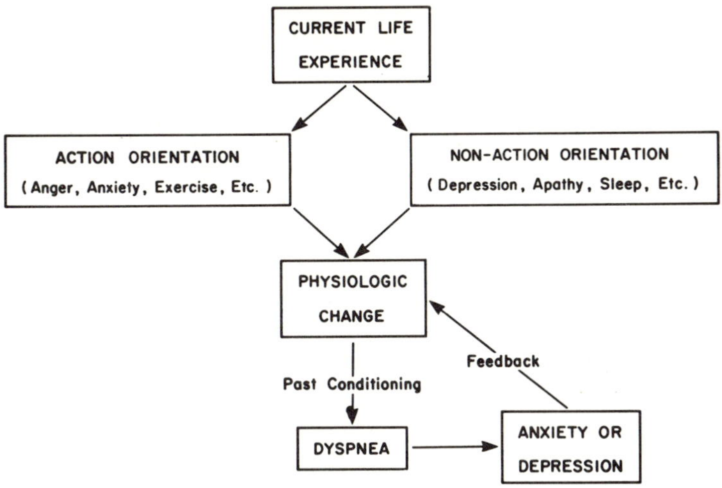

Fig. 1. Postulated mechanism by which disability is produced and perpetuated in many patients with diffuse obstructive pulmonary syndromes. Some naturally occurring change (current life experience) produces change in activation which is associated with physiologic change. These changes lead to symptom production which in turn provides input for further changes in activation and further physiologic change. Symptoms are thereby perpetuated. Past conditioning experiences are thought to be of importance as many patients do not experience symptoms despite identical psychologic and physiologic changes.

up a reasonable exercise program, limit their activity to their abilities, remove themselves from air pollutants such as tobacco smoke and industrial fumes, and learn good bronchial hygiene. More common, however, is a response of resentment, anger, anxiety, fear, or depression. Usually the disorganization that a heavy dose of these emotions produces is enough to upset a therapeutic program. The patient may be too anxious and fearful to see his physician or carry out a good therapeutic program, or he may be too depressed and thereby lack the motivation or energy to take adequate care of himself. He may also become self-destructive and actively attempt to thwart the therapeutic efforts of the physician.

The emotions themselves produce physiologic change over and above the social consequences which increase discomfort and decrease productivity. As shown in previous chapters, dyspnea can be produced with any emotional change, and is also associated with dynamic changes in respiration.

IRREVERSIBLE DOPS

The picture presented by the patient with emphysema who is in trouble is, in many ways, frightening and overwhelming. There is the realization by the patient, his physician, and his friends and relatives that he has an incurable, eventually fatal disease which is in many ways worse than a cancer. This kind of hopeless picture has many aspects, not the least of which is the negative attitude of the physician when he deals with a patient to whom he feels he has little to offer. The patient who accepts the hopelessness of his position and the negative response of those around him may simply wait to die, with little or no effort expended in a realistic treatment program.

As noted, the disease itself leads to the production of a vicious cycle of emotional and physiologic change. Once affective changes and their physiologic counterparts have occurred, the resulting symptomatic expression of this change tends to perpetuate the cycle. Harmful feedback may be provided at all levels in the cycle; this perpetuates the disability, insufficiency, and probably the disease process itself. The response of friends, relatives, and health personnel feeds into this cycle of events and can be either helpful or destructive.

The acute illness treatment model, in which the ill person becomes a source of concern and intense work over a short period of time after which he is prepared to shoulder his responsibilities again, cannot be used with a chronic debilitating disease. The end clinical result must be coordinated with realistic expectations on the part of the community. In addition, the acute concern, anxiety, and/or depression of those close to the patient in response to an acute illness are relatively easy to deal with as they are self-limiting. However, if these feelings go on for years about the patient with a chronic disease, they may be destructive for all concerned. If the family remains anxious or depressed, the patient is placed in the position of having to comfort them at a time when he may be unable to face his own psychologic needs. In addition, his own need for medical care, actual dependence on others for his life, and decreasing physiologic effectiveness lead to special problems.

He can no longer afford to get angry, anxious, or depressed because of symptom production and the fear of alienating key treatment personnel. He thereby tends to isolate himself from others and to avoid psychologic stimulation as much as possible. This is often misunderstood and provides the nidus for emotional upsets with those near to him. As the disease progresses his need for medical care becomes continuous, and his feeling that he cannot afford to alienate people who may be important in his gaining access to medical help is enhanced. This leads to an inability to express properly his emotional responses because of fear of isolation from help, and the realization that emotional change increases his disability. At the same time, he is isolating himself from those around him in order to avoid emotional stimulation. The methods left for dealing with emotional change are denial and repression.

As this occurs it becomes clear to those around him that emotional change is somehow associated with increasing symptomatology and disability. An attempt is made to avoid upsetting the patient. As the patient's symptoms produce more concern and guilt in those near him there appears to develop a relationship which is signified by increasing dependence on the part of the patient owing both to his realization of his need for care and the need of those around him to grant his wishes and to avoid being responsible for increasing symptoms and possible death. This can have many ramifications, but one of the most common appears to be an ever-increasing amount of dependency from the patient and an ever-increasing need to fill this dependency from those around him until complete disability occurs and/or those around him reject him.

Dependency is a fact of life to these people; however, it is also a fact of death. If the patient cannot learn techniques to handle emotions, keep up a reasonable therapeutic program, and retain some degree of independence, the chance of long-term productive survival is very small.

In trying to protect himself from disturbing psychologic inputs which produce increases or decreases in activation, and thereby place demands on the respiratory system which may lead to decompensation, he uses the three main psychologic defenses mentioned previously. The isolation is obvious and is aimed at insulating the patient from environmental changes which lead to changes in activity levels. Some of these patients literally cannot be pried from their rooms, and will completely ignore activities in the home, other parts of the hospital, or in the next room. The denial and repression are also clinically evident, but can be demonstrated experimentally as well. If normals and those with severe emphysema are exposed to noxious stimulation of the head, the normals become activated and complain bitterly of pain. The patients with emphysema deny pain and do not become activated (see Chapter 18). The denial and repression are, therefore, seen as effective in protecting the pulmonary system from change which might be severe enough to cause decompensation.

REVERSIBLE DOPS

Differences in response to psychiatric therapy in patients with reversible and irreversible DOPS are mainly secondary to the existence of an intermittent versus a fixed physiologic deficit. If the asthma patient develops a fixed deficit or is in status asthmaticus his psychologic reactions are generally those of the patient with emphysema.

Little is known of the predisposing personality structure in irreversible DOPS. In asthmatics, however, definite personality attributes have been described. In general, asthmatics are seen as immature, egocentric, seclusive, impulsive, and dependent—with decreased ability to adapt to unfavorable life situations, disturbed psychosexual development, and delayed maturation. Graham has described an attitude which he sees as being responsible for or associated with most asthmatic attacks. The attitude is described by the patient as "being left out in the cold" and being unable to do anything about it.

Asthmatic attacks are often preceded by emotional change and conditioning is known to play a role in some. Symptomatic relief of the bronchospasm, edema of bronchial wall, and viscid sputum causing the airway obstruction can be obtained with adrenergic and parasympatholytic agents. More prolonged relief in some can be obtained by desensitization to antigenic agents. Psychotherapy is also effective in the treatment of this disease. Both individual and group therapy have proved to be effective in the control of asthmatics. The temporary response of the patient when he is removed from the stressful environment of the home is well known. A recent study of chronic asthmatic children demonstrating this phenomenon used substitute mothers in the home. Every attempt was made to keep the physical environment identical to that which was present with the parents in the home. Sixty percent of the children expected to improve on the basis of psychologic evaluation did improve, while only 25 percent of the subjects predicted to be nonresponders showed improvement. Suggestion will increase airway resistance in asthmatics. According to Knapp, an asthmatic attack can probably be predicted by using biologic predisposition and three additive factors of equal weight. These factors are emotional arousal, preceding social stress, and impaired psychologic defenses. This approach may enable the clinician of the future to advise patients when they are in danger of having an asthma attack. The physician can then provide the patient with the means of decreasing social stress and emotional arousal and increasing his psychologic defenses.

Therapeutic rules for these patients are much the same as those for the patients with irreversible DOPS. The patients need access to the physician at all times and must be dealt with in an understanding, supportive manner. They need time to ventilate on stressful subjects, and to learn about the emotional changes that accompany their asthmatic attacks. Once they have learned of these psychological stresses they are often able to avoid asthma-producing situations or develop more effective ways of coping with them. As with irreversible DOPS, good psychologic treatment is as necessary as good medical treatment, but neither should be used to the exclusion of the other.

Unlike the patient with severe irreversible DOPS who is unable to tolerate group therapy, most asthmatics do as well in group as in individual therapy. Asthmatics are not constantly disabled—a fixed physiologic defect is not present and they do not experience increasing disability with minimal emotional change. The patient with irreversible DOPS requires much more support than is possible in a group therapy situation.

INITIAL EXAMINATION AND COMMENTS ON PSYCHOTHERAPY

Along with the initial medical history, physical examination, and laboratory tests, a psychophysiologic and psychosocial evaluation of the patient should be made. This initial contact will form the basis for future therapeutic contacts, and it is exceedingly important that the patient develop the proper attitude toward the physician. If a feeling of mutual understanding and rapport is established in the initial evaluation, the patient will develop a sense of confidence and assurance in the physician which will be of lasting value. The effectiveness of future psychotherapeutic measures depends mainly upon the degree of rapport and trust initially established. This can best be attained by allowing the patient to express himself and tell his story from the beginning. A confident relationship may then be established which will enable the examiner to ask specific questions later without arousing antagonism. In addition, the initial free expression of the patient's difficulties may bring considerable relief from pent-up emotions and may actually be the most therapeutic interview which is possible. Through his manner and willingness to listen, the physisian can set the patient at ease so that he can tell the important story which he came to discuss. Mechanically going through a set of questions gives the impression that the physician is a cross-examiner rather than an understanding, interested human being. Questions may be injected in order to clarify the problem and cover the patient's background. Eventually the physician should arrange the material chronologically, in order to get an integrated picture of the development of the personality and the related illness.

Regardless of the initial approach, the patient may need time to adjust to the idea of psychotherapy, and may need several interviews before he is comfortable with the physician and can trust him sufficiently to relate feelings or events which are of importance to him. Also important may be his current medical condition, which may make it impossible to work on psychologic problems until the acute crisis is over. On the other hand, he may need active psychiatric intervention in order to survive the medical crisis. Regardless, it must be remembered that the patient and not the diagnosis is being treated, and the evaluation of the patient's needs at any particular time depends entirely on his verbal and nonverbal cues which in times of crisis need expert evaluation. There are no general formulas for this kind of therapy; however, it is usually possible for an expert to work out a psychotherapeutic formula which is applicable to the specific patient. Many patients are taken care of psychotherapeutically by the paramedical staff. This is particularly so in rehabilitation units. These professionals generally do a very good job, and it is probably the exceptional patient who needs psychiatric evaluation. However, it should be kept in mind that the paramedical personnel need support and reassurance when they are dealing with particularly difficult patients. Ignoring the psychologic needs of staff members may make it very difficult for them to function effectively. On the other hand, they support and reassure the psychiatrist when a particularly difficult patient is being treated and make the psychiatrist's job much more comfortable and effective.

A detailed account of the daily pattern from waking time to waking time is useful. Note under what circumstances the patient feels at his worst and at his best. How do the symptoms affect the patient? Do they fluctuate from day to day, from morning to evening, from hour to hour? Are they affected by eating, sleep, exercise, work, social, emotional, or other special situations? What brings relief, temporary or otherwise? Are there known precipitating factors such as worry, accidents, disappointments, bereavements, financial concerns, or other strain? Has there been any previous period of similar difficulty? Did anyone frighten him about his illness? What did other physicians say? Has he been depressed, elated, angry or apprehensive? Does overall worry affect the symptoms?

The reaction of the patient to various parts of the history and the physical examination may give a clue to his personality conflicts. What are his spontaneous remarks, his mode of response to questions, and his gestures? If the patient shows any evidence of increasing tension, a particular line of questioning should not be pursued at the time but may be resumed when there is an opportunity later. In taking the personal history, significant data should be obtained in regard to the patient's early development and behavior, schooling, occupational record, habits, recreations, religion, and economic situation. It is important to know his concept of success and how nearly he has satisfied his personality needs. His interpersonal relationships in the home and in the community are of great significance. (To be specifically noted are his needs in regard to food and sex.) His behavior and attitudes should be evaluated as well as the information obtained because of the necessity of knowing about the whole person in action. The examiner needs both to observe and participate. The aim of the history and examination should be to understand and modify disordered patterns of behavior rather than to classify, so that the knowledge obtained may be constructively used in modifying unhealthy patterns. Thus, for psychophysiologic treatment, a dynamic formulation is the most significant part of the total examination.

Psychotherapy

Psychotherapy is based on the mutual exchange of verbal and nonverbal cues between two persons, one of whom is designated the therapist and the other the patient. The exchange of information is designed to help the patient solve interpersonal and intrapersonal maladjustments, and to discharge emotional energy. This does not mean just talking. It implies a structured disciplined interview of 5 to 60 min in length, depending on the time available and the patient's tolerance. During the interview the therapist listens, watches, and stimulates through verbal and nonverbal cues in a manner designed to assist the patient. Depending on the patient's needs, the interviews may be conducted daily or once every several months. Regardless, it is not a time of socialization or of intellectualization, but one of concentration on problem-solving and emotional discharge in which the therapist must work hard to maintain the therapeutic format. Many times this must be done against the patient's wishes.

The goals of psychotherapy can best be achieved by helping the patient understand the motivations and mechanisms of disturbed function so that he may achieve more adequate utilization of his capacities toward greater satisfaction and more salutary integration. Not only is a changed attitude usually necessary for modification of his pattern of behavior, but also repeated application of the patient's new understanding to practical aspects of his daily life so that his improved manner of meeting his needs will become reinforced and part of his life pattern. When the physician has an understanding of the emotional reactions and behavior patterns of the patient under varying life situations, which can be correlated with the physiologic changes, an explanation can be given to the patient concerning what has been happening to him in order that perplexity may be replaced by a grasp of dynamic psychophysiologic mechanisms. Past experiences and reactions obtained from the history can be integrated with the present in order to increase insight into life adaptation. Although a knowledge of the hypotheses of others affords a useful orientation to the physician, he must be cautious in applying it to the individual patient or he may fall into error. For example, the physician may be intrigued by the importance of the concept of unfulfilled dependency needs in one patient, and may try to base his formulation of an individual case on this theoretical concept when the facts do not warrant it. Such lack of emotional objectivity with resultant inability to appraise the patient on the basis of facts obtained from him is prejudicial to the adequate evaluation of the individual on which good treatment is based.

FREE EXPRESSION

Free expression of conflicts and feelings through verbalization promotes a release of tension and often results in relief from the disturbing emotion. Such a release through expression of conflicts also may aid in developing a useful understanding. Not permitting the patient to talk causes him to leave the physician's office with his inner tension unalleviated and the feeling that his problems are not understood. There is no satisfactory short cut for allowing the patient to find out about himself by discussing himself frankly with a tolerant physician. When he is allowed to talk at his own pace, relevant conflicts and traumatic situations can usually be brought out. Encouragement to discuss the advantages and disadvantages of different approaches to a given situation helps the patient to make constructive decisions. Independent action may then be taken with a greater feeling of security and capacity to deal with ensuing problems.

ADVICE

At certain times when the psychodynamics have been clarified, practical advice is helpful in enabling the patient to break away from unhealthy fixed habit patterns. Such advice coming from a physician can relieve the patient of feelings of responsibility and guilt so that he can make constructive plans which might otherwise have been delayed indefinitely.

CONFRONTATION

It is undesirable to confront the patient with unpleasant facts about himself unless he has supplied information which may substantiate the concept given to him. Whenever possible the patient should formulate his own problems and possible solutions. When he is not able to do this and progress is not being made, it may be necessary to confront him with a dynamic formulation which should be based on evidence supplied by the patient rather than on preconceived hypotheses or speculation by the physician. Such speculation, if given, is likely to be unacceptable, to arouse resentment, and further to build up a defensive barrier.

DREAM ANALYSIS AND NARCOANALYSIS

An analysis of the emotional development during infancy, childhood, and adult life is elicited by the biographical review and by allowing the patient to associate freely about the significant life events and his reactions to them. Recall and interpretation of dreams through spontaneous association by the patient facilitate the uncovering of emotional conflicts. If the physician is experienced in interpreting them, dreams may be of greatest importance in clarifying the fundamental emotional forces. Intravenously administered sodium amytal when given by a physician trained in the technique of narcoanalysis is of value in the alleviation of symptoms, in the elucidation of dynamic mechanisms, and in gaining therapeutic leverage.

Problems recalled under the influence of the drug serve as a basis for further analysis of emotional conflicts and personality reactions in subsequent interviews. The drug itself should not be considered a specific agent but rather a tool to induce in the patient a special state by its action on the highest integrative functions.

As long as the physician maintains respect for and a kindly appreciation of the patient's basic problems without falling into traps which may be laid by the patient, he will be able to control the treatment situation and make progress in psychotherapy.

INSIGHT

Frequently considerable improvement may be achieved with the verbal expression of insight. However, many patients who appear to have developed some comprehension of the psychophysiologic dynamics of their illness express it rarely or not at all. In some of these people, pride and a need for a feeling of self-sufficiency interdict an admission of improved integration which may be conveyed indirectly to the physician. The evaluation of physiologic disturbances and the correlation of them with emotional reactions and behavior in varying life situations serve to promote an understanding of the total biologic response. This method is often especially helpful to patients who are puzzled and apprehensive about the nature of their disorder.

REASSURANCE AND SUPPORT

Reassurance and emotional support utilize the human warmth of the physician as therapeutic tools and are helpful in enhancing the strength, courage, and determination of the patient. They imply an understanding and tolerant attitude on the part of the physician and involve an unswerving interest and concern for whatever problem or question may be brought to him. Recognition and praise for assets and achievements promote a feeling of self-esteem and security in the patient. The physician should have an awareness of his reaction to the patient and his emotional conflicts and should avoid injecting his own prejudices and moral convictions into the patient's problem. An understanding, tolerant attitude toward the patient's shortcomings does not necessarily imply personal approval on the part of the physician. Integrity, flexibility, maturity, sincerity, and sufficient knowledge of himself are necessary in the physician for the development of the best doctor-patient relationship. Although he needs to be sympathetic, he must avoid an undue identification with the patient which may lead to activation of anxiety and a loss of objectivity. When the patient is allowed the freedom of self-expression, repressed emotion may be unleashed, and occasionally reactions of unprovoked hostility or professions of love may be expressed. Such attitudes can usually be understood on the basis of past experiences, with the physician currently representing a significant individual in the patient's past life.

DEPTH OF TREATMENT

The depth of treatment attempted may depend on the ability of the patient to use his resources in developing improved patterns of reaction rather than on the frequency of the interviews or on the duration of the treatment. As the response in different patients is variable, flexibility in devising the best approach is indispensable. When the physician is aware that he cannot deal with the problems which arise or when the response to treatment is poor, he may need to consult with a psychiatrist for advice on his treatment of the patient. In other cases it may be advisable to refer the patient to a psychiatrist for more intensive treatment. However, whenever it is possible, it is desirable to have one physician care for the complete health needs of the individual.

PROGNOSIS

Insight into the patient's life adaptation with integration of past experiences and reactions with the present promote successful treatment. The prognosis is favorably influenced by the following circumstances: recognition of failure of present patterns of adjustment and desire for help; confidence in and ability to cooperate with the physician; flexibility of personality structure; disorder of recent origin; long interval between attacks; capacity and willingness to assume responsibility in treatment; past record of constructive interpersonal relationships; past record of ability to derive satisfaction from occupation, religion, sports, lodge memberships, and other activities; willingness of family to cooperate. The greater the lack of these assets, the poorer the outlook for improvement. Some patients have such a strong front of independence that they block any attempts to give them help. Others cling to an immature dependency relationship as a mode of adaptation. When powerful therapeutic forces stemming from the ability of the physician to inculcate in the patient faith in himself and the capacity to recognize and deal constructively with his problems can be employed, it is possible for him to abandon costly, inappropriate emergency patterns and manage the threats and challenge of day to day living.

SPECIFIC STEPS IN PATIENT MANAGEMENT

Education

The first and most important task is the education of the patient and his family. This process consists of frank, open discussions with the patient and his family about the nature of the disease, its social implications, and its prognosis with good medical treatment. Care must be taken to ensure that all significant family members understand the basic anatomic and physiologic defects and how they can be managed. The same care must be taken in a discussion of the psychophysiology of respiration and how it can be manipulated to aid in the treatment of the patient. The more information available to the patient and significant persons, the fewer desperate telephone calls the physician will receive. The above is self-evident; however, it is seldom practiced. With a primitive knowledge of the disease, the unknown factors provide the background for disabling fears on the side of both the patient and his family.

Identification of Problem Areas

The next step is the identification of psychologic and social situations which tend to perpetuate disability and insufficiency. This is best done by visiting the patient's home. In this regard it is important to ask oneself the question, "Who does what for whom and why?" Is the patient placed in a position of forced dependency? Is he hovered over and waited on regardless of his wishes? If it is enforced dependency on the part of the family, therapeutic attention should be directed mainly at the family.

If, despite attempts to educate the family, they continue to overcontrol the patient's activities, the therapist must deal directly with their fear and guilt at the possible decompensation or death of the patient. Brief psychotherapy or appropriate medications for individual family members are indicated. Once the family realizes that their fears are based on the faulty premise that independence equals increasing illness, guilt and fear are readily resolved and the patient can begin a more active interaction with his environment.

If the patient himself is unable to accept independence because of excessive dependency needs, depression, or anxiety, these conditions will have to be treated before the patient can mobilize his energies toward constructive goals.

Dealing with Dependency

If the problem is one of severe lifelong dependency, efforts to change this ongoing life style will likely be met with extreme resistance as the patient is literally getting what he has always wanted. Such patients appear almost impossible to treat realistically from a psychiatric or medical point of view. The best that can be done is to help the family or individuals caring for him to force the patient to accept more independence despite his rage and protestations. This at least leads to increased interaction with his environment, but the amount of good if any that can be accomplished is debatable. Perhaps a better use of psychiatric help in these cases is to help the staff and family maintain a comfortable attitude as the patient destroys himself through refusal and inability to accept realistic therapeutic manipulations.

Dealing with Specific Emotions

Patients with depression, anxiety, or anger may need appropriate symptomatic treatment before therapeutic measures can be effective. Anxiety can be treated with minor tranquilizers, psychotherapy, or perhaps with simple relaxation techniques. A clenched-fist technique used in light hypnosis or a modification of psychologic desensitization works frequently and requires almost no experience on the part of the therapist. With the clenched-fist technique the patient is first asked to clench his fist as tightly as he can and to concentrate on the fist. He is then told repeatedly to note the tension in his hand, arm, and shoulder. After several minutes he is told to relax his fist and to note that the relaxation extends over his hand, arm, shoulder, neck, and, in fact, his whole body. After repeating this process several times, he is told that clenching his fist is symbolic of his ability and determination to overcome his anxiety or anger, and relaxation of his fist is associated with bodily relaxation. Prior hypnosis is not required and many patients respond remarkably well after one session.

Another technique which is useful follows more closely the techniques developed by Wolpe. With this method the therapist identifies upsetting experiences and suggests them during periods of learned muscular relaxation. This is repeated until the patient can stay relaxed despite thinking of the upsetting experience. When the situation is no longer effective in producing emotional change, the patient is said to be deconditioned or desensitized to that particular situation.

There are many variations of the above treatment techniques and the individual physician can easily work out those which best suit him. One approach which should not be used is simply telling the patient to "just relax and everything will be all right" or a similar expression. This solves nothing and if anything aggravates the condition because the patient is told to do something that the physician has not bothered to give him the tools to do.

The symptomatic treatment of mild depressive reactions should be limited to the amphetamines or similar types of central nervous system stimulants and psychotherapy. If the patient does not respond to such techniques, a psychiatric evaluation should be requested. The patient needs support and reassurance that depression is amenable to treatment, and is many times self-limiting.

Hypnosis

In some patients, dyspnea can be partially alleviated with hypnotic suggestion. This requires more sophistication on the part of the therapist, but it can be very useful. Patients who are very neurotic or psychotic, have unrealistic expectations, or are overly fearful of the technique, either should not be treated by hypnosis or the hypnosis should be done by an expert. After induction, hypnotic suggestion should be limited to the suggestion of relaxation and possibly that the patient's breathing will become easier as he relaxes. Prior to the patient's being awakened, the suggestion should be made that he will awaken with a sense of well-being and will remember everything that went on during the hypnotic session. Some patients learn hypnotic techniques rapidly and find that self-hypnosis is an excellent tool in controlling many of their symptoms. However, if the dyspnea is removed completely, an important danger signal is lost.

Psychopharmacology

The same rules apply to drug therapy in this group of patients that apply to patients in general. As mentioned earlier, symptoms of anxiety can be treated with the minor tranquilizers or light sedation. Depression can be treated with the tricyclic compounds or amphetamines, but a prior evaluation by a psychiatrist should be done if anything other than a mild depression is suspected. Monoamine oxidase inhibitors are falling out of favor and should not be used without psychiatric supervision.

Psychotic patients with chronic lung disease need evaluation and treatment by trained psychiatric personnel. Initial evaluation and treatment of these people by nonpsychiatric personnel are not recommended and may be harmful to the patient.

Of particular importance when one is treating the psychotic chronic-lung-disease patient with psychoactive medications is an awareness of the side-effects. All of the phenothiazines commonly used in psychiatry have autonomic blockade as a major side effect, or directly affect the bronchial tree in a manner which may lead to difficulty with bronchial drainage. The patient using these drugs may need added aerosols, mucolytic agents, or other specific therapies aimed at promoting good bronchial drainage. In addition, the major tranquilizers commonly produce symptoms similar to those seen in Parkinsonism. These extrapyramidal symptoms can be managed with commonly utilized anti-Parkinsonism medications. However, these medications may make bronchial drainage even more difficult. Also seen are anxiety reactions, potentiation of depression, drowsiness, listlessness, and orthostatic hypotension. These effects may not be easily treated, and withdrawal of the medication may be necessary. A particularly dangerous side-effect of most of the phenothiazines is the production of a paradoxical hypotension with the use of epinephrine. Patients should be warned against this possible side-effect and should avoid bronchodilators that contain epinephrine. Other possible side-effects of the phenothiazines fill a good sized monograph, and there is no substitute for having expert consultation available if the use of these medications is deemed necessary.

The phenothiazines represent the model for the major tranquilizers. As indicated above, there are numerous problems with their use which limit clinical effectiveness in patients with chronic lung disease. The major antidepressants in common use at this point are the tricyclic compounds. Like the phenothiazines, there are many problems with their use. Again, poor bronchial drainage may result. In addition, orthostatic hypotension, tachycardia, extrapyramidal symptoms, anxiety, aggravation of glaucoma, urinary retention, pyloric stenosis, and possibility of suicide may be side-effects. Special problems include the production of a first-degree atrioventricular block, and the potentiation of the pressor effects of norepinephrine.

The monoamine oxidase inhibitors are also effective in certain types of depression, but they present even more severe side-effects in lung-disease patients who require the constant use of sympathomimetic agents.

The above information is designed to introduce the subject of drug therapy in patients who suffer from psychotic reactions, and it illustrates a small number of the problems which are built into the therapeutic effects of these agents. Unless the proper medication is selected for the proper symptom, the physician may be left with the side-effects of the drug as the only effect produced. A psychiatric evaluation is mandatory in psychotically ill patients before such medications are used. In most cases, alternative therapy can be arranged.

Electroconvulsive Therapy

Electroconvulsive therapy is an effective method of treatment in many depressive reactions and other psychiatric disease states. However, a discussion of this treatment modality is outside the scope of this monograph.

COORDINATION OF TREATMENT

In general, one physician needs to coordinate all aspects of treatment in these patients, and be ready to meet psychologic as well as medical emergencies. If this is not done the patients are generally unable to solve problems and increase mobilization because of a realistic fear of what happens to them when they do. An example of this is provided by the attempts at formal group therapy with patients with severe irreversible DOPS. These patients literally interpreted the psychophysiologic trauma of psychologic problem-solving as killing them. They were uncomfortable enough so that none of the severely ill patients was able to stay in the group. This reaction was in contrast with individual therapy, which was acceptable. With the individual therapy, it was clear to the patient that when difficulty arose his medical needs would be immediately met. In this way the fears of decompensation secondary to affect mobilization in severely ill patients were overcome and they were able gradually to increase their activity levels.

SUMMARY

Psychiatric aspects of the treatment of the diffuse obstructive pulmonary syndromes can be placed into two categories. The first is concerned with the care and treatment of the disease itself, and the psychologic and social problems it produces. The second is concerned with the treatment of psychiatric disorders which may exist along with the respiratory disease.

The aim in the first case is the complete education of the patient about his disease, avoidance of negative feelings about himself or his disease, respect for his psychologic defenses, and the maintenance of open lines of communication at all times. In addition, the family needs to be brought into the therapeutic arena and given an adequate amount of information and support to enable them to tolerate and assist the patient. This type of treatment can be given by any informed, interested physician.

The treatment of psychotic disorders which may coexist with the respiratory disease is another matter. Before treatment is begun the patient should have a careful evaluation by a psychiatrist. The treatment can then often be carried out by another physician or by paramedical personnel. Failure to call in qualified psychiatric personnel in the treatment of these people may lead to disastrous medical results.

REFERENCES

Bastiaans, J., and Groen, J. Psychogenesis and psychotherapy of bronchial asthma, in Modern Trends in Psychosomatic Medicine, O'Neill, D. ed. London, Butterworth and Company, Ltd., 1955.

Dekker, E., Barendregt, J. T., and De Vries, K. Allergy and neurosis in asthma, in Advances in Psychosomatic Medicine, I. Jores, A. and Stokvis, B. eds. Basel/New York, Karger, 1960.

——— and Groen, J. Reproducible psychogenic attacks of asthma, J Psychosom Res, 1:58, 1956.

——— Pelser, H. E., and Groen, J. Conditioning as a cause of asthmatic attacks, J Psychosom Res, 2:97, 1957.

Grace, W. J., and Graham, D. T. Relationship of specific attitudes and emotions to certain bodily diseases, Psychosom Med, 14:243, 1952.

Graham, D. T., Lundy, R. M., Benjamin, L. S., Kabler, J. D., Lewis, W. C., Kunish, N. O., and Graham, F. K. Specific attitudes in initial interviews with patients having different "psychosomatic" diseases, Psychosom Med, 24:257, 1962.

Knapp, P. H. Acute bronchial asthma: II Psychoanalytic observations on fantasy, emotional arousal and partial discharge, Psychosom Med, 22:88, 1960.

——— and Nemetz, J. S. Acute bronchial asthma: I Concomitant depression and excitement, and varied antecedent patterns in 407 attacks, Psychosom Med, 22:42, 1960.

——— Mushatt, C., Nemetz, S. J., Constantine, H., and Friedman, S. The context of reported asthma during psychoanalysis. Presented at the annual meeting of the American Psychosomatic Society, Boston, 1968.

Luparello, T., Lyons, H. A., Bleecker, E. R., and McFadden, E. R., Jr. Influences of suggestion on airway reactivity in asthmatic subjects, Psychosom Med, 30:819, 1968.

Purcell, K., Brady, K., Hyman, C., Muser, J., Gordon, N., and Molk, L. The effect of experimental separation from the family on asthma in children. Presented at the Annual Meeting of the American Psychosomatic Society, Boston, 1968.

Stein, C. Practical Psychotherapeutic Techniques. Springfield, Ill., Charles C Thomas, Publisher, 1968.

Treuting, T. F., and Ripley, H. S. Life situations emotions and bronchial asthma, J Nerv Ment Dis, 108:380, 1948.

Wolpe, J. The desensitization treatment of neuroses, J Nerv Ment Dis, 132: 189, 1961.

22

Rehabilitation

The death rate from irreversible DOPS (clinical emphysema) has risen more than 600 percent between 1953 and 1963, and it continues to rise. It has become one of the most important health problems of our time. The financial loss is measured in the hundreds of millions of dollars. In terms of personal suffering and productivity loss, it is even higher.

Despite these sobering facts there are very few centers actively engaged in the rehabilitation and treatment of these patients. It does not appear to be one of the "fashionable" diseases and is not subject to the intensive investigation and care found in such conditions as coronary artery disease or valvular heart disease. It is seldom a dramatic disease in the sense that a number of unpredictable attacks occur which subside after treatment, with a grateful and admiring patient as the result. Emphysema and chronic bronchitis patients are unattractive as a group.

The physician is presented with a middle-aged male, with few funds, who chronically complains, does not respond well to treatment, and who may constantly cough and spit. With an office full of such patients, most physicians would go broke. Even if the physician could tolerate the financial loss and decreased patient load these patients might produce, most physicians seem poorly equipped to deal with them both psychologically and physiologically. The patient gratification which physicians need in order to be able to face disease and death is very often lacking.

PSYCHOSOCIAL AND PSYCHOPHYSIOLOGIC VARIABLES

Psychosocial and psychophysiologic variables have relevance and pertinence to prognosis, treatment, and rehabilitation in patients with chronic obstructive lung disease. The ability to respond to treatment and maintain oneself outside a hospital setting is determined by psychosocial assets as well as by the basic biologic format presented by the patient. Treatment failures and patients with poor prognosis are seen to have few psychosocial and physiologic assets, and thereby inadequate defenses against environmental inputs (see Chapter 18).

The significance of psychosocial variables lies in part in their influence on the psychophysiology of respiration. From a psychologic point of view, the respiratory system is very reactive. This means that people who have a great number of affective changes are also going to have great variability in the dynamics of respiration. This variability is almost always associated with increased disability in the patient who has chronic obstructive lung disease. People with few psychosocial assets—or, in other words, a limited number of coping behaviors—experience more affective changes than subjects with many psychosocial assets. This is another way of saying that people who do not know how to adapt are more likely to get angry, anxious, or depressed in their attempt to adapt, and are likely to find therapeutic orders difficult to follow.

When these patients get angry or anxious (activated) they increase ventilation and metabolism; when they are depressed or apathetic (inhibited) they decrease ventilation and metabolism. These changes in respiration make the balance between the supply and demand of oxygen even more precarious than it already is. This leads to increased hypoxia and may precipitate hypercarbia with or without acidosis.

Patients with many psychosocial assets are more effective in protecting themselves from dangerous symptoms or behaviors and are more likely to proceed with a realistic appropriate treatment program. They are therefore better able to cope with an unprotected (nonhospital) environment. From the data presented previously, psychosocial assets are seen to be as important as the physiologic assets in treatment and prognosis.

The resistance of the low-psychosocial-asset patient to therapeutic attempts in rehabilitation is seen to be directly proportional to the amount of change required. Social changes of any kind are tremendous threats as these patients have few or no alternative behaviors. Lack of compliance to a therapeutic program seems to be directly proportional to the amount of behavioral and vocational change required. Learning to deal with the patient with few psychosocial assets is important because they seem to constitute the great majority of problem patients or those needing rehabilitation. Patients with high psychosocial assets, in general, do not need rehabilitation or can rehabilitate themselves with little or no assistance.

If an excellent rehabilitation record is desired, patients should be chosen who are under 50; are happily married; have at least a high school education; were previously steadily employed; had good emotional support from both parents; have good emotional support from siblings, spouse, and children; have an adequate salary and adequate housing; are goal-directed and not overly sensitive; are satisfied with life; are flexible, congenial, reliable, and show good judgment; are willing to change; and are willing to shoulder responsibility. These variables may have little to do with physiology, but they do have a great deal to do with rehabilitative potential. If they are not accounted for one could expect a great deal of variability in the efficacy of a given rehabilitative method in different hands. Thus psychosocial variables may account for many diverse results obtained with seemingly identical techniques in the hands of different investigators.

One rehabilitative technique deserves special mention at this point, as it illustrates the interaction of psychologic and physiologic factors in rehabilitation. This is the "exercise therapy" currently in vogue. It has been shown that increasing efficiency of muscular performance can be obtained in some emphysema patients by using this technique. However, the results would seem to be better explained by a combination of psychologic and physiologic means than by physiologic ones alone.

It should be evident that many if not most patients with severe chronic obstructive lung disease are very anxious about exercise. Increase in activity increases their anxiety—the anxiety in turn increases disability, ventilation, and oxygen consumption—which in turn increases anxiety. Anxiety also decreases the efficiency of respiration and muscular function in that it takes more oxygen to perform work if one is anxious. This cycle can continue to the point that the patient has severely increased hypoxia, hypercarbia, and acidosis. One of the things most of the therapies seem to offer is deconditioning to anxiety and other significant emotions. In the eyes of the behavioral therapist it would go something like this:

1. Anxiety associated with activity

   ↓

2. Constant exposure to activity in a setting conducive to reassurance, confidence, and relaxation

   ↓

3. The association of activity with confidence, reassurance, and relaxation (Anxiety and reassurance, confidence, and relaxation are mutually exclusive.)

Exercise or other treatment which does not use the above would likely be ineffective because it does not supply the necessary ingredients for deconditioning. Regardless of how one views the therapeutic effectiveness of exercise therapy, it would appear that properly done it is a relatively easy method of deconditioning, and it is doubted if formal deconditioning of any kind could be better structured. In addition, it is doubted that this method would be as effective in patients with low psychosocial assets as in those with high psychosocial assets.

GENERAL REHABILITATIVE PROCEDURES

Evaluation of each patient should consist of: (1) the clinical workup, including history, physical, routine laboratory studies and chest x-rays; (2) pulmonary function evaluation; (3) a vocational re-evaluation; and (4) a psychosocial and psychophysiologic evaluation. Following such an evaluation, a decision can be made as to the direction the patient shall take. Patients with bronchitis, but without DOPS, should be advised on their tracheobronchial hygiene, particularly significant air pollutants, and the care of infections. They need clinic appointments for follow-up at six months or shorter intervals with repeated screening pulmonary function studies and x-rays.

Mild DOPS

A mild diffuse obstructive pulmonary syndrome (see Chapter 4), whether reversible or irreversible, provokes little disability in the patient on moderate activity (walking and stair climbing, mowing lawns, etc.). A maximal voluntary ventilation greater than 80 percent of the predicted provides sufficient reserve for all ordinary tasks without shortness of breath. These patients need no rehabilitation if they keep physically fit. If not ordinarily active, they should have an exercise program involving 15 to 20 min of workout twice daily.

These patients should be followed in an outpatient clinic at three-month or shorter intervals. If the patient is stable over a period of one year, clinic visits can be lengthened to three- or six-month intervals. Repeat flow rate testing should be done on each visit.

It is this group of patients that holds the most interest. These patients can be found by objective means and preventative medicine may stop the progression that ordinarily takes place. Toward this end some of these patients with active tuberculosis associated with DOPS have been treated with steroids, with an early reversal of their infection, a weight gain, a rapid clearing of x-ray findings, and other clinical benefits. The course of the obstructive syndrome in these patients, however, has not been appreciably different from that in a control group in a one-year follow-up. In the clinics, patients with mild DOPS tend to be stable for the most part as indicated by their flow rates. At present, it is not possible to predict those who will deteriorate, nor do there appear to be means presently available to prevent deterioration.

Moderate DOPS

Patients with moderate DOPS without subjective disability can also be treated in an outpatient clinic. Tracheobronchial hygiene—which includes aerosol therapy—should be emphasized. These patients should be given advice on maintaining an exercise regimen. Patients with moderate and severe DOPS with severe disability usually need admission to an inpatient program. The inpatient program should have a more formal scheme for instruction of the patient in tracheobronchial hygiene.

Severe DOPS

Patients with severe reversible DOPS or unremitting bronchial asthma limit their activity and develop the attitudes of the chronically ill. These patients need inpatient evaluation. Patients with irreversible DOPS occurring at middle age have dwindling physical capacities anyhow, but they further restrict physical activity to avoid shortness of breath. Their contacts with the world about them diminish and their interests become more and more focused on their disability. Social intercourse is limited to those who take care of them. In severe DOPS the muscular inefficiency from the lack of exercise combined with mental depression and a hopeless outlook accelerate the deterioration of the patient. With these patient's inactivity and low air flows, sputum is not moved in the respiratory tract and they suppress any cough that might be generated. (The observer is prompted to cough for these patients as he hears the sputum rattling in the chest.) Any hypoxia and hypercarbia present will be aggravated as a result of this sputum retention. Hypoxia results in insomnia, loss of appetite, mental confusion, and memory loss. Marked irritability and unpleasant personality traits may be uncovered and the patient is considered to be "senile." The physician may view this patient as a cranky, forgetful, ungrateful old man with a hopeless disease.

Physiotherapy techniques may be used to promote the production of sputum and a sense of well-being. This requires that the physical therapist position the patient so that the various segments of lung can be drained. In each of these positions, clapping or deep percussion of the chest is performed with vibration of the chest wall as well. A few minutes of such therapy, particularly with adequate drainage of the base of the lung, is of benefit in the debilitated patient who is not coughing and raising his sputum. This quite often should be preceded by adequate aerosol therapy to humidify the tracheobronchial tree and liquefy that sputum which can be reached.

Reversal of this condition requires the attention of a team of occupational, physical, and inhalation therapists. The goals of this team are those of reversing the deteriorating trend by demonstrated accomplishment in a program which improves muscular efficiency. Throughout the program the patient must be stimulated, and social contacts encouraged. The patient can be conditioned to his symptoms so that shortness of breath is accepted as natural to his condition and not feared. He must be taught to exercise to the limit of his ability, rest, catch his breath, and go on. Our grandmothers considered heat, humidification, and hydration to be important years ago, and we agree. The patient and his family are instructed about keeping the home moist and above 65°F. The patient is told to drink ten glasses of water a day. Removal of sticky secretions is aided with steam inhalation in the hospital and this is carried into the posthospital period. Grandmother did not like cigarettes and other air pollutants, and we concur with her on this. Patients should be advised to avoid smoke-filled rooms and to get an electrostatic air filter if they can afford it. We have not seen any specific benefit from the use of filtered air. Patients should be advised of those agents that cause ciliary suppression so that they may be avoided. Intermittent Positive Pressure Breathing (IPPB) machines are an efficient but expensive way of administering aerosol that can be given as well with a small compressor and nebulizer system. However, patients who need hyperventilation—that is, those with carbon dioxide retention—need IPPB several hours a day. Most of these patients can be treated with a simple valve and do not need models that cost several hundred dollars. Good aerosol therapy includes water and a bronchodilator consisting of Isoproteranol, and a decongestant such as Neo-Synephrine. Aminophyllin may be of particular benefit. Postural drainage is emphasized in those who raise sufficient sputum. Oxygen therapy is provided for those who need it—in the hospital or in the home. The large tanks with a long tube for nasal oxygen are best for use inside the hospital, and the oxygen cane or a small tank are best for use outside the hospital.

PHYSICAL REHABILITATION

A program for muscular conditioning with the psychotherapeutic benefits described includes exercises in different stages.

Stage 1 Exercises

Patients who have deteriorated to a chair or bed existence must have the exercise regimen limited in scope so that they can receive the satisfaction of accomplishing an outlined task. Diaphragmatic and slow, deep breathing patterns can be taught and are useful in the early stages of rehabilitation. The use of pursed lips breathing to overcome dyspnea is practiced and explained. The value of prolonging expiration so that the obstructive check valve mechanism is not activated is discussed. Isometric exercises are added when the patient is thought to be ready for them. As the patient's physical condition improves, candle blowing or bottle blowing is added.

Stage 2 Exercises

When the patient can be up and about in his room a second stage of exercises is introduced. The physical therapist stresses shoulder and arm relaxation exercises, body and toe curls, as well as pelvic tilt with thigh abduction and adduction exercises. These exercises are routine to most physical therapists.

Stage 3 Exercises

The patient may be ordered to Stage 3 exercises after he has passed through Stages 1 and 2. If he begins the program at this stage, the exercises above must still be discussed and practiced. At the Stage 3 level the patient should have a standing tolerance of several minutes. Shoulder exercises are then begun by using a target marked on the wall or a large wheel with a handle. This activity rotates the arm and shoulder through full motion and prevents freezing of the shoulders. A sense of accomplishment is particularly noticed in those who are able to walk. Walking in the hall to tolerance is started as early as possible. If oxygen is available, the patient is encouraged to exercise and then use the oxygen for relief when needed. The distance walked is increased with tolerance. The goal is to get the greatest amount of exercise a day at the best pace that can be mustered. Many patients who enter the hospital confined to their chair are able to get up and walk a mile a day after suitable training. Some of these exercises are more easily accomplished if special equipment is available. Bicycle riding and treadmill walking can be used as substitutes for hiking in the hall. Oxygen therapy is more easily administered by using the stationary equipment.

The exercises outlined in Stage 3 and many of those in Stage 2 can be conducted by a therapist in a group situation. An esprit de corps develops among these patients in such groups. Rivalry and banter in the group may arouse competitive efforts. The therapist can stimulate discussions on breathing difficulties and their relief. In this setting more formal lectures or movies on the obstructive syndrome can be offered. A cheerful, aggressive outlook is maintained by the staff in their attempts to get all patients into the group function.

The family must be educated about the nature of this syndrome. The limits of physical activity must be outlined so that too much is not expected of the patient and, on the other hand, the family should not take over the functions that the patient can easily accomplish. The patient's identity must be preserved, and complete dependence upon others should be avoided. His responsibility for certain activities that are beyond his physical capabilities should be unobtrusively removed.

Comment. With good cooperation approximately 75 percent of patients will have some decrease in dyspnea in response to a standard exercise input, and perhaps 50 percent will have some increase in pulmonary function after the initial intensive treatment. However, over the long run, there does not appear to be any change in resting gross pulmonary function studies after the patient has stabilized.

EMOTIONAL REHABILITATION

Formal psychiatric group therapy on respiratory cripples has proved to be of little use. In fact, for the severe cripple it tended to produce physiologic and psychologic decompensation. It did help the staff to understand the problems of the patients better and to understand themselves and the attitudes of rejection that are often exhibited toward these people. However, the therapy seriously threatened the stability of many of the respiratory cripples, and in place of desensitizing them to their symptoms, it aggravated them. We have found that an informal approach by the staff to inform the patient of his disease, to assure him that the shortness of breath is not damaging to his lungs, that he will not die, that he will be self-sufficient, is more useful. Also, didactic lectures with educational materials on emphysema—particularly those educational materials that are not alarming in their content—are very useful. The nursing, occupational, and physical therapy staff should look for opportunities to discuss the patient's progress with him. The support of the family should be sought by educating them to the needs of the patient. We continuously attempt to build a friendly supportive milieu in the company of others similarly affected. We feel that this is aided by the physical, inhalation, and occupational therapy arena's being located on the cripple ward. Ward rounds should be conducted once or twice a week which include all the paramedical services involved in patient care. With the patient and the paramedical personnel the physician discusses the progress in inhalation therapy and physical therapy, etc. If a misunderstanding has arisen it can be settled with everyone concerned.

VOCATIONAL REHABILITATION

If the goal is to increase productivity and produce financial independence, the techniques utilized are somewhat different from those that would be involved if the goal is simply to increase mobility and comfort. The rehabilitative procedures mentioned previously do increase mobility and comfort; however, they often have little to do with vocational rehabilitation. Getting job retraining and returning to productive employment are a very different matter than attaining relative physical and emotional comfort. Most people want to feel comfortable, but a good many people do not enjoy working unless the return is high enough to make it worth while. Thus it may be relatively easy to motivate people to aim at a goal of increasing comfort, but when the goal is that of increasing economic productivity which of necessity may also involve discomfort, the job of motivation may be much harder. In addition, returning to work or changing jobs involves a great deal of life change. This kind of change is seldom comfortable, as it involves adjustment to a new way of life. Most people resist change as a result. This is borne out by the fact that many rehabilitation programs get 95 percent complete cooperation with inhalation therapy, educational therapy, and general psychotherapeutic measures, but only 10 percent cooperation with vocational rehabilitation for those who need it. The amount of cooperation received is directly related to the amount of life change required by the patient. The significance of this life change to the patient can be quantified by the Schedule of Recent Events developed by Holmes.

The first goals of clinical medicine (increasing comfort, decreasing disability, and halting disease progression) appear at least partially attainable. However, once attained, complete rehabilitation requires a return to productive employment or job retraining. This is seldom possible. The reasons vary. For patients still working the loss of income required to retrain may be too much to take. For those not working, vocational rehabilitation requires a change in a well-entrenched life style, and at least a temporary decrease in comfort. Whatever the reason there are few "takers" in terms of good vocational readjustment.

In evaluating patients for vocational rehabilitation four areas are used to determine if retraining is warranted: (1) the age of the patient and the medical prognosis, (2) the exertional level feasible with maximal therapy; (3) individual motivation and interest; and (4) skills and aptitudes. In general, emphasis is placed on Categories 3 and 4. In other words, a well-motivated, interested patient with highly developed skills and with a poor medical prognosis and low exercise tolerance is a better bet than a poorly motivated patient with no skills, a good medical prognosis, and relatively high exercise tolerance.

This is illustrated by a 69-year-old male, who had a vital capacity of 0.9 (29 percent of normal), a maximal breathing capacity of 15 (18 percent of normal), a maximal expiratory flow rate of 50, a pH of 7.38, a Pa_{CO_2} of 50, a Pa_{O_2} of 51, and a Sa_{O_2} of 83. He "should" have been completely disabled. This patient, however, walked several miles each day, took care of his home and garden and, in general, conducted his life in a manner not unlike his unaffected neighbors. Despite severe dyspnea on mild exercise he could not be considered disabled. He had an enormous interest in life and, in general, as his disease had progressed he had increased this interest and his activities. He used several interesting techniques for dealing with dyspnea. The most evident technique was his denial of distress except when it got to the point that he literally could not stay on his feet. At that point, he would drop to the ground or sit on a curb until he caught his breath. He was not concerned with what those around him thought, and was as likely to rest on a busy downtown sidewalk as on his front porch. This was the technique used to rototill his garden. He would complete one row, turn the machine off, fall to the ground as though dead, get up in 3 or 4 min, do one more row, and then repeat the process. When walking he precisely matched his pace with his ability and could literally walk for miles. Perhaps the most remarkable characteristic was his ability to handle emotions. He stated that fear of death by suffocation was a primary motivating factor behind most of his dyspnea and he dealt with fear in part by taking mild tranquilizers or bourbon. Another technique he used to avoid having emotional change affect him was full immediate expression of the emotion. He immediately informs you of the way he feels and expresses it appropriately. Weeping was a very common emotional outlet for him and it was not uncommon for him to begin weeping several times during the course of an interview if he was experiencing emotion of any kind. He was completely frank and honest about his emotions and said that as a result emotions never became strong enough to affect his breathing.

COMMENT. This patient is an example of high motivation and high skills in an elderly man with almost no physiologic assets. He did not require rehabilitation despite his severe disease as he had never been disabled. There may be many people such as this, who do not come to the attention of specialists because of their drive and motivation. On the other hand, patients lacking in insight, interest, and motivation may be completely incapacitated with much less or no physiologic insufficiency.

ACCEPTANCE OF THE PROGRAM

On an inpatient program, 90 to 95 percent of the patients will not object to inhalation therapy, medication, or the educational routine. This acceptance may vary from the experience of other institutions as patients are not all voluntarily assigned to the program. Patients found to have a moderately severe obstructive pulmonary syndrome on admission to the hospital for tuberculosis may not be convinced of the presence of this other disease. They may wish to believe that it is all a result of tuberculosis. Therefore, any attempts to treat any disease other than the tuberculosis is met with resistance. Because of the nature of tuberculosis in this day and age, some of the resistance is a product of the social strata of the people being treated. These patients are unwilling to socialize and will not exert themselves. These symptoms are not only exhibited in the patients' failure to enter this treatment program but are also exhibited in their life adjustments as well. Complete cooperation in the whole program—particularly for the physical and occupational therapy portions of the program—does not exceed 75 percent of the patients. Incomplete cooperation occurs in 15 percent more. Outright rejection of this portion of the program occurs in about one of ten individuals. Acceptance of individual psychotherapy when indicated is better than 90 percent, but acceptance of group psychotherapy is less than 50 percent. As noted previously, the lower the level of pulmonary function and the lower the level of psychosocial assets, the lower the level of acceptance of group psychotherapy. On the other hand, acceptance of didactic lectures from the ward physician is about 100 percent.

The vocational rehabilitation division has had the most consistently poor results. These staff members take a dim view of working with patients who have an expected mortality of 7 out of 10 within five years and who would be expected to have repeated work absences and severe limitations from their physical incapacity. A few of these patients have succeeded at part-time bench work, particularly in corporations aimed at helping the handicapped, but the availability of this type of work is limited. Vocational rehabilitation has also had a very difficult time with patients with mild DOPS. Such patients—with few or no symptoms—cannot bring themselves to change their jobs, lose seniority, start a low-income retraining program, and enter a new position at low pay. They tend to put off making a decision about this to sometime in the future.

IMPROVEMENT

What evidence is there that the condition of the disabled patient is improved? An account of the exercise tolerance exhibited daily on the ward is particularly pertinent. Patients are discharged when they reach a plateau in their exercise improvement and it is believed that they have satisfactorily mastered therapeutic techniques. These patients are then followed in outpatient clinics where clinical and functional evaluation is repeated at first every three months, and then every six months. The clinical and physiologic variables that can be measured are not changed by the program. The increase in exercise tolerance in this group of patients, however, is most rewarding—indicating a substantial increase in efficiency. Respiratory cripples who are essentially confined to a chair get up and go out to get the mail daily. By simple means their outlook is improved, the burden of living is somewhat relieved, and their ability to see friends and family is improved.

Is there any evidence that the course of the disease in patients with severe disability is changed? With the use of gross ventilation or blood gas studies, it does not appear to be possible to predict which patients will do well and which will do poorly within this group. There is no functional, roentgenologic, medical, or therapeutic criterion that designates the patient who will walk out of the hospital and the one who will not. At present there is no evidence that the natural history of DOPS is materially changed. However, as shown in Chapter 18, psychosocial plus physiologic variables may offer good predictive data.

SUMMARY

Treatment failures and patients with a poor prognosis are generally those with few psychosocial assets and thereby inadequate protection from environmental inputs. The patients with few coping behaviors—i.e., few psychosocial assets—are constantly experiencing emotional changes which increase or produce disability, and they are unable to recognize or effectively deal with danger signals in the form of symptoms or environmental change. In addition, they have a difficult time understanding what is expected of them or complying when they do understand. Social changes of any kind are tremendous threats as these patients have few or no alternative behaviors.

Learning to deal with the patients with few psychosocial assets is important because they seem to constitute the great majority of patients needing rehabilitation. Patients with high psychosocial assets, in general, do not need rehabilitation or can rehabilitate themselves with little or no assistance.

If psychosocial variables are not accounted for one could expect a great deal of variability in the efficacy of a given rehabilitative method in different hands. Thus psychosocial variables may account for many diverse results obtained with seemingly identical techniques in the hands of different investigators.

REFERENCES

The Health Consequences of Smoking: A Public Health Service Review. United States Department of Health, Education and Welfare, 1967, p. 90.

Holmes, T. H., and Rahe, R. H. The social readjustment rating scale, J Psychosom Res, 11:213, 1967.

Petty, T. L., and Nett, L. M. For Those Who Live and Breathe with Emphysema and Chronic Bronchitis. Springfield, Ill., Charles C Thomas, Publishers, 1967.

Pierce, A. K., Taylor, H. F., Archer, R. K., and Miller, W. F. Responses to exercise training in patients with emphysema, Arch Intern Med, 113:28, 1964.

Section V

Integration

This section attempts to integrate the varied data presented in the preceding chapters. It is important to understand that general psychophysiologic principles of respiration are similar in normal individuals and in those with clinical emphysema, asthma, tuberculosis, or other diseases. However, specific differences in response secondary to the respiratory abnormalities found in a particular disease and to psychologic protective mechanisms may be present. In other words, if a patient with severe emphysema can be provoked to anger—despite his psychologic defenses—ventilation and metabolism are increased as they are in the normal person. However, the increase in ventilation is limited and costly in the work required to maintain it, so that the oxygen available for other work is limited. With a level of ventilation that is unable to provide enough oxygen or to remove enough carbon dioxide to support the new activity level, hypoxia and hypercarbia may be initiated or caused to progress. In normal subjects without the limited ability to change ventilation and without a high oxygen cost of breathing, this does not occur. The physiologic response of the patient with clinical emphysema, however, does not represent a difference in the psychophysiologic mechanism. It is the consequence of a normal psychophysiologic response directed at a failing organ system.

23

Discussion and Formulation

An integrated medical, psychiatric, and physiologic approach provides the greatest number of therapeutic modalities possible in the treatment and evaluation of respiratory problems. It leads to the fullest understanding of the patient. With this understanding the patient can be aided to achieve optimal use of his impaired respiratory system.

PSYCHOPHYSIOLOGIC CONSIDERATIONS

It is fashionable to speak in terms of differentiating emotions in specific ways with complex and sophisticated formulations. In the final analysis, however, simple answers are often found to complex questions. The following is no exception.

The experimental data presented in this monograph indicate that the ventilatory and metabolic responses to incoming stimuli are modified by psychological orientation. The hyperventilation or hyperpnea observed with action-orientation is interpreted as preparation for an increase in metabolism. Conversely, the hypoventilation or decreased ventilation with non-action-orientation is the preparation for a decrease in metabolism. This relationship is independent of the functional status of the pulmonary system. Action-oriented behavior was said to be present when action or desire for action formed the major component of the psychologic reaction. Nonaction-oriented behavior was said to be present when a lack of desire for action or withdrawal formed the major component of the psychologic reaction.

In the experiments described here as well as elsewhere, the ventilatory response to the suggestion of exercise has been shown to be as marked as the reaction to the exercise itself. Furthermore, the suggestion of sleep produced ventilatory changes similar to those which occurred during naturally occurring sleep. A close parallel exists between the respiratory changes occurring during sleep, depression, and apathy, and those occurring during exercise, anger, and anxiety, respectively. Sleep, depression, apathy, and related states, fall into the nonaction-oriented category. Exercise, anger, anxiety, and related states fall into the action-oriented category. It is thought that all behavior and emotion can be placed in one of the above categories or in a neutral category. This formulation has been investigated in detail by Gellhorn, with neurophysiologic techniques.

A variety of inputs have been shown to play roles in the control of respiration (see Chapter 3). Of the various factors providing signals to the respiratory center, carbon dioxide has been the most intensively investigated. As the carbon dioxide concentration in the blood increases and the pH falls, ventilation increases; and as the carbon dioxide concentration falls and the pH rises, ventilation falls. During conditions such as exercise and sleep—when the respiratory center appears to have a high and low sensitivity to carbon dioxide, respectively—cerebral inputs into the respiratory center are seen to be in operation. This is a simplified view and is useful as a heuristic device in the expositions to follow. Although the chemical role in the control of respiration is appreciated, it is thought that the respiratory changes illustrated in this communication result from inputs from cortical elements. Metabolic changes occur in association with the same psychologic stimulation but are not thought to play a role in producing the respiratory changes. During the hyperventilation associated with action-orientation, the carbon dioxide concentration of the alveolar air falls, and, therefore, the arterial carbon dioxide concentration must also fall. During the hypoventilation associated with nonaction-orientation, the carbon dioxide concentration in the alveolar air rises, and thus the carbon dioxide concentration in the arterial blood must also rise. The chemical changes are in the direction opposite to their usual action on ventilation. Central (cerebral) stimuli must, therefore, be counteracting the chemical stimuli, or the sensitivity of the respiratory center to carbon dioxide must vary widely in response to inputs from cerebral sources.

With normal pulmonary function short-term changes in ventilation (minutes) associated with psychologic change cause the carbon dioxide concentration in the alveolar air to fall with an increase and to rise with a decrease in the alveolar ventilation. When the psychologic reactions persist for hours, days, or weeks, the carbon dioxide content of the alveolar air tends to return to normal levels. There is an adjustment of metabolism to ventilation. Once again, if chemical inputs are responsible for sustaining the level of ventilation after metabolic adjustment has occurred, it is probably through a centrally induced increase or decrease in the sensitivity of the respiratory center.

Patients with pulmonary disease may get into serious difficulty by reacting in either of the patterns described. A patient with borderline or abnormal blood-gas values and whose ventilation is severely taxed may not be able to increase ventilation to meet the metabolic demand when he is reacting to a stimulus with the action-oriented pattern. He becomes more hypoxic and hypercarbic because of the increased work of breathing and skeletal muscle tension, as well as the failure of his ventilation to compensate by increasing the supply of oxygen and removing excess carbon dioxide. On the other hand, the patient reacting with nonaction-orientation has a metabolic change in the downward direction. The change in ventilation is postulated to lead the change in metabolism. The subject is pushed into hypoxia and hypercarbia because ventilation is decreased more than the oxygen requirements by a reduction in the respiratory center sensitivity.

PSYCHOSOCIAL CONSIDERATIONS

Patients with many psychosocial assets are more effective in protecting themselves from dangerous symptoms or behaviors and are more likely to proceed with a realistic appropriate treatment program. They are, therefore, better able to cope with an unprotected (nonhospital) environment. From the data presented, psychosocial and physiologic assets are found to be of equal importance in the treatment of respiratory disease.

The importance of being able effectively to deal with the environment cannot be overemphasized. People with a great number of emotional changes also have great variations in the dynamics of respiration. This variability is almost always associated with increased disability. People with few psychosocial assets and, consequently, a limited number of coping behaviors, experience more emotional changes than subjects with many psychosocial assets.

Patients with few psychosocial assets also have difficulty understanding what is expected of them or complying when they do understand. They are more likely to resist therapeutic attempts. This is particularly so when some change in behavior or occupation is required during rehabilitation procedures. Social changes of any kind are tremendous threats because these patients have few or no alternative behaviors. Lack of compliance to a therapeutic program seems to be directly proportional to the amount of behavioral and vocational change required. Learning to deal with patients with few psychosocial assets is important as these people seem to constitute the great majority of problem patients or those needing rehabilitation.

Patients with high psychosocial assets, in general, do not need rehabilitation or can rehabilitate themselves with little or no assistance.

DYSPNEA

Dyspnea is commonly experienced with emotional and physiologic changes independently of pulmonary insufficiency. Dyspnea initiates a feedback mechanism which can produce further psychologic and physiologic change and increased disability. In this regard it is interesting to note that patients with severe pulmonary disease isolate themselves from interpersonal contacts. Such contact almost always leads to some kind of emotional response. This response is associated with a change in ventilation and metabolism which may lead to dyspnea. The dyspnea in turn produces more emotional change, ventilatory change, and metabolic change. These factors may initiate or aggravate hypoxia and hypercarbia, and lead eventually to acidosis. In treating these people, it is important to recognize the psychophysiologic mechanisms in operation. Otherwise the therapist may unwittingly be an additive factor in perpetuating the above cycle.

In addition, it should be noted that removal or reduction of a symptom such as dyspnea is a complex operation which may involve major changes in life adjustment. Conditioning, psychologic problems, psychosocial variables, and underlying lung pathology all contribute to the development and perpetuation of dyspnea and must all be considered in treatment.

DIFFUSE OBSTRUCTIVE PULMONARY SYNDROME (IRREVERSIBLE)

Clinical emphysema (DOPS) is described in detail elsewhere (Chapter 4). The structural defect in DOPS is unknown. The mechanism producing the airway obstruction is one of unequal pressures that acts across bronchial walls, tending to collapse them. Following the loss of the elastic recoil of the lungs, the intrapleural pressure rises, expiration is no longer a passive event (as in the normal lungs), and the chest cage must increase pleural pressure to empty the lungs. The increased pressures act to collapse airways as well as to empty alveoli. Such obstructive mechanisms accompany centrilobular emphysema, panlobular emphysema, and chronic bronchitis, and occur in normal-looking lungs. The change in elastic recoil does not necessarily accompany emphysema or bronchitis. A defect in the mechanical properties of tissues is probably responsible for the loss of the elastic recoil.

Clinical emphysema is best identified with the use of a measure of expiratory flow such as a peak flowmeter, a timed vital capacity, or a maximal breathing capacity. The increase in static compliance in these syndromes can also be measured, as well as an unequal distribution of inspired gas in the lungs (as measured by the nitrogen washout). Ventilation-perfusion abnormalities that accompany these changes result in hypoxemia and hypercapnia. As hypercapnia progresses respiratory acidosis may occur, and cor pulmonale may appear in the course of these physiologic changes.

As these physiologic changes progress the patient is less and less able to react to environmental stress with the respiratory system. The eventual setting in which he finds himself is marked by increasing dependency and increasing attempts to control his environment. Emotional upsets lead to increased disability and discomfort and this soon becomes obvious to the patient and those caring for him. The patient responds by utilizing repression, denial, and isolation to insulate himself from emotional change. On the other hand, the doctor, nurse, relative, or friend, tries hard to fulfill the patient's wishes—partly because of the traditional role sick people play and partly because of anxiety over being responsible for the decompensation and possible death of the patient. The patient recognizes this and responds by exerting more environmental control in order to extend periods of comfort and to keep in contact with people who are vital to his care.

Eventually he may dictate his total care. As a result, it may be extremely difficult to mobilize these people. Each time they are forced to increase their activity against their wishes they decompensate. In this way the patient is able to decrease considerably the total amount of stress, but this paves the way for continued debility because of the reluctance of those around him to take a chance on increasing his activities and because of his own dependency needs. The patient's dependency is related to his anxieties about impending decompensation and death. As he suffers periodic crises in keeping with the natural history of the disease, he is literally dependent on specific people to save his life. He feels that in order to be assured of proper medical attention during a crisis, he must not be separated from or alienate some vital person who would then not respond to his needs during the crisis. By his continued dependency, he insures that these people will be there and will respond to his needs—but this also produces much antagonism. The patient thus places himself in a position of always knowing what to expect, and he walks a narrow path in which he must satisfy his needs without producing undue antagonism from the people on whom he is dependent. The patient becomes very compulsive and will insist on accounting for every minute of the day in order to satisfy his need for security.

Anxiety and anger also serve as an added stimulus to respiration in severely ill patients. Physiologic decompensation with hypercapnea, hypoxia, acidosis, and even death has occurred with a reduction in anxiety and anger through drugs and psychotherapy. Thus anxiety and anger play a dual role—some amount is beneficial, but a large amount may be fatal. At the opposite extreme, depression is seen as reducing respiratory drive, and may also lead to decompensation and death.

Dying with Emphysema

Dying behavior is the patient's realistic response to the total life situation. This is usually triggered by specific social events which are difficult or impossible for the patient to accept. Dying is seen to be a goal-directed behavior which is accompanied by a variety of emotions and their physiologic counterparts. These emotions are usually related to environmental situations and not to the dying behavior itself. Dying is described by the articulate patients as comfortable and relaxing. It is exceedingly difficult to give up once begun. As described by one particularly verbal patient: "It's like getting ready for something; like curling up for a long winter's nap." This patient also described her feelings when this behavior was halted by the doctors as among the most uncomfortable she had ever had: "I felt like screaming."

Although the actual process of dying is relatively comfortable, the emotions generated by the patient's interaction with those around him can be very distressing. Interestingly, these emotions are often related to fear of what the doctors would do in terms of resuscitative procedures, and to power struggles between the patient who insists on dying and the hospital staff and relatives who refuse to grant the patient the right to die or even to talk about death.

DIFFUSE OBSTRUCTIVE PULMONARY SYNDROME (REVERSIBLE)

Asthma is usually divided into atopic (extrinsic) and nonatopic (intrinsic). Extrinsic asthma often occurs secondary to specific antigens and is more common in the younger population. Intrinsic asthma often occurs secondary to respiratory infections and is more common in older individuals (see Chapter 4). In many patients the asthma attack is ushered in by bronchoconstriction secondary to excessive parasympathetic discharge. This is supported by the facts that mecholyl precipitates asthma attacks in many asthmatics, sympathomimetic agents generally afford prompt relief, and the adrenal medulla appears to hypofunction in some asthmatics. Depending on individual bias, infectious, allergic, psychologic, or genetic factors are emphasized in discussions of this disease. In addition, histamine and serotonin contribute to asthma attacks in a few patients.

There is evidence that asthmatic attacks can be produced by psychologic factors alone in susceptible individuals. Also, many asthmatics have specific psychologic attitudes which are associated with the symptomatic periods. A combination of psychologic and physiologic treatment methods seems most effective in dealing with a patient's symptoms. An intimate relation between psychologic factors and asthma is suggested by the fact that the so-called functional illnesses (such as psychoses) are sometimes substituted for asthma or vice versa. Also interesting are the low incident rates of asthma in some chronic care hospitals. It has long been observed in the institution where these studies were carried out that asthmatics seldom have attacks in the hospital even though constantly plagued on the outside. The shifting from one disease to another or the complete absence from a previously unremitting disease under specific psychosocial circumstances has been studied extensively by Groen.

Asthma is usually diagnosed on the basis of wheezing, great subjective discomfort, and agitation, along with changes in pulmonary function which are completely reversible. Clinical measurements which are readily available for assessing the severity of an attack are the vital capacity and the maximal expiratory flow rate, both of which fall during attacks. The static compliance, however, remains normal. More sensitive measures of airway resistance can be obtained from the body plethysmograph. However, this device is rarely available to the clinician who is treating the patient.

Evidence has been provided by Dekker that collapse of the posterior wall of the trachea and main bronchi is responsible for asthmatic wheezing in some patients. He found that a positive pressure of 2 cm of water is necessary to collapse the posterior wall of the major airway in vitro. He proposes that an intrathoracic pressure head of this amount during the forced expiration of asthmatic breathing collapses the posterior airway wall and leads to the wheezing. Whether major airway compression is a main factor causing asthmatic wheezing is debatable. Most certainly, however, major airway obstruction can be a secondary result of bronchiolar constriction which allows the buildup of intrathoracic pressure. The role of conditioning in the production of some asthmatic attacks has also been elucidated by Dekker.

The chronic asthmatic develops defensive mechanisms which are similar to those discussed for the patient with clinical emphysema. The psychophysiologic and psychosocial variables discussed as being significant in the understanding of the emphysema patient also apply to the chronic state in asthma. The patient with intermittent acute attacks does not experience social and physiologic disorganization and thereby leads an unencumbered life. Knapp has studied the natural history of some acute asthma attacks. He found that many attacks were preceded by emotional change, which led directly into acute asthma. Acute asthma is necessary to the life style of many people, but it does not interfere with adequate adjustment.

Regardless of other factors, once an asthma attack is in process an important clinical goal is the maintenance of the patient without undue amounts of anger, anxiety, or depression. All such affects will lead to clinical deterioration. Anxiety and anger operate by increasing the metabolic need and the struggle to breathe, and depression decreases the drive to maintain adequate oxygenation. However, as mentioned previously, a little anxiety or anger may be beneficial—but a lot may be fatal.

HYPERVENTILATION AND HYPOVENTILATION

Hyperventilation syndrome is probably the most commonly made psychophysiologic diagnosis. Essentially it represents an accentuation of the normal respiratory response to anxiety, fear, anger, or a combination of these action-oriented emotions. Because, as mentioned previously, ventilation precedes metabolic processes in short-term psychophysiologic respiratory reactions, the above emotions are initially correlated with a reduced arterial carbon dioxide tension. In most subjects, however, the arterial carbon dioxide tension does not fall to symptom-producing levels because of the concomitant increase in metabolism or because the emotional reaction is not sufficiently severe. Patients with the hyperventilation syndrome appear to lose control of their emotional response, and the increase in metabolism is not adequate to keep the arterial carbon dioxide tension out of the symptom-producing range. As the carbon dioxide tension is reduced, the patient becomes dyspneic and lightheaded, and has paresthesias, vertigo, chills, chest pain, and excess sweating. These symptoms provide the inputs for further emotional and physiologic change and thereby increased disability. Treatment depends upon reducing the psychologic stimulus to breathing. This can be accomplished immediately by reassurance, sedation, or tranquilization. In certain cases, inhalation of low levels of carbon dioxide is also helpful. Long-term control depends upon problem-solving and perhaps low doses of a minor tranquilizer or sedative.

Possibly the most common diagnostic mistake made is confusion of the hyperventilation syndrome with what should be described as the hypoventilation syndrome. It is not uncommon to find that a patient will complain of dyspnea with depression and shallow slow breathing. The word dyspnea has been firmly associated with hyperventilation and the possibility of hypoventilation with dyspnea has been largely ignored. Sedation in the hypoventilating patient will often increase his symptoms. Low doses of central nervous system stimulants may be of value.

PHYSIOLOGIC VARIABLES

From a biological point of view the purpose of the respiratory system is to supply oxygen and remove carbon dioxide in order to support varying activity levels. The high degree of uniformity found in the response of ventilation and gas-exchange variables to symbolic or real changes in activity is consistent with this role. As different variables reflect different aspects of function, all respiratory variables would not be expected to follow the pattern exhibited by gas-exchange and ventilation variables. For example, although the alveolar ventilation is consistently increased during action-orientation and decreased during nonaction-orientation, the respiratory rate showed no such consistency. It remained unchanged or went up or down largely independent of the alveolar ventilation. Although frequency is an important variable, its significance lies in the efficiency with which a change in it can alter alveolar ventilation. Some subjects may accomplish an increase in alveolar ventilation by decreasing frequency and increasing tidal volume, while others may increase frequency and tidal volume. Other combinations are possible, but the point is that an increase or decrease in alveolar ventilation is not dependent on any particular change in frequency. Alveolar ventilation is the significant variable, as it directly reflects the amount of air available at the alveolar level for gas exchange.

The same concept applies to the cardiovascular system, in which one of the significant variables reflecting basic cardiac function is the cardiac output. Changes in cardiac output can be produced by changing rate or stroke volume. An increase in cardiac output does not necessarily correlate with an increased rate or stroke volume, and vice versa. Also, increased cardiac output does not necessarily correlate with other variables such as blood pressure, velocity of blood flow, galvanic skin response, or skin temperature, as the values of these variables depend upon multiple factors, one of which is the cardiac output. The variable selected to represent the function of a particular organ or organ system must be one which reflects basic function. Otherwise significant correlations with basic human biology cannot be made. This probably accounts for the lack of correlation between different variables found in Chapter 11.

PSYCHOLOGIC VARIABLES

Emotional change was the independent variable and time and intensity of stimulation the dependent variables in the experimental work described in this monograph. When emotional change is the independent variable, largely comparable data are obtained for all subjects. This has the advantage of taking into consideration the fact that a standard stimulus is not the same stimulus to two different subjects. The use of this approach depends on the research aim being that of attaining comparable psychologic changes in all subjects for correlation with simultaneously occurring physiologic changes.

A variety of stimuli were used to elicit psychologic change. These consisted of naturally occurring events, suggestion of naturally occurring events (with and without hypnosis), and experimental head stimulation. From the data presented it would seem that the best stimuli for producing psychologic and physiologic change are naturally occurring events, or an actual experimental event (e.g., noxious head stimulation). The next best is hypnotic suggestion of the event, and the least effective is suggestion without hypnosis. If naturally occurring events do not always produce the most pronounced psychologic or physiologic change, they represent an experiment of nature and indicate what to expect in the real world. Therefore, other methods should be evaluated in the light of their ability to mimic the naturally occurring event. Hypnosis seems to do this to a better degree than suggestion without hypnosis and is considered the next best thing.

It is important to have a good definition of various emotional states, and to have some idea of how they fit into the biological world. For example, some patients with the diagnosis of depression may be retarded and withdrawn and display physiologic hypofunction. This is the kind of condition called "conservation withdrawal" by Engel. It is characterized by hopelessness. The patient feels there is nothing that he can do to help himself, and nothing anyone else can do for him. He has stopped struggling. The emphasis is on conservation of energy and on nonparticipation. Other patients with a diagnosis of depression present with anxiety or anger mixed with feelings of self-depreciation. This is a very different picture from that presented by the hopeless patient. This depressed patient is hyperfunctioning psychologically and physiologically.

Cannon's "fight or flight" responses—such as anger and anxiety—are those in which the individual is mobilized for physical activity, whether it be aggressively attacking, holding ground, or running. The emphasis is on expending energy in physical activity. Anxiety conveys to the individual the idea of danger and is characterized by increased bodily tension and feelings of apprehension. When confronted with the actual danger he may run, fight, do nothing, remain anxious, or withdraw into a depressive reaction. Anxiety can thereby be seen as the primary response and anger or depression the secondary response. Depression and anger, however, are also primary responses to incoming signals. When the immediate situation is seen as being appropriately dealt with by withdrawal and nonparticipation, depression may be the initial response. When the immediate situation is seen as requiring destructive activity, anger may be the initial response.

Once a sustained psychologic reaction has developed, homeostatic mechanisms come into play. Thus depression—with its opposing affect and physiology—may overlie anger and anxiety, or vice versa. An agitated depression represents a combination of anger, anxiety, and depression which may have originally started as a pure state of anxiety, anger, or depression and become mixed as the individual attempted to return to equilibrium. Relatively pure anger, anxiety, or depression would therefore be seen as conditions in which opposing physiologic and affective responses were overwhelmed.

The words action-orientation and nonaction-orientation were used rather than the terminology of Cannon or Engel because of the inclusion of normal everyday behaviors such as exercise and sleep in the two categories. An analogy is drawn between emotions and fluctuations in activity. This would appear to be consistent with the real world, in which certain emotions are associated with participation in activity and others are associated with withdrawal from activity. It is important to note that the nonaction-oriented response is seen as an active change to a lower energy state, just as action-orientation is seen as an active change to a higher energy state. This may seem a highly simplified concept of complex behavior, but it serves the purpose of providing common physiologic and psychologic bonds between biologic conditions which may otherwise seem very different.

REFERENCES

Bannister, R. G., Cunningham, D. J. C., and Douglas, G. G. The carbon dioxide stimulus to breathing in severe exercise, J Physiol, 125:90, 1954.

Bastiaans, J., and Groen, J. Psychogenesis and psychotherapy of bronchial asthma, in Modern Trends in Psychosomatic Medicine. O'Neill, D., ed. London, Butterworth and Co., Ltd., 1955.

Bates, D. V., and Christie, R. V. Respiratory Function in Disease. Philadelphia, W. B. Saunders Co., 1964.

Birchfield, R. I., Sieker, H. O., and Heyman, A. Alterations in respiratory function during natural sleep, J. Lab Clin Med, 54:216, 1959.

Cannon, W. B. Bodily Changes in Pain, Hunger, Fear and Rage, 2nd ed. Boston, Charles T. Branford Co., 1953.

Cobb, L. A., Ripley, H. S., and Jones, J. W. Role of the nervous system in free fatty acid mobilization as demonstrated by hypnosis, in Physical Activity and the Heart: Proceedings of a Symposium, Helsinki, Finland. Karvonen, M. J., and Barry, A. J., eds. Springfield, Ill., Charles C Thomas, Publisher, 1967.

Dekker, E. Further experiments on the origin of asthmatic wheezing, in Advances of Psychosomatic Medicine. Jores, A. ed. New York, Brunner, 1961.

——— Barendreet, J. T., and De Vries, K. Allergy and neurosis in asthma, in Advances in Psychosomatic Medicine, Vol. I. Jores, A. and Stokvis, B. eds. Basel/New York, S. Karger, 1960.

——— and Groen, J. Reproducible psychogenic attacks of asthma, J. Psychosom Res, 1:58, 1956.

——— Pelser, H. E., and Groen, J. Conditioning as a cause of asthmatic attacks, J Psychosom Res, 2:97, 1957.

Engel, G. L. Psychologic Development in Health and Disease. Philadelphia, W. B. Saunders Co., 1962.

Gellhorn, E. Principles of Autonomic-Somatic Integrations. Minneapolis, Univ. of Minnesota Press, 1967.

Grace, W. J., and Graham, D. T. Relationship of specific attitudes and emotions to certain bodily diseases, Psychosom Med, 14:243, 1952.

Graham, D. T., Lundy, R. M., Benjamin, L. S., Kabler, J. D., Lewis, W. C., Kunish, N. O., and Graham, F. K. Specific attitudes in initial interviews with patients having different "psychosomatic" diseases, Psychosom Med, 24:257, 1962.

——— Stern, J. A., and Winokur, G. Experimental investigation of the specificity of attitude hypothesis in psychosomatic disease, Psychosom Med, 20:446, 1958.

——— and Wolf, S. The relation of eczema to attitude and to vascular reactions of the human skin, J Lab Clin Med, 42:238, 1953.

Groen, J., Bastiaans, J., and Van Der Valk, J. M. Psychosomatic aspects of syndrome shift and syndrome suppression in Psychosomatics. Booij, F. ed. New York, Elsevier Publishing Co., 1957.

Harrison, T. R., Ed. Principles of Internal Medicine. 4th ed. New York, McGraw-Hill, 1962.

Knapp, P. H. Acute bronchial asthma: II. Psychoanalytic observations on fantasy, emotional arousal, and partial discharge, Psychosom Med 22:88, 1960.

——— and Nemetz, S. J. Acute bronchial asthma: I. Concomitant depression and excitement, and varied antecedent patterns in 406 attacks, Psychosom Med 22:42, 1960.

Lowry, T. P. ed. Hyperventilation and Hysteria: The Physiology and Psychology of Overbreathing and Its Relationship to the Mind-Body Problem. Springfield, Ill., Charles C Thomas, Publisher, 1967.

Masuda, M., Notske, R. N., and Holmes, T. H. Catecholamine excretion and asthmatic behavior, J Psychosom Res, 10:255, 1966.

Robin, E. D., Whaley, R. D., Crump, C. N., and Travis, D. J. Alveolar gas tensions, pulmonary ventilation and blood pH during physiologic sleep in normal subjects, J Clin Invest, 37:981, 1958.

Ruch, T. C. and Fulton, J. F. Medical Physiology and Biophysics, 18th ed. Philadelphia, W. B. Saunders Co., 1960.

Sieker, N. O., Heyman, A., and Birchfield, R. I. The effects of natural sleep and hypersomnolent states on respiratory function, Ann Intern Med, 52:500, 1960.

Treuting, T. F., and Ripley, H. S. Life situations, emotions and bronchial asthma, J Nerv Ment Dis, 108:380, 1948.

24

Summary

This monograph has been concerned with the role of the respiratory system in human adaptation to naturally occurring, suggested, and experimentally induced changes. It was found that regardless of the method of stimulation the respiratory system responds consistently with one of two general categories of function. When action or desire for action (anger, anxiety, exercise, and related states) formed a major component of the reaction, the subjects experienced hyperventilation or hyperpnea and increased oxygen consumption. This was called action-orientation. When lack of desire for action or inaction (depression, apathy, sleep, and related states) formed a major component of the reaction (nonaction-orientation), the subjects experienced hypoventilation or decreased ventilation, and decreased oxygen consumption. These responses were seen as consistent in an organ system which supplies oxygen and removes carbon dioxide in the face of consistently varying activity levels.

An attempt was made to correlate changes in blood pressure, pulse rate, skin temperature, and catecholamine excretion (3-methoxy-4-hydroxymandelic acid, normetadrenaline, and metadrenaline) with the changes in respiration. With the exception of blood pressure these variables did not appear to be closely associated with changes in the respiratory variables.

The role that these changes in activity levels played in the production of symptoms and perpetuation of respiratory disease processes was explored. In general, emotional changes of any kind were found to change levels of activation. These changes in activation were found to produce or increase symptoms. In patients with pulmonary insufficiency, as reflected in gross ventilatory studies and blood gases, the physiologic changes accompanying the changes in activation were sometimes sufficient to produce respiratory decompensation. In addition, the symptoms produced often acted as positive feedback which produced more emotional and physiologic changes in a "vicious cycle," the end result of which was psychologic and physiologic decompensation.

The patients attempted to protect themselves from changes in activation by using isolation, denial, and repression. These psychologic defense mechanisms often led to misunderstandings with medical personnel and other individuals who were important to the patient's well-being. Respect for the patient's defense system was seen to be very important in organizing the treatment program. With a breakdown in the defense system, rapid psychologic and physiologic decompensation often followed.

Prediction of outcome in patients with severe clinical emphysema was equally dependent upon psychosocial and physiologic variables. Psychosocial assets were found to be important in aiding the patient to maintain good defensive measures and to get optimal use of a failing respiratory system. The patients with low psychosocial assets experienced more disability in relation to the physiologic impairment and were less able to cope with the environment.

The end expression of disease (death) was seen to be a comfortable, specific, goal-directed behavior. The distressing emotions which sometimes accompanied death were related to the reactions of those around the dying person. Most often these responses were actuated by someone significant in the patient's life, who was threatened by his death. This person was unable to face the death of the patient and reacted by ignoring the patient or by relating to the patient in a manner which was upsetting. The same behavior directed at the patient when he was not dying would produce similar emotional upsets.

INDEX